Septic Bone and Joint Surgery

Reinhard Schnettler, MD
Professor and Director
Department of Orthopedic Trauma Surgery
University Hospital Giessen and Marburg
Giessen, Germany

Hans-Ulrich Steinau, MD
Professor and Director
Department of Plastic Surgery
University Hospital Bergmannsheil
Ruhr University Bochum
Bochum, Germany

With contributions by
Stefan Adams, Volker Alt, Henning Breithaupt,
Lars Frommelt, Thorsten Gehrke, Volkmar Heppert,
Gustav Hoer, Siegfried Hofmann, Heinz-Herbert
Homann, Ralf Kraus, Michael Kroetz, Marcus Lehnhardt,
Ulrich Linsenmaier, Klausdieter Parsch, Martin Pietsch,
Maximilian Reiser, Urs Schiefer, Hergo G. K. Schmidt,
Reinhard Schnettler, Hans-Ulrich Steinau,
Christoph Wenisch

530 illustrations

Thieme
Stuttgart · New York

Library of Congress Cataloging-in-Publication Data
Septische Knochenchirurgie. English
  Septic bone and joint surgery / [edited by] Reinhard
Schnettler, Hans-Ulrich Steinau ; with contributions by Stefan
Adams ... [et al.] ; [translator, Barbara Herzberger ; illustrators,
Christiane and Michael von Solodkoff].
     p. ; cm.
  Includes bibliographical references and index.
  ISBN 978-3-13-149031-5 (alk. paper)
  1. Osteomyelitis--Handbooks, manuals, etc. 2. Bones--
Infections--Surgery--Handbooks, manuals, etc. 3. Joints--
Infections--Surgery--Handbooks, manuals, etc. I. Schnettler,
Reinhard. II. Steinau, Hans-Ulrich. III. Adams, Stefan, Dr. IV. Title.
  [DNLM: 1. Knee Joint--pathology. 2. Knee Joint--surgery. 3.
Osteomyelitis--surgery. 4. Surgical Procedures, Operative--
methods. WE 870 S479s 2010a]
  RC931.O7S4713 2010
  617.5'82059--dc22
                          2009035823

This book is an authorized and revised translation of the
German edition published and copyrighted 2004 by Georg
Thieme Verlag, Stuttgart, Germany. Title of the German
edition: Septische Knochenchirurgie.

Translator: Barbara Herzberger, MD, Munich, Germany

Illustrators: Christiane and Dr. Michael von Solodkoff,
Neckargmünd, Germany

We wish to thank

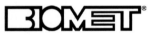

for the kind support.

© 2010 Georg Thieme Verlag,
Rüdigerstrasse 14, 70469 Stuttgart, Germany
http://www.thieme.de
Thieme New York, 333 Seventh Avenue,
New York, NY 10001, USA
http://www.thieme.com

Cover design: Thieme Publishing Group
Typesetting by medionet, Berlin, Germany
Printed in China by Everbest Printing Co. Ldt, Hong Kong
ISBN 978-3-13-149031-5

Important note: Medicine is an ever-changing science undergoing continual development. Research and clinical experience are continually expanding our knowledge, in particular our knowledge of proper treatment and drug therapy. Insofar as this book mentions any dosage or application, readers may rest assured that the authors, editors, and publishers have made every effort to ensure that such references are in accordance with **the state of knowledge at the time of production of the book.**

Nevertheless, this does not involve, imply, or express any guarantee or responsibility on the part of the publishers in respect to any dosage instructions and forms of applications stated in the book. **Every user is requested to examine carefully** the manufacturers' leaflets accompanying each drug and to check, if necessary in consultation with a physician or specialist, whether the dosage schedules mentioned therein or the contraindications stated by the manufacturers differ from the statements made in the present book. Such examination is particularly important with drugs that are either rarely used or have been newly released on the market. Every dosage schedule or every form of application used is entirely at the user's own risk and responsibility. The authors and publishers request every user to report to the publishers any discrepancies or inaccuracies noticed. If errors in this work are found after publication, errata will be posted at www.thieme.com on the product description page.

1 2 3 4 5 6

Contributors

Stefan Adams, MD
Clinic for Radiology and Nuclear
Medicine
Ruhr University Bochum
Bochum, Germany

Volker Alt, MD
Department of Orthopedic
Trauma Surgery
University Hospital Giessen and
Marburg
Giessen, Germany

Henning Breithaupt, MD
Professor Emeritus
Department of Internal Medicine
University Hospital Giessen and
Marburg
Giessen, Germany

Lars Frommelt, MD
Private Practice
Hamburg, Germany

Thorsten Gehrke, MD
Medical Director
Endo-Clinic Hamburg
Hamburg, Germany

Volkmar Heppert, MD
Clinic for Accident Surgery
Director
Department of Posttraumatic
Osteomyelitis
Ludwigshafen, Germany

Gustav Hoer, MD
Professor Emeritus
Department of Nuclear Medicine
J.-W.-Goethe-University Frankfurt
Frankfurt, Germany

Siegfried Hofmann, MD
General and Orthopedic Clinic
Stolzalpe
Stolzalpe, Austria

Heinz-Herbert Homann, MD
Professor and Chief Physician
Department of Plastic Surgery
University Hospital Bergmannsheil
Ruhr University Bochum
Bochum, Germany

Ralf Kraus, MD
Department of Orthopedic
Trauma Surgery
University Hospital Giessen and
Marburg
Giessen, Germany

Michael Kroetz, MD
Private Radiology Practice
Heilbronn, Germany

Marcus Lehnhardt, MD
Senior Physician
Department of Plastic Surgery
University Hospital Bergmannsheil
Ruhr University Bochum
Bochum, Germany

Ulrich Linsenmaier, MD
Institute for Clinical Radiology
University Hospital Munich
Munich, Germany

Klausdieter Parsch, MD
Professor and Former Medical
Director
Orthopedic Clinic Olgahospital
Stuttgart, Germany

Martin Pietsch, MD
General and Orthopedic Clinic
Stolzalpe
Stolzalpe, Austria

Maximilian Reiser, MD
Professor and Director
Institute for Clinical Radiology
University Hospital Munich
Munich, Germany

Urs Schiefer, MD
Department of Orthopedic
Trauma Surgery
University Hospital Giessen and
Marburg
Giessen, Germany

Hergo G. K. Schmidt, MD
Head Physician
Septic Bone Surgery, Eilbek-Clinic
Hamburg, Germany

Reinhard Schnettler, MD
Professor and Director
Department of Orthopedic
Trauma Surgery
University Hospital Giessen and
Marburg
Giessen, Germany

Hans-Ulrich Steinau, MD
Professor and Director
Department of Plastic Surgery
University Hospital Bergmannsheil
Ruhr University Bochum
Bochum, Germany

Christoph Wenisch, MD
Professor and Medical Director
Department of Infectiology and
Tropical Medicine
Kaiser-Josef-Spital
Vienna, Austria

Obituary

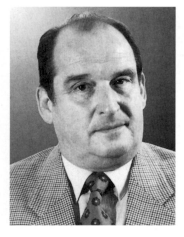

Dr. Klaus Klemm was chief of the unit for the treatment of septic cases at the BG Trauma Hospital in Frankfurt am Main, Germany for the last three decades of the 20th century. Dr. Klemm was born in May 1932 in Frankfurt am Main. He studied in Frankfurt and Freiburg before taking a position in Mount Kisco, NY in 1958 for 2 years. He received his license in Germany in 1962 and began working as an assistant to Professor Junghans at the new Frankfurt Workman's (BG) Hospital, where he became head of the septic unit.

Klaus Klemm is recognized internationally as an innovator for the development of antibiotic implants placed in wounds and for the interlocking nailing of long bone fractures. Both of these methods significantly reduce the morbidity of infected fractures. In his science, in his clinic, and in his life Klaus was a team player. He worked with Helmut Wahlig and Elvira Dingeldein of Darmstadt to establish the scientific basis for antibiotic leaching from antibiotic bead chains and with Dieter Schellmann in the improvement of Küntscher's medullary nailing by interlocking screws. In the hospital Klaus performed much of his own surgery and worked hard with hospital staff to promote a healing atmosphere. The walls of his office were decorated with patient art, his former patients sent letters about their activities from around the world, and strands of antibiotic bead chains hung from the rear view mirror of his car. Dr. Klemm invested heavily in his students. Dinners were festive. He promoted careers, arranged for international fellowships, knew his assistants' families and helped and believed in them even when they faced adversity. Klemm liked a good meal and went to great trouble to find the best ingredients, the best wines, and the best tables.

Dr. Klemm travelled, and lectured and wrote extensively. Above all, he is remembered for his humanism. From Klaus Klemm his students learned to accept the complexity and the imperfections inherent in the treatment of bone infection. Klemm developed specific algorithms for patient care so he was able to document the success of his strategies and improve his treatment plans. Thus, he helped patients over decades to control, not cure, their disease, which allowed them to continue with their lives. He was a practical and amiable person who grew up under difficult and changing circumstances. His art focused on making people better, including all those whom he treated, and with whom he worked and studied. Ironically, after a short retirement, Dr. Klemm died in August 2001 of a skeletal infection in the hospital where he had worked.

David Seligson, MD
Louisville, Kentucky, USA

Foreword

The treatment of bone and joint infections has remained the orphan stepchild of orthopedic surgery for the past 60 years. It has been confined to a rather small group of surgeons, who often fell upon this type of work accidentally or by assignment from a superior. The task of treating such problems was resultantly confined to teaching and government-run hospitals, to where such cases could be transferred.

Over the past 15 years this has slowly been changing, with an evolution and renaissance in understanding the treatment of osteomyelitis. Pioneers like Klaus Klemm and his work with antibiotic beads (*local antibiotic delivery systems*), and George Cierny with his work on the comprehensive classification of osteomyelitis including the role of the host, have helped change the mystique of this entity.

Better antibiotics have also added to the care of these infections. However, with this has also come the dreaded plague of ever greater resistance among organisms. It is now becoming an ever-increasing battle for drug manufacturers to keep up with the rate of development of antibiotic-resistant organisms. Hence the need for better understanding of the pathophysiology of bone and soft tissue infections, as well as the need for clear and reliable surgical treatment methods.

This superb text represents a major step in providing a clearer understanding of osteomyelitis and its treatment, which has been sorely lacking in the literature until now. It should serve as the basic reference for residents and fellows in their training, as well as a key reference text for the practicing orthopedic surgeon faced with a case of osteomyelitis. The book covers in a clear and concise manner not only the basis of the disease process, but also appropriate diagnostic techniques as well as treatment techniques and options based on the type of osteomyelitis or joint infection present. This is the first text in recent memory that has successfully accomplished this for the care of osteomyelitis.

The reader is further assisted by key learning points, highlighted in blue boxes, and tips and tricks, highlighted in yellow boxes, throughout the text. This helps the surgeon at all levels of experience better comprehend the important points in the diagnosis, pathology, and treatment of osteomyelitis. This feature is especially useful to residents and surgeons early in their career, as nothing comparable currently exists in this subfield of orthopedics.

Hopefully works such as this will represent a new era of synthesizing data on the care of bone and joint infections into a resource available to all orthopedic surgeons, which should also help take some of the mystery out of the treatment of this often debilitating condition. Its translation into English represents a giant step in this direction, and is greatly appreciated by all of us involved in the treatment and *the education of treatment* of osteomyelitis.

David Loewenberg, MD
Orthopedic Surgeon
San Francisco, CA, USA

Preface

Bone and joint infections are of great relevance to the fields of orthopedics and orthopedic trauma surgery worldwide, and it is with great pleasure that we present this first English edition of the textbook *Septic Bone and Joint Surgery*, translated from the first German edition. This textbook enables colleagues from all over the world to deepen their knowledge of this fascinating field of medicine.

The principle aim of this textbook is to provide both fully trained specialists and residents and fellows with the fundamental concepts of the diagnosis and therapeutic field of bone and joint infections.

The essential principles governing everyday practice are presented here without long theoretical debates or discrepant didactic opinions. The textbook combines the experience of experts in the fields of orthopedic and orthopedic trauma surgery, plastic surgery, radiology, and infectiology, together representing all disciplines involved in the care of patients with bone and joint infections including infections of indwelling devices.

The English edition of the textbook required the help of many colleagues and we are particularly grateful for the kind support of Professor D. Seligson, Louisville, Kentucky, USA, Professor D. Lowenberg, San Francisco, California, USA, and Thieme Publishers for their excellent manuscript preparation.

We hope that the presented concepts will improve both the treatment and outcome for many patients with bone and joint infections all over the world, which is the one and only purpose of this book.

Reinhard Schnettler

Contents

1

Historical Background

V. Alt, R. Schnettler

"Aside from maintaining the greatest possible distance from the source of infection when drilling into the medullary cavity or removing the affected bone segment, a special dressing technique is used for immobilization and elevation of the involved extremity."

This therapeutic advice is not from a current textbook, but was written by Johannes Scultetus (1595–1645), a surgeon from Ulm (Germany), who described this technique in his book *Armantarium Chirurgicum*, thus confirming that osteomyelitis has plagued mankind for many centuries.

The history of chronic bone infection actually goes back millions of years. Findings from the age of dinosaurs display obvious signs of inflammatory processes in fractured dinosaur vertebrae. Remainders of hominid skeletons also show lesions indicating the presence of osteomyelitic processes. The approximately 500 000-year-old femur of Java man (Homo erectus) shows possible signs of fracture healing complicated by osteomyelitis.

Cases are even described among Neanderthals (approximately 50 000 years ago), like the case of osteomyelitis of the clavicle found in the Shanidar region of Iraq. The Smith papyrus from Ancient Egypt (approximately 1550 BCE) is considered the oldest written report of a bone disease. It also contains descriptions of bone infections. Radiographs of Egyptian mummies identified remains of osteomyelitic processes.

In ancient times the Greek physician Hippocrates recommended "conservative therapy" of affected skeletal regions. In his opinion, necrotic bone and soft tissue should not be removed, but should be left to spontaneous rejection. He attributed great importance to treatment by rest and immobilization of the affected limb. Already in the first century the Roman physician Celsus recognized the importance of debridement and of vital bone tissue. In his view, one should only stop scraping the bone when blood appeared, which he considered to be a sign of vital bone tissue.

During the following centuries little new knowledge appeared in the theory and treatment of bone infections. In the 16th century, Paracelsus (approximately 1493–1541) recommended a consistently hygienic procedure to keep the wound free from contamination.

The history of posttraumatic osteomyelitis is closely connected with combat surgery, since the invention of firearms led to a multitude of open fractures caused by gunshot wounds. For example, Baron Larrey (1766–1842), a military surgeon in the Napoleonic army, reported that amputation was the preferred therapeutic treatment of gunshot wounds with bone involvement and performed more than 300 amputations on wounded soldiers in one day during Napoleon's invasion of Russia.

John Hunter (1728–1793) developed the first scientifically based concepts about the origin of sequestra in bone infections based on experiments performed in his animal laboratory. These theories can be considered the first milestone in understanding the pathophysiologic processes in osteomyelitis.

Leading works by Semmelweis, Pasteur, Koch, and Lister from the middle of the 19th century led to pioneering conclusions in the theory and treatment of infection. The observations of Ignaz Semmelweis (1818–1865) in the 1840s that not only body parts left over from autopsies, but also pus on physicians' hands, were responsible for puerperal sepsis, are considered the origins of antisepsis. Twenty years later Louis Pasteur (1822–1895) succeeded in discovering bacteria and identifying them as the cause of disease. He pinpointed staphylococci as the causative agent in osteomyelitis. Joseph Lister (1827–1912) asked himself why open fractures usually produced pus, but closed fractures did not, and what the critical difference was between an open and a closed fracture. Lister's familiarity with the work of his contemporary Pasteur induced him to combat the organisms responsible for wound and bone infections to prevent them occurring. He used carbolic acid (phenol) for the disinfection of contaminated wounds in the 1860s. Carbolic acid was applied directly to the wound and was also used to saturate the dressings applied afterwards, which led to the term "Lister dressing."

The discovery of penicillin by the Scot, Alexander Flemming (1881–1955), in 1928 revolutionized the whole field of medicine, as well as the treatment possibilities for osteomyelitis. In the 1930s, hematogenous osteomyelitis was responsible for 75 % of all bone infections, which before the era of antibiotics led to a mortality rate of 20 %. The introduction of penicillin reduced this mortality rate to less than 3 %.

Lorenz Böhler (1885–1973), founder of the field of orthopedic trauma surgery, recognized the danger of osteomyelitis in the operative treatment of fractures, especially when placing internal fracture fixation devices, and issued the following warning in 1930: "The most dangerous innovation in the treatment of fresh fractures is the fundamental operative approach, especially when practiced by novices, without the appropriate indication and with insufficient asepsis and inadequate materials." He emphasized the importance of disinfecting both instruments and hands, which had already been called for by Semmelweis, Pasteur, and Lister. Robert Koch (1843–1910) ushered in modern sterilization by recommending the use of heat and steam, which is safer and more reliable than disinfection with acid.

In the late 1950s Hans Willenegger (1910–1998) modified the practice of irrigation drainage (**Fig. 1.1**), which had been in use since World War I, by adding chloramphenicol to the irrigation fluid and draining it through a second drain. This often led to better healing of chronic osteomyelitis. This procedure, however, required intensive nursing care, and patients had to remain in bed beyond the treatment duration, which lasted several weeks.

In 1970 Hans-Wilhelm Buchholz, a surgeon with extensive knowledge for that time in the field of total joint prosthesis, published a paper in which he reported a reduction in the rate of infections occurring with the placement of hip prostheses when the antibiotic gentamicin was added to the bone cement consisting of polymethylmethacrylate (PMMA).

Klaus Klemm (1932–2000), a surgeon from Frankfurt, Germany, adapted this concept by forming small beads molded from the malleable gentamicin-PMMA cement. After several experiments, in 1972 he first placed these in the medullary space of a patient's infected bone following classical surgical debridement. This was the birth of the concept of operative local antibiotic treatment. At the same time, Verhoeve and colleagues used gentamicin-cement seals for local antibiotic treatment. This, however, proved unsuccessful. Until 1976 Klemm produced his gentamicin-PMMA beads himself in the operating theater and achieved very good treatment results. In November of the same year, Merck Pharmaceuticals (Darmstadt, Germany) overcame the fundamental problems in the industrial production of these beads. Klemm thus introduced a new, albeit controversial, therapeutic concept which demonstrated unprecedented treatment success combined with patient comfort. Patients were no longer confined to their bed, and the treatment duration was considerably reduced in comparison to the suction/irrigation drainage procedure.

Despite available therapeutic possibilities, chronic osteomyelitis still presents both the patient and the doctor in charge with a serious situation. The increasing number of multidrug-resistant organisms over the past years, above all in bone and soft-tissue defects, complicates therapy considerably and calls for united efforts on the part of involved physicians, microbiologists, and industry to come up with new antimicrobial substances and/or new therapeutic approaches.

Further Reading

Bishop W. The Early History of Surgery. London: Hale; 1960

Buchholz HW, Engelbrecht H. Depot effects of various antibiotics mixed with Palacos resins. [Article in German] Chirurg 1970;41(11):511–515

Janssens PA. Palaeopathology. London: John Baker; 1970

Klemm K. Gentamicin-PMMA-beads in treating bone and soft tissue infections (author's transl). [Article in German] Zentralbl Chir 1979;104(14):934–942

Pasteur, L. La théorie des germes et ses applications à la medicine et à la chirurgie. Compt rend Acad sc 1878;86:1037–1043

Pickett JC. A short historical sketch of osteomyelitis. Ann Med Hist 1935;7:183–191

Popkirov PG. Behandlung der hämatogenen und der traumatischen Osteomyelitis. Berlin: VEB Verlag Volk und Gesundheit; 1971

Povacz F. Geschichte der Unfallchirurgie. Berlin: Springer; 2000

Scultetus J. Armentarium Chirurgicum. Ulm: Kühnen; 1655

Thomann KD, Rauschmann M. Der Krankheit den Schrecken genommen. Osteosynth. Int. 2000;8(Suppl. 1):S23–S27

Trinkaus E, Zimmerman MR. Trauma among the Shanidar Neandertals. Am J Phys Anthropol 1982;57(1):61–76

Wenz W, Spranz B, Kosack W. View of the past: Roentgenography of an Egyptian mummy. [Article in German] Radiologe 1975;15(2):45–49

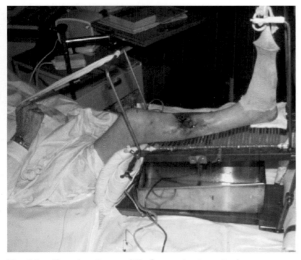

Fig. 1.1 Chronic osteomyelitis, former treatment scheme applying mechanical toilet.

2

Pathophysiology and Classification of Osteomyelitis

R. Schnettler, V. Alt

Introduction

Postoperative and posttraumatic infections of bones, soft tissues, and joints still present a large problem and are among the most serious complications despite rapid advances in the field of medicine.

Osteomyelitis basically means inflammation of bone and bone-marrow components. This could be of bacterial origin, but may also result from tuberculosis or syphilis and, depending on the immune status of the host, may even be of fungal or parasitic (echinococci, toxoplasma) origin.

The infectious organisms reach the bones either through the bloodstream (endogenous) or by direct colonization (exogenous). The bacteria reach the bones through skin lesions, soft-tissue necroses, or operation wounds. The term osteomyelitis has achieved worldwide acceptance.

From a pathologic-anatomical point of view, osteomyelitis can be differentiated into a focal form—referred to as a bone abscess—and one with diffuse spread.

Pathophysiology of Osteomyelitis

Bone provides supportive tissue consisting of an organic matrix and cellular elements. Because of the morphology of bone structure, osteomyelitis is not limited to the bone surface, but extends to all components of the infected osseous area. Osteocytes are distributed throughout the bone matrix and are connected to neighboring cells and blood vessels through cytodendrites in tiny canals (**Fig. 2.1**).

This canal system is of central importance for metabolic processes. Longitudinal vascular canals (haversian canals) run through the center of each bone lamella, and Volkmann's canals run through the compact layer. These two systems are interconnected, thus when bone infection occurs the inflammatory process usually affects all osseous components. Moreover, inflammatory resorptive processes create wide connecting canals between the individual osteons.

Surgical implantation of foreign materials, for example plates, nails, screws, and fixator pins, as well as joint prostheses and bone cement, is associated with a higher infection rate than operative procedures in which no foreign material is implanted (Southwood et al. 1985, Gristina 1987).

After implantation, a "battle" evolves for colonization of the surface of the foreign body in which cell or tissue integration and bacterial adhesion simultaneously compete. This is referred to as the "race for the surface" (Gristina 1987, 1990).

The bacteria stick to the surfaces in order to survive, whereby approximately 90% of the physiologic bacteria survive in the adherent biofilm (Gristina 1987).

For the manifestation of an infection, for example following wound contamination, the first 5 hours are decisive, during which the invading organisms are attacked by the immune cells. Antibiotics help reduce the number of pathogens during this phase (Gristina et al. 1989, König et al. 1998).

Since healthy bone tissue is highly resistant to infection, additional factors other than contamination must be present to promote an infection (Andriole et al. 1973, Burri 1979, Klemm 1979). Implants reduce the natural resistance of bones to infection by a factor of 1000, whereby the threshold number of pathogens/infectious dose which can cause an infection in healthy bone tissue is reduced from 10^8 to 10^5 pathogens (Rüter et al. 1995).

If the pathogens have initially reached or entered the bone, specific mechanisms enable them to adhere to the surface of the implants. These include bacterial factors, surface characteristics of the implants, and host factors. Adherence of the pathogens is achieved by polysaccharides in their capsules and surface components resembling fimbria. Electrostatic and hydrophobic interactions (van der Waals forces) between bacteria and the implant surface also play an important role.

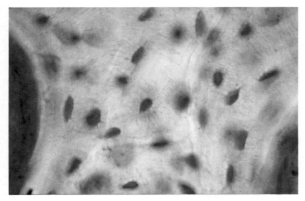

Fig. 2.1 Osteocytes with cytoplasmatic projections.

On the part of the host, the function of fibronectin is particularly important in pathogen adhesion to plates, nails, and screws (Fischer et al. 1996).

Bacterial adhesion to the surface of implants is a decisive prerequisite for the development of a biofilm. The term biofilm can be defined as a structured collection of bacteria (microcolonies) which produces a glycocalix through the synthesis of an extracellular slimy substance or exopolysaccharides and can be found on the surface of both vital and inert structures. This resultant slime protects the pathogens from the body's own immune defenses and also from antibiotics (Peters et al. 1982). The biofilm can be mono- or polymicrobial and is considered a potential source of spread of infection (Berendet 1999, Costerson et al. 1999, O'Gara et al. 2001, Donlan 2002; **Fig. 2.2**).

This creates the foundation for the proliferation of pathogens in bone tissue or on the implant covering the bone. Local ischemia and devitalized bone fragments following an operation or trauma decisively promote the proliferation of bacteria (Norden and Kennedy 1970, Emslie and Nade 1983).

Microembolisms, endotoxin release, and granulation tissue further decrease blood circulation and can disturb

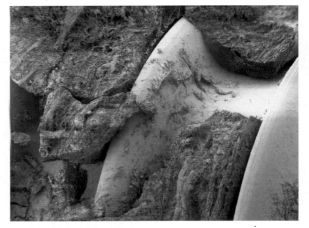

Fig. 2.2 Biofilm formation by *S. aureus* on a screw.

the medullary and periosteal circulation and lead to sequestration (Khouri and Shaw 1989).

Sequestra constitute an ideal nutrient medium for the further spread of bacteria, which can evade endogenous immune defenses and antibiotic therapy in this necrotic tissue (Notzli et al. 1989, Klemm 1993).

Pathogens

Staphylococci are the most common pathogens detected in connection with osteomyelitis, and they often appear in mixed infections (Gentry 1988, Perry et al. 1991, Haas and McAndrew 1996, Schnettler et al. 1997; **Table 2.1, Fig. 2.3**). *Staphylococcus aureus* is the most common species, accounting for 30% (Gentry 1988) to 70% (Perry et al. 1991, Haas and McAndrew 1996, Schnettler et al. 1997) of bone infections; however, coagulase-negative staphylococci, like *Staphylococcus epidermidis*, also deserve mention. *Staphylococcus epidermidis* is found in up to 90% of bone infections following intraoperative implantation of foreign material, like joint prostheses and internal fracture fixation devices (Quie and Belani 1987, Mahan et al. 1991). This is normally a nonvirulent bacillus which colonizes the skin, but its common ability to form a biofilm predestines it to colonize implants and endanger the patient (von Eiff et al. 2002). Besides staphylococci, *Pseudomonas* species and other Gram-negative pathogens are detected, though less frequently (Gentry 1988, Perry et al. 1991, Haas and McAndrew 1996, Schnettler et al. 1997).

During the past years, an increasing number of multi-resistant pathogens have been identified as causative agents for infections in many medical fields. In one study in the USA the proportion of nosocomial infections with

methicillin-resistant *S. aureus* (MRSA) increased from 2.4% in 1971 to 29% in 1991 (Panlilio et al. 1992). In the same study, this figure exceeded 38% in large hospitals with over 500 beds. The incidence of MRSA infections is increasing, especially in intensive care units. In 1995 a European prevalence study reported that up to 60% of infections in intensive care units were caused by MRSA (Vincent et al. 1995).

The fields of emergency and orthopedic surgery have also witnessed an increase (not only in absolute terms,

Table 2.1 Confirmed pathogens in osteomyelitis (Gentry 1988).

Pathogen	1987 (n = 192)	
Staphylococcus aureus	57	(30%)
Pseudomonas aeruginosa	18	(9%)
Mixed infection	70	(36%)
Other Gram-positive pathogens	17	(9%)
Other Gram-negative pathogens	25	(13%)
Unclassified bacteria	5	(3%)

but also in terms of percentage) in infections with multiresistant pathogens, for example, of joint prostheses (Kilgus et al. 2002). Treating infections with multiresistant pathogens is much more difficult and costly than infections with nonmultiresistant pathogens (Kilgus et al. 2002, Herr et al. 2003).

Staphylococcal resistance to methicillin and all other β-lactam antibiotics is associated with the production of the penicillin-binding protein PBP2a, which is not found in methicillin-sensitive *Staphylococcus* species (Pierre et al. 1990, Chambers 1997). The PBP2a protein is encoded by the mecA gene, whose regulation is controlled by the mecR1-mecI inducer-repressor system (Matuhashi et al. 1986, Tesch et al. 1990, Hackbarth and Chambers 1993, Sharma et al. 1998). The mecR1 gene encodes a β-lactam-detecting transmembranous signal protein; the mecI gene encodes a repressor protein for the mecA gene. Loss or inactivation of the mecI gene removes the inhibition of the mecA gene, thereby leading to resistance to methicillin and other β-lactam antibiotics (Suzuki et al. 1993, Shimaoka et al. 1994, Weller et al. 1999).

For a detailed discussion of antibiotic treatment and special precautions against MRSA and other multiresistant pathogens, see Chapter 4.

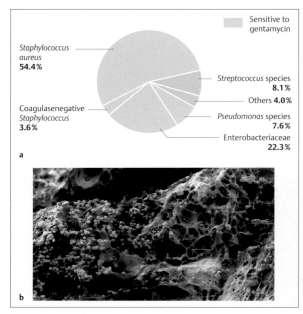

Sensitive to gentamycin

Staphylococcus aureus **54.4%**

Streptococcus species **8.1%**

Others **4.0%**

Coagulasenegative *Staphylococcus* **3.6%**

Pseudomonas species **7.6%**

Enterobacteriaceae **22.3%**

a

b

Fig. 2.3a, b Pathogen spectrum. *S. aureus*

Risk Factors

Local:
- Disturbances in arterial and venous circulation
- Tissue damaged by radiation
- Extensive exposure of the operation site
- Extensive soft-tissue defects
- Extensive hematomas
- Remaining hollow spaces

Systemic:
- Diabetes mellitus
- Nicotine and drug use
- Disturbances of liver and kidney function
- Severe infections with immunosuppression

Besides bacteria–host interactions, there exist interactions between the host and implants, independent of bacterial colonization. Polymorphonuclear neutrophilic leukocytes are part of endogenous immunity and are activated not only by bacteria, but also by implant surfaces. With the aid of the enzymes in their cell membranes they produce not only nitrogen and intermediate oxygen products, but also hypochloric acid and proteases and release antibacterial peptides, also known as defensins, for antimicrobial resistance. These aggregate, integrate into the pathogens' cell membranes, and perforate them (Kaplan et al. 1999, Schiefer 2003).

Colonization with pathogens on the surface of implants, prostheses, and/or bones causes infection with a typical pathologic appearance:
- Acute, inflammatory reaction around the implant or bone with all signs of infection
- Chronic inflammatory reaction with loss of bone on the surface in contact with the implant caused by activation of osteoclasts and recruiting of cells originating from monocytes

NOTE

The main characteristic of an infected implant or bone is the presence of an inflammatory infiltration.

In principle, the disease can be categorized according to:
- Clinical symptoms (acute or chronic)
- Infective mechanism (exogenous or endogenous-hematogenous)
- Wound status (simple wound, chronic ulcer, multiple fistula with and without contact with the body surface)
- Host reaction (abscess formation or not)

Forms of Osteomyelitis

Acute:
- Hematogenous
- Iatrogenous (postoperative, posttraumatic, disseminated)

Chronic:
- Inactive
- Active

Osteomyelitis is classified into a purulent and a nonpurulent form. On the basis of the clinical findings, the purulent form can be classified into an acute, subacute, and chronic (active and inactive) form (Simon and Stille 1997; **Table 2.2**).

Because of the prognostic and therapeutic relevance of differentiating the purulent form into acute, subacute, and chronic osteomyelitis, this classification will be used in the following text.

Acute Osteomyelitis

A hematogenous spread of pathogens is usually present in the bone. The patient presents with general malaise and a painful, swollen, localized lesion. The majority of cases

Table 2.2 Classification of osteomyelitis according to the duration of symptoms, origin of infection, and host factors (Gentry 1988).

	Acute	Chronic
Duration	Symptoms < 4 weeks	Symptoms > 4 weeks
Source of infection	Spread from infectious focus Secondary bacteremia	Posttraumatic or postoperative spread from neighboring skin ulcer
Host factors	Rare	Often with diabetes mellitus (arterial occlusive disease)

involve children and adolescents between 2 years of age and skeletal maturity. Acute osteomyelitis is referred to as the juvenile form of hematogenous osteomyelitis.

Another age peak is described in infants after an infection of the umbilicus and inflammations of the ears, nose, and throat. These occur mostly between 1 and 10 months; boys are more often affected than girls (Lamprecht 1997).

Because the arteries in the epiphyses are terminal, the capillaries enter wide sinusoids located just in front of the growth plates. Thrombi caused by bacteria or an embolus can occlude these vessels and lead to a significant decrease in perfusion of this region. As a result, necroses can develop in the transition zone between metaphysis and epiphysis and provide an ideal nutrient medium for osteomyelitis (Morgan 1959, Trueta 1959, Dich et al. 1975).

The infection first establishes itself in the bone marrow and then spreads via the haversian and Volkmann's canals along the thrombosed capillaries and through the cortex below the periosteum.

This leads to the classic metaphyseal abscess. As soon as the periosteum has been raised from the bone, reduced periosteal perfusion together with reduced cortical perfusion resulting from thrombosed capillaries leads to the typical cortical sequestrum. This may be surrounded by periosteal new bone formation and is then referred to as bone cavity (**Figs. 2.4 and 2.5**).

The epiphyseal plate serves as a barrier to infection, preventing the infection from spreading to the epiphysis. Exceptions are anatomical variants among small children up to 18 months of age. During this period, blood vessels can cross the growth plate (Trueta 1959, Ogden 1979). The epiphysis may also be affected after completion of skeletal growth, where there is no more epihyseal plate and, therefore, no infection barrier (Perry 1996; for a detailed discussion see Chapter 5, Hematogenous Infection of Bones and Joints, p. 152).

Direct inoculation of germs in the bones, for example after trauma or surgery, can also lead to acute osteomyelitis. This is then called acute exogenous osteomyelitis. (The treatment of an early infection is described in Chapter 5, Acute and Chronic Posttraumatic Osteomyelitis, p. 94.)

Subacute Osteomyelitis

The subacute form of osteomyelitis differs from the acute form in that it lacks systemic disease manifestations and begins gradually. This can be explained by a good immune system and/or low virulence of the pathogen (Gledhill 1973, Bergmann and Levenberg 1990). The frequent lack of pain and unremarkable laboratory parameters of-

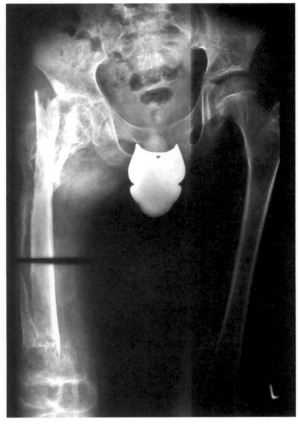

Fig. 2.4 Sequestrum.

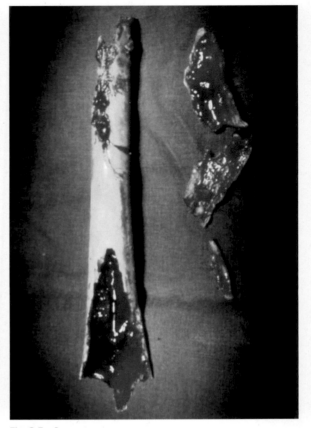

Fig. 2.5 Sequestrum.

ten cause diagnosis to be delayed by months (Cottias et al. 1997). The most common manifestation of subacute osteomyelitis is a Brodie abscess (**Fig. 2.6**), which is a circumscribed osteomyelitic lesion surrounded by granulation tissue in the metaphysis of a tubular bone.

Differential diagnosis of an abscess, which is usually discovered by chance in the distal femoral metaphysis or the distal or proximal tibial metaphysis, should exclude an enchondroma, bone cyst, or osteosarcoma. (Treatment is described in Chapter 5, Hematogenous Infection of Bones and Joints, p. 152.)

Chronic Osteomyelitis

Chronic osteomyelitis arises primarily from a posttraumatic or postoperative infection, but can also develop from acute hematogenous osteomyelitis. After an arbitrary time period of over 4 weeks, it should be referred to as a chronic inflammation (Gentry 1988, Perry 1996). This persisting, productive form of bone inflammation is characterized by chronic purulent fistulous discharge (**Fig. 2.7**).

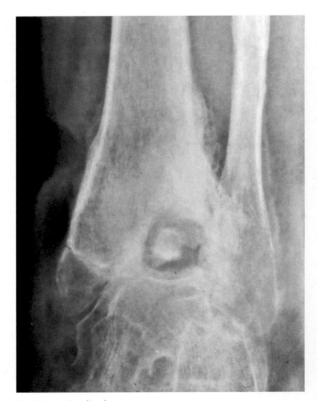

Fig. 2.6 A Brodie abscess.

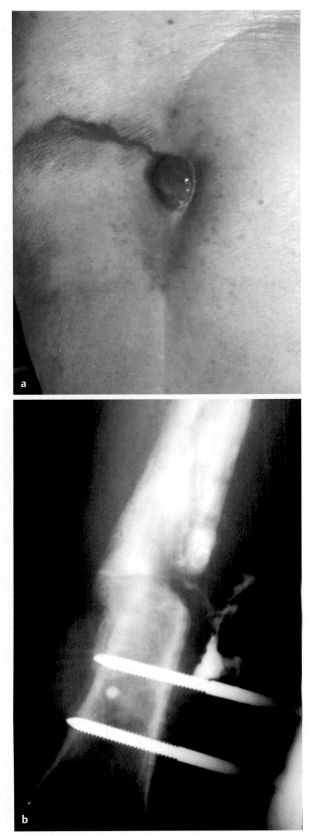

Ulcerous soft-tissue defects above the affected bone provide important indications of chronicity. After months or years of quiescence, the local infection can flare up again. This is defined as an acute attack of chronic postoperative or posttraumatic osteomyelitis.

Chronic osteomyelitis rarely presents as generalized malaise, but an acute flare-up can cause general illness (Perry 1996). Implants constitute a risk factor for persistence of osteomyelitis (**Fig. 2.8**).

Chronic osteomyelitis is pathologically characterized by infected osseous necroses (Klemm 1979 and 1993, Cierny 1987, Perry 1996, Mader 1997). A further important prerequisite for the appearance of chronic osteomyelitis is the virulence of the pathogen. We know that *S. aureus* can assume a reduced metabolic state, the so-called small-colony variant. This allows it to effectively evade antibiotics (Hoffstadt and Youngmann 1932, Nair et al. 1996, von Eiff et al. 1998).

Osteolyses and the development of infected nonunions are two important pathophysiologic processes in posttraumatic or postoperative chronic osteomyelitis. Osteolyses are caused by bacteria, either directly by their endotoxins—lipopolysaccharides and N-acetylmuramin dipeptides (Hausmann et al. 1970, Dewhirst 1982, Ishmi et al. 1980, Nair et al. 1996) or by IL-1, IL-6, and tumor necrosis factor (TNF) (Stashenko et al. 1987).

Osteolysis is responsible for the lack of bony consolidation and the development of nonunions. The same mechanisms also cause septic loosening of prostheses (Ciampolini and Harding 2000).

Infected nonunion, a special form of chronic osteomyelitis, is a combination of two severe, local, mutually potentiating complications—**instability and infection**.

A fundamental problem in the treatment of osteomyelitis is the fact that neither a uniform terminology exists, nor an agreement on when certain terms are to be used (Gordon and Chiu 1988).

Fig. 2.7a, b **a** Secreting fistula. **b** Fistulography with visualization of the fistulous channel.

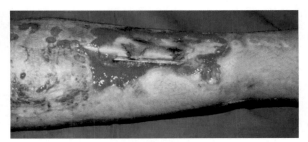

Fig. 2.8 Chronic osteomyelitis after internal plate fixation.

Cierny et al. (1985) classified chronic osteomyelitis into 12 groups, whereby four types are differentiated according to the location of the infection (**Fig. 2.9**).

Gordon and Chiu (1988) defined their classification according to the severity of the bony injury:

Type A: defect in the tibia and nonunion without significant bone loss

Type B: defect in the tibia >3 cm with intact fibula

Type C: defect in the tibia <3 cm with fractured fibula

May et al. (1989) founded their classification based on the size of the defects in the tibia and fibula (**Fig. 2.10**).

Since this classification includes neither the different forms of nonunion nor the degree of soft-tissue injury, it is of limited value for clinical application. Further classifications are based on the type of infected tissue (Ger 1970), the etiology and affected regions (Waldvogel et al. 1980, Kelly 1984), or the size of the infected area (Weiland et al. 1984).

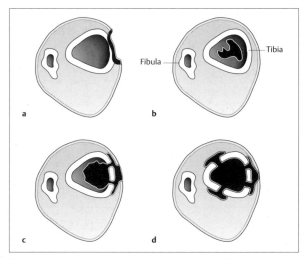

Fig. 2.9a–d Location: **a** superficial, **b** intramedullary, **c** local, **d** diffuse.

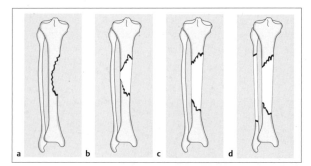

Fig. 2.10a–d Spread of infection. Type I: intact tibia and fibula, stable on weight bearing (not shown). **a** Type II: intact tibia that requires a bone transplant for structural support. **b** Type III: Defect in tibia that is 6 cm or less with an intact fibula. **c** Type IV: Defect in tibia of more than 6 cm with intact fibula. **d** Type V: Defect in tibia of more than 6 cm with nonintact or useless fibula.

Bibliography

Andriole VT, Nagel DA, Southwick WO. A paradigm for human chronic osteomyelitis. J Bone Joint Surg Am 1973; 55(7):1511–1515

Berendt AR, McLardy-Smith P. Prosthetic joint infection. Curr Infect Dis Rep 1999;1(3):267–272

Bergman AT, Levenberg R. Brodie's abscess of the tibia. Orthop 1990;11:1316–1317

Blyth MJ, Kincaid R, Craigen MA, Bennet GC. The changing epidemiology of acute and subacute haematogenous osteomyelitis in children. J Bone Joint Surg Br 2001;83(1):99–102

Bonnaire F, Hohaus T, Cyffka R, Lein T. Bone infections. [Article in German] Unfallchirurg 2002;105(8):716–731, quiz 731, 733

Burri C. Posttraumatische Osteitis. Bern: Verlag Hans Huber; 1979

Chambers HF. Methicillin resistance in staphylococci: molecular and biochemical basis and clinical implications. Clin Microbiol Rev 1997;10(4):781–791

Christensen GD, Parisi JT, Bisno AL, Simpson WA, Beachey EH. Characterization of clinically significant strains of coagulase-negative staphylococci. J Clin Microbiol 1983;18(2):258–269

Ciampolini J, Harding KG. Pathophysiology of chronic bacterial osteomyelitis. Why do antibiotics fail so often? Postgrad Med J 2000;76(898):479–483

Cierny G III, Mader JT, Pennick JJ. A clinical staging system of adult osteomyelitis. Contemp Orthop 1985;10:17–37

Costerton JW, Stewart PS, Greenberg EP. Bacterial biofilms: a common cause of persistent infections. Science 1999;284(5418):1318–1322

Cottias P, Tomeno B, Anract P, Vinh TS, Forest M. Subacute osteomyelitis presenting as a bone tumour. A review of 21 cases. Int Orthop 1997;21(4):243–248

Craigen MA, Watters J, Hackett JS. The changing epidemiology of osteomyelitis in children. J Bone Joint Surg Br 1992;74(4):541–545

Dewhirst FE. N-acetyl muramyl dipeptide stimulation of bone resorption in tissue culture. Infect Immun 1982;35(1):133–137

Dich VQ, Nelson JD, Haltalin KC. Osteomyelitis in infants and children. A review of 163 cases. Am J Dis Child 1975; 129(11):1273–1278

Donlan RM. Biofilms: microbial life on surfaces. Emerg Infect Dis 2002;8(9):881–890

Emslie KR, Nade S. Acute hematogenous staphylococcal osteomyelitis. A description of the natural history in an avian model. Am J Pathol 1983;110(3):333–345

Espersen F, Clemmensen I. Isolation of a fibronectin-binding protein from Staphylococcus aureus. Infect Immun 1982;37(2):526–531

Fischer B, Vaudaux P, Magnin M, et al. Novel animal model for studying the molecular mechanisms of bacterial adhesion to bone-implanted metallic devices: role of fibronectin in Staphylococcus aureus adhesion. J Orthop Res 1996;14(6):914–920

Gentry LO. Osteomyelitis: options for diagnosis and management. J Antimicrob Chemother 1988;21(Suppl C):115–131

Ger R. The management of open fracture of the tibia with skin loss. J Trauma 1970;10(2):112–121

Gledhill RB. Subacute osteomyelitis in children. Clin Orthop Relat Res 1973;96(96):57–69

Gordon L, Chiu EJ. Treatment of infected non-unions and segmental defects of the tibia with staged microvascular muscle transplantation and bone-grafting. J Bone Joint Surg Am 1988;70(3):377–386

Gristina AG. Biomaterial-centered infection: microbial adhesion versus tissue integration. Science 1987;237(4822): 1588–1595

Gristina AG, Webb LX, Barth E. Microbial adhesion, biomaterials and man. In: Coombs R, Fitzgerald RH Jr, eds. Infection in the Orthopaedic Patient. London: Butterworths; 1989

Gristina AG, Naylor PT, Webb LX. Molecular mechanisms in musculoskeletal sepsis: The race for the surface. In: Greene WB, ed. Park Ridge, IL: AAOS Instructional Course Lecture XXXIX; 1990:471–482

Gustilo RB, Anderson JT. Prevention of infection in the treatment of one thousand and twenty-five open fractures of long bones: retrospective and prospective analyses. J Bone Joint Surg Am 1976;58(4):453–458

Gustilo RB, Mendoza RM, Williams DN. Problems in the management of type III (severe) open fractures: a new classification of type III open fractures. J Trauma 1984;24(8):742–746

Gustilo RB, Merkow RL, Templeman D. The management of open fractures. J Bone Joint Surg Am 1990;72(2):299–304

Haas DW, McAndrew MP. Bacterial osteomyelitis in adults: evolving considerations in diagnosis and treatment. Am J Med 1996;101(5):550–561

Hackbarth CJ, Chambers HF. blaI and blaR1 regulate beta-lactamase and PBP 2a production in methicillin-resistant Staphylococcus aureus. Antimicrob Agents Chemother 1993;37(5):1144–1149

Hausmann E, Raisz LG, Miller WA. Endotoxin: stimulation of bone resorption in tissue culture. Science 1970;168(933): 862–864

Hayes CS, Heinrich SD, Craver R, MacEwen GD. Subacute osteomyelitis. Orthopedics 1990;13(3):363–366

Herr CEW, Heckrodt TH, Hofmann FA, Schnettler R, Eikmann TF. Additional costs for preventing the spread of methicillin-resistant Staphylococcus aureus and a strategy for reducing these costs on a surgical ward. Infect Control Hosp Epidemiol 2003 24(9):673–678

Hoffstadt RE, Youngman GP. Staphylococcus aureus dissociation and its relation to infection and immunity. J Infect Dis 1932;51:216

Ishimi Y, Miyaura C, Jin CH, et al. IL-6 is produced by osteoblasts and induces bone resorption. J Immunol 1990; 145(10):3297–3303

Kahn DS, Pritzker KP. The pathophysiology of bone infection. Clin Orthop Relat Res 1973;96(96):12–19

Kaplan SS, Heine RP, Simmons RL. Defensins impair phagocytic killing by neutrophils in biomaterial-related infection. Infect Immun 1999;67(4):1640–1645

Kelly PJ. Infected nonunion of the femur and tibia. Orthop Clin North Am 1984;15(3):481–490

Kilgus DJ, Howe DJ, Strang A. Results of periprosthetic hip and knee infections caused by resistant bacteria. Clin Orthop Relat Res 2002;404(404):116–124

König DP, Schierholz JM, Hackenbroch MH. Häufung und Prophylaxe von Staphylococcus-epidermis-Infektionen in der Endoprothetik. Hyg Med 1998;23:274–279

Kuusela P. Fibronectin binds to Staphylococcus aureus. Nature 1978;276(5689):718–720

Lamprecht E. Acute osteomyelitis in childhood. [Article in German] Orthopade 1997;26(10):868–878

Lopes JD, dos Reis M, Brentani RR. Presence of laminin receptors in Staphylococcus aureus. Science 1985;229(4710): 275–277

Mackowiak PA, Jones SR, Smith JW. Diagnostic value of sinus-tract cultures in chronic osteomyelitis. JAMA 1978; 239(26): 2772–2775

Mader JT, Shirtliff M, Calhoun JH. Staging and staging application in osteomyelitis. Clin Infect Dis 1997;25(6):1303–1309

Mahan J, Seligson D, Henry SL, Hynes P, Dobbins J. Factors in pin tract infections. Orthopedics 1991;14(3):305–308

Matsuhashi M, Song MD, Ishino F, et al. Molecular cloning of the gene of a penicillin-binding protein supposed to cause high resistance to beta-lactam antibiotics in Staphylococcus aureus. J Bacteriol 1986;167(3):975–980

May JW Jr, Jupiter JB, Weiland AJ, Byrd HS. Clinical classification of post-traumatic tibial osteomyelitis. J Bone Joint Surg Am 1989;71(9):1422–1428

Morgan JD. Blood supply of growing rabbit's tibia. J Bone Joint Surg Br 1959;41-B(1):185–203

Nair SP, Meghji S, Wilson M, Reddi K, White P, Henderson B. Bacterially induced bone destruction: mechanisms and misconceptions. Infect Immun 1996;64(7):2371–2380

Norden CW, Kennedy E. Experimental osteomyelitis. I. A description of the model. J Infect Dis 1970;122(5):410–418

Nötzli HP, Swiontkowski MF, Thaxter ST, Carpenter GK III, Wyatt R. Laser Doppler flowmetry for bone blood flow measurements: helium-neon laser light attenuation and depth of perfusion assessment. J Orthop Res 1989;7(3): 413–424

O'Gara JP, Humphreys H. Staphylococcus epidermidis biofilms: importance and implications. J Med Microbiol 2001; 50(7):582–587

Ogden JA. Pediatric osteomyelitis and septic arthritis: the pathology of neonatal disease. Yale J Biol Med 1979;52(5): 423–448

Panlilio AL, Culver DH, Gaynes RP, et al. Methicillin-resistant Staphylococcus aureus in U.S. hospitals, 1975-1991. Infect Control Hosp Epidemiol 1992;13(10):582–586

Patti JM, Boles JO, Höök M. Identification and biochemical characterization of the ligand binding domain of the collagen adhesin from Staphylococcus aureus. Biochemistry 1993;32(42):11428–11435

Perry CR, Pearson RL, Miller GA. Accuracy of cultures of material from swabbing of the superficial aspect of the wound and needle biopsy in the preoperative assessment of osteomyelitis. J Bone Joint Surg Am 1991;73(5):745–749

Perry CR. Bone and Joint Infections. London: Martin Dunitz; 1996

Peters G, Locci R, Pulverer G. Adherence and growth of coagulase-negative staphylococci on surfaces of intravenous catheters. J Infect Dis 1982;146(4):479–482

Pierre J, Williamson R, Bornet M, Gutmann L. Presence of an additional penicillin-binding protein in methicillin-resistant Staphylococcus epidermidis, Staphylococcus haemolyticus, Staphylococcus hominis, and Staphylococcus simulans with a low affinity for methicillin, cephalothin, and cefamandole. Antimicrob Agents Chemother 1990;34(9):1691–1694

Quie PG, Belani KK. Coagulase-negative staphylococcal adherence and persistence. J Infect Dis 1987;156(4):543–547

Rüter A, Trentz O, Wagner M. Unfallchirurgie. Munich: Urban and Schwarzenberg; 1995

Scheman L, Janota M, Lewin P. The production of experimental osteomyelitis. JAMA 1941;117:1525–1529

Schiefer U. Antibiotikahaltige Knochenzemente: In vitro Untersuchungen der Freisetzungskinetik und antimikrobiellen Wirkung. Gießen: Inauguraldissertation; 2004

Schnettler R, Lieser H, Klemm K. Chirurgische Behandlung der posttraumatischen chronischen Osteomyelitis. Akt Chir 1997;32:18–22

Sharma VK, Hackbarth CJ, Dickinson TM, Archer GL. Interaction of native and mutant MecI repressors with sequences that regulate mecA, the gene encoding penicillin binding protein 2a in methicillin-resistant staphylococci. J Bacteriol 1998;180(8):2160–2166

Shimaoka M, Yoh M, Segawa A, Takarada Y, Yamamoto K, Honda T. Development of enzyme-labeled oligonucleotide probe for detection of mecA gene in methicillin-resistant Staphylococcus aureus. J Clin Microbiol 1994;32(8):1866–1869

Simon C, Stille W. Antibiotika-Therapie in Klinik und Praxis. 9th ed. Stuttgart: Schattauer; 1997

Southwood RT, Rice JL, McDonald PJ, Hakendorf PH, Rozenbilds MA. Infection in experimental hip arthroplasties. J Bone Joint Surg Br 1985;67(2):229–231

Stashenko P, Dewhirst FE, Peros WJ, Kent RL, Ago JM. Synergistic interactions between interleukin 1, tumor necrosis factor, and lymphotoxin in bone resorption. J Immunol 1987;138(5):1464–1468

Suzuki E, Kuwahara-Arai K, Richardson JF, Hiramatsu K. Distribution of mec regulator genes in methicillin-resistant Staphylococcus clinical strains. Antimicrob Agents Chemother 1993;37(6):1219–1226

Swiontkowski MF, Hanel DP, Vedder NB, Schwappach JR. A comparison of short- and long-term intravenous antibiotic therapy in the postoperative management of adult osteomyelitis. J Bone Joint Surg Br 1999;81(6):1046–1050

Tesch W, Ryffel C, Strässle A, Kayser FH, Berger-Bächi B. Evidence of a novel staphylococcal mec-encoded element (mecR) controlling expression of penicillin-binding protein 2′. Antimicrob Agents Chemother 1990;34(9):1703–1706

Trueta J. The three types of acute hematogenous osteomyelitis, a clinical and vascular study. J Bone Joint Surg Br 1959;41:671–680

Vincent JL, Bihari DJ, Suter PM, et al; EPIC International Advisory Committee. The prevalence of nosocomial infection in intensive care units in Europe. Results of the European Prevalence of Infection in Intensive Care (EPIC) Study. JAMA 1995;274(8):639–644

von Eiff C, Lindner N, Proctor RA, Winkelmann W, Peters G. Development of gentamicin-resistant Small Colony Variants of S. aureus after implantation of gentamicin chains in osteomyelitis as a possible cause of recurrence. [Article in German] Z Orthop Ihre Grenzgeb 1998;136(3):268–271

von Eiff C, Peters G, Heilmann C. Pathogenesis of infections due to coagulase-negative staphylococci. Lancet Infect Dis 2002;2(11):677–685

Waldvogel FA, Medoff G, Swartz MN. Osteomyelitis: a review of clinical features, therapeutic considerations and unusual aspects. 3. Osteomyelitis associated with vascular insufficiency. N Engl J Med 1970;282(6):316–322

Waldvogel FA, Papageorgiou PS. Osteomyelitis: the past decade. N Engl J Med 1980;303(7):360–370

Weiland AJ, Moore JR, Daniel RK. The efficacy of free tissue transfer in the treatment of osteomyelitis. J Bone Joint Surg Am 1984;66(2):181–193

Weller TMA. The distribution of mecA, mecR1 and mecI and sequence analysis of mecI and the mec promoter region in staphylococci expressing resistance to methicillin. J Antimicrob Chemother 1999;43(1):15–22

Widmer AF. New developments in diagnosis and treatment of infection in orthopedic implants. Clin Infect Dis 2001;33(Suppl 2):S94–S106

Zimmerli W, Waldvogel FA, Vaudaux P, Nydegger UE. Pathogenesis of foreign body infection: description and characteristics of an animal model. J Infect Dis 1982;146(4):487–497

Zimmerli W, Lew PD, Waldvogel FA. Pathogenesis of foreign body infection. Evidence for a local granulocyte defect. J Clin Invest 1984;73(4):1191–1200

3 Diagnosis of Osteomyelitis

Radiologic Imaging

M. Kroetz, U. Linsenmaier, M. Reiser

Imaging Procedures

Conventional Radiography

Principle

Radiation from a point source passes through an object according to the principle of central projection. The x-rays are attenuated according to the properties of the irradiated material. A radiograph is created when the emerging x-rays strike a detector, which is usually a film–screen combination, digital storage screen or, more recently, a solid-state detector (Laubenberger and Laubenberger 1999).

Indications

Conventional radiographs have numerous indications, including the detection of osteolysis, osteonecrosis, and fractures; the identification of intra-articular loose bodies; the assessment of joint instabilities, dislocations, nonunions, degenerative changes, and reflex sympathetic dystrophy; and for evaluating fracture reduction and the placement of internal fixation devices (Reiser and Peters 1995, Freyschmidt 1997, Bohndorf and Imhof 2001).

Contraindications

There are no absolute contraindications to radiography, but the potential benefit should always be weighed against the risks of radiation exposure.

Pregnancy is a relative contraindication, and very rigorous criteria should be applied to patient selection. Magnetic resonance imaging (MRI) may be performed initially as an alternative to radiography.

Other relative contraindications are limited storage capacity and superimposed shadows from dressing materials, splints, fixation devices, or oral contrast medium following abdominal computed tomography (CT) or gastrointestinal radiography (Kauffmann and Rau 2001).

Indications for conventional radiography:
- Standard procedure for bone imaging when trauma, inflammation, or tumors are suspected
- Visualization of osteolysis, osteonecrosis, and demineralization
- Assessment of joint instabilities and dislocations and evaluation of reduced fractures

- Evaluation of bone healing, placement of internal fixation devices, and nonunions
- Detection of intra-articular loose bodies, reflex sympathetic dystrophy, and primary and secondary osteoarthritis

Contraindications to conventional radiography:
No absolute contraindications exist.
- Pregnancy (very strict selection criteria, especially in the first trimester)
- Children and adolescents (primary MRI may be considered as an alternative)
- Superimposed shadows from dressings, splints, fixation devices, and oral contrast medium

Quality Control

The German Medical Association has published quality control guidelines for conventional radiography (German Medical Association 1995). They include recommendations on exposure technique, film–screen systems, and radiation safety. Gridless projections without automatic exposure control, preferably with a 200-speed film–screen system, should be used for imaging the hand, ankle, and foot. Radiographs of the knee, hip, and axial skeleton should be performed on a Bucky table with grid using a 400-speed film–screen system. A leaded rubber shield should cover adjacent body regions while the films are exposed.

In pediatric examinations a 1-mm aluminum and 0.1-mm copper filter should additionally be used. Knee radiographs and other selected views may be taken without a grid, depending on the age of the child. Film–screen systems with a sensitivity of 400 or 800 are recommended for children. It should be noted that changing from 200 to 400 speed, for example, reduces the necessary radiation dose by half (German Medical Association 1995, Laubenberger and Laubenberger 1999).

Long Tubular Bones

Technique

Standard radiographic films of the long bones are taken in two mutually perpendicular planes. Images should include the adjacent joint to permit the accurate localization of abnormalities. Spot radiographs or fluoroscopy may be necessary for special investigations (Linsenmaier et al. 2000).

Interpretation

Surrounding soft tissues should always be evaluated along with the bony skeleton. Pay close attention to the contours and structure of the bones. Associated findings such as calcifications (e.g., vascular) and superimposed densities should also be assessed.

Interference Factors

Interpretation may be hampered due to difficulties of patient positioning or superimposed shadows from dressings, splints, or internal fixation devices.

Quality Control

Quality control includes checking the indication for the examination, the selection of a suitable imaging procedure, accurate collimation, and the centering of all films.

Use lead aprons to shield the rest of the body from exposure. This may include gonadal protection with a testis capsule in males and a lead shield over the ovaries in females (German Medical Association 1995).

Whenever possible remove dressings, splints and the like to eliminate superimposed shadows. It is best to take radiographs before dressing changes or before the application of a new splint or cast. If uncertainties arise, consult the person who ordered the radiograph prior to the examination (Linsenmaier et al. 2000).

Joints

The wrist, shoulder, elbow, hip, knee, and ankle joints are examined as described below.

Technique

As a rule, the joints should be imaged in two mutually perpendicular projections. If this is not possible due to adjacent body parts, as in the hip or shoulder region, the limb should be rotated 90° so that at least a portion of the joint—the femoral head or humeral head—will be at right angles to the initial plane (Linsenmaier et al. 2000, Bohndorf and Imhof 2001).

Interpretation

The articular surfaces, cortical and cancellous bone, marginal osteophytes, joint-space width, intra-articular calcifications, joint capsule, and tendons should all be evaluated (Dihlmann and Bandick 1995, Reiser and Peters 1995,

Freyschmidt 1997, Bohndort and Imhof 1998, Greenspan 1999).

Interference Factors

Interpretation may be hampered due to difficulties of patient positioning or superimposed shadows from dressings, splints, or internal fixation devices

Quality Control

Key aspects in quality control are precise beam collimation and centering, plus radiation shielding for the rest of the body (see Long Tubular Bones, p. 16).

If interpretation is hampered by superimposed shadows or artifacts from internal fixation devices, spiral CT (SCT) or multidetector-row spiral CT (MSCT) may be considered. The image data can be processed to generate nonsuperimposed multiplanar reconstructions (MPRs) in any desired plane (Linsenmaier et al. 2000).

Cervical Spine

Technique

Biplane radiographs are obtained. To obtain nonsuperimposed views of the upper cervical spine in the anteroposterior (AP) projection, instruct the patient to move his or her lower jaw during the scan so that superimposed bone structures are blurred. Oblique views display the intervertebral foramina when the longitudinal body axis is rotated approximately 45° to the left and right. Here it is important to rotate the whole patient, not only the head, to enable examination of the entire cervical spine and intervertebral foramina. For functional imaging of the cervical spine, lateral flexion/extension views are obtained with the patient in the sitting or standing position.

A dens view is obtained by taking an AP projection through the open mouth.

Radiographs of the cervical spine are used to evaluate for degenerative and inflammatory changes; to evaluate the intervertebral foramina in neurologic disorders involving the upper half of the body, shoulders, and arms; and to check for segmental laxity and functional disorders of the cervical spine (Bohndort and Imhof 1998, Linsenmaier et al. 2000).

Interpretation

Pay close attention to the position of the cervical spine, the width of the intervertebral disk spaces, and the shape of the vertebral bodies. Degenerative changes are often manifested by thickening of the uncinate processes in uncovertebral arthrosis, marginal spurring in ankylosing spondylitis, intervertebral disk-space narrowing in osteochondrosis, and irregularities with increased facet-joint sclerosis in spondylarthrosis.

Inflammatory changes in rheumatic diseases are often manifested by alterations in the joints between the dens and atlas, the facet joints at the craniocervical junction, and the facet joints between the atlas and axis.

Malalignments and functional changes can be appreciated in functional views, paying particular attention to a reference line connecting the posterior margins of the vertebral bodies (Bohndorf and Imhof 2001, Dihlmann and Bandick 1995, Freyschmitt 1997, Greenspan 1999, Reiser and Peters 1995).

Interference Factors

If the patient is of heavy build or has restricted mobility, the lower segments of the cervical spine may be poorly visualized in the lateral projection because the shoulders are superimposed. This problem can be solved by drawing the shoulders downward and forward when the radiograph is taken (e. g., by placing weights in both hands).

Quality Control

Check the indication and necessary views (oblique views, functional views, special dens views). Protect the rest of the body from radiation exposure with a lead shield. Accurate beam collimation reduces scattered radiation and overall exposure (German Medical Association 1995).

Thoracic Spine

Technique

Biplane radiographs can be obtained with the patient lying down or standing upright in front of a wall cassette holder. Special oblique projections for defining the cervicothoracic junction (swimmer's views) are rarely necessary.

Indications are degenerative and inflammatory diseases of the spine (Bohndorf and Imhof 1998, Linsenmaier et al. 2000).

Interpretation

Pay particular attention to the position, shape, and structure of the vertebral bodies and to the intervertebral disk spaces. Evaluate the facet joints with rib attachments, the pedicles, and the spinous processes.

Also take note of any calcification or ossification at the ligamentous attachments of individual vertebral bodies: spondylophytes, parasyndesmophytes, and bamboo spine in ankylosing spondylitis (Bandick 1995, Reiser and Peters 1995, Dihlmann and Freyschmidt 1997, Greenspan 1999, Bohndorf and Imhof 2001).

Interference Factors

See Cervical Spine, page 17.

Quality Control

Accurate beam collimation eliminates scattered radiation and reduces the radiation dose. Use a flexible compensating filter (German Medical Association 1995).

Lumbar Spine

Technique

Radiographs of the lumbar spine are taken in the recumbent position. Oblique views can also be obtained with the patient rotated approximately 45° to the right and left to assess the foramina and vertebral arches in spondylolisthesis and check for vertebral arch defects. Standing and functional flexion/extension views are added when evaluating patients for spondylolisthesis and segmental instabilities (Linsenmaier et al. 2000, Bohndorf and Imhof 2001).

Interpretation

See Thoracic Spine above. For functional imaging, also check for laxity and increased motility of individual vertebral segments that would indicate spondylolisthesis. The height of the intervertebral disk space provides evidence of disk pathology (Dihlmann and Bandick 1995, Reiser and Peters 1995, Freyschmidt 1997, Greenspan 1999, Bohndorf and Imhof 2001).

Interference Factors

Lateral projections of the lumbar spine require a high radiation dose due to the thickness of the interposed soft tissues. Thus, accurate positioning and collimation are particularly important for lateral lumbar views.

Quality Control

Accurate beam collimation is essential. Views at lower levels should include only a small portion of the sacrum. Recumbent views require the use of lead shielding for gonadal protection (German Medical Association 1995).

Standard Pelvic Radiograph

The standard pelvic radiograph consists of an AP projection in the supine patient.

Technique

The AP view should cover the entire pelvis. In examinations of the sacroiliac joint, the sacrum is imaged with the beam collimated on both sacroiliac joint lines (Linsenmaier et al. 2000, Bohndorf and Imhof 2001).

Indications are degenerative and inflammatory diseases of the sacroiliac and hip joints. Pelvic radiographs are also used to screen for metastases and bone tumors.

Interpretation

Pay particular attention to bony contours and osseous structure. Other findings such as calcifications and superimposed densities should also be evaluated (e.g., calcification of the iliac vessels (Dihlmann and Bandick 1995, Reiser and Peters 1995, Freyschmidt 1997, Greenspan 1999, Bohndorf and Imhof 2001).

Interference Factors

Image interpretation may be hampered by overlying bowel gas, which can mimic osteolytic lesions, and by superimposed oral contrast medium in the bowel.

Quality Control

Key aspects are accurate beam collimation and gonadal shielding (testis capsule for males and lead shield over the ovaries for females) (German Medical Association 1995).

Ultrasound

Principle

Ultrasound waves propagate through tissue by causing the tissue molecules to vibrate. The waves are partially or completely reflected at interfaces between different organs. The degree of reflection depends on the wave resistance or *impedance* of the particular organ (acoustic impedance = product of density times sound velocity). The propagation velocity of sound waves in tissue is relatively low, thus the different organs can be localized in relation to one another by measuring the transit time of the sound waves based on the time–distance principle (Laubenberger and Laubenberger 1999).

Technique

In the pulse-echo technique, ultrasound waves are transmitted into the tissue, and the time taken for the echo to return from an interface is measured (topographic mapping). This is achieved technically by utilizing the piezo-electric effect. When an alternating voltage is applied to ceramics or certain crystals, it alters the shape of the material at a microscopic level, giving rise to ultrasound waves. These piezoelectric materials can also receive reflected acoustic pressure waves and transform them back into electric energy. The frequency range of diagnostic ultrasound is between 2 and 30 MHz. The shorter the wave frequency, the higher the resolution and the smaller the depth of sound penetration. As the frequency increases, the waves penetrate more deeply but provide less resolution.

The basic principle of ultrasound imaging is to detect the sound waves reflected from interfaces (impedance) and process them into an ultrasound image corresponding to the structures encountered by the beam. Very dense tissue like bone reflects all of the incident sound. It appears hyperechoic (white) on the image display and obscures underlying structures. Less dense tissue appears hypoechoic (black) on the display. Sound waves pass completely through water and other fluids (transmission), which then appear hypoechoic (black) on the display while underlying structures appear hyperechoic in relation to the surrounding tissue.

Not all transmitted sound waves are reflected because they are subject to physical effects such as scatter, refraction, and absorption.

The returning sound waves detected by the transducer are electronically amplified. The echo return from a particular depth can be selectively amplified (time-gain compensation, TGC), or the entire image can be uniformly amplified (gain) (Laubenberger and Laubenberger 1999).

Indications

The main indication for ultrasound scanning in osteomyelitis is to detect and evaluate associated soft-tissue changes. A diffuse, edematous imbibition of the soft tissues surrounding the bone can be reliably diagnosed sonographically by comparing the left and right sides. Circumscribed fluid collections such as abscesses, hematomas, lymphoceles, or joint effusions can be clearly and completely visualized with ultrasound. A subperiosteal fluid collection may be detectable in acute osteomyelities, especially in children and adolescents (Heuck 1997, Bohndorf and Imhof 2001, Resnick 2002).

Indications for ultrasound:
- Visualization of soft-tissue edema
- Visualization of circumscribed fluid collections and abscesses
- Visualization of joint effusion
- Visualization of subperiosteal fluid

Contraindications

According to the findings of a World Health Organisation (WHO) Commission, the acoustic intensity of low-energy diagnostic ultrasound (10 mW/cm²) is harmless to biological tissues. Hence there are no contraindications to ultrasonography.

Interpretation

Ultrasound provides good soft-tissue contrast. Its spatial resolution is better than that of SCT. Another advantage is the ability to perform dynamic imaging. Muscles and tendons can be examined during motion, especially near joints. Cooperation from the patient, for example by indicating the most painful point in the region of interest (ROI) when transducer pressure is applied, can aid in the detection of pathology and shorten the examination time (Bohndorf and Imhof 2001, Resnick 2002).

Computed Tomography

Principle

Detectors measure the intensity loss in focused x-rays that pass through the patient from a radiograph tube rotating around the longitudinal body axis. Complex calculations yield a raw dataset, which is then computer processed to produce 2D sectional images (Laubenberger and Laubenberger 1999, Reiser et al. 2001).

Technique

Today only SCT should be used in the diagnosis of axial and peripheral skeletal changes. Thin slices (0.5–1.0 mm) should be used for the examination of joints, especially small ones. MPRs should be routinely obtained by reformatting the image date in sagittal and coronal planes. The original dataset is available for evaluating the axial plane. If necessary, sophisticated secondary reconstruction techniques can also be performed for more specialized studies.

The introduction of multidetector-row SCT technology has further advanced the diagnostic capabilities of CT. Since the scan time can be shortened to approximately one-eighth (4-slice CT) with otherwise equal scan parameters, motion artifacts are largely eliminated and slice thicknesses of 0.5–1.0 mm can be achieved. This generates near-isotropic volume elements (voxels) that greatly improve resolution along the longitudinal body axis (Z axis), while multiplanar (MPR) and 3D reconstructions (shaded surface display, virtual reality) can be produced with excellent image quality (Reiser et al. 2001).

IV contrast administration is recommended for the investigation of inflammatory soft-tissue processes, abscesses, and tumors

Interpretation

CT provides exceptionally high contrast resolution of bony structures and calcifications. Soft-tissue contrast is considerably higher than on conventional radiographs but lower than on MR images. CT can easily provide nonsuperimposed views of bones and joints, osteolytic lesions, bone fragments, sequestra, and fracture fragments.

Indication

The indications for skeletal imaging by CT include the visualization of bone fragments and sequestra; the determination of their number, size, and location; the evaluation of complex fractures; follow-up (especially of fracture consolidation); the detection of nonunions; and the detection or exclusion of osteonecrosis. All these indications coincide with the traditional indications for conventional tomography. In our view, conventional tomography should be performed only if a modern CT system is not available (Linsenmaier et al. 2000, Bohndorf and Imhof 2001).

Because MRI is more sensitive than CT, it is better for the detection of occult fractures and bone contusions and for assessing the viability of bone. CT is also becoming increasingly important in preoperative planning, especially for the acquisition of preoperative datasets for image-guided navigation and for postoperative follow-up (Linsenmaier et al. 2000, Bohndorf and Imhof 2001).

Indications for computed tomography:
- Visualization of bone fragments, sequestra, and intra-articular loose bodies
- Evaluation and follow-up of complex fractures (bone healing, fracture consolidation, nonunion, etc.)
- Preoperative planning, including determination of the number, size, and position of bone fragments
- Postoperative follow-up, including the position of fragments and internal fixation device

Contraindications

There are no absolute contraindications to CT, but the therapeutic benefit should always be weighed against the risks of radiation exposure. Pregnancy is a relative contraindication that calls for rigorous selection criteria. If necessary, primary investigation by MRI should be considered.

Quality Control

Positioning constraints are a limitation, especially if the patient cannot be positioned at the center of the gantry. Resulting image deficiencies can be partially offset by obtaining MPRs. Key elements are careful planning of the examination, careful patient positioning, and the possible need for limb fixation and padding.

Image quality may be degraded by metal implants. The more metal there is in the beam path, the greater the image distortion. Beam hardening, scattered radiation, absorption, and the resulting photon deficit can produce characteristic streak artifacts, registration errors, and deletions. Implants made of metal with a low atomic number, such as titanium and carbon, cause fewer artifacts than metals with a higher atomic number (steel). Various strategies are available for reducing metallic artifacts. Good practical solutions are to increase the window width (>3000 HU) and process very thin primary slices into secondary MPRs. Increasing the tube voltage or tube current is of no advantage (Link et al. 2000). Metal external fixation rods also cause artifacts. These devices may be removed before the examination or replaced by carbon rods. Plaster casts do not degrade image quality.

The examination protocol and scan volume should be based on clinical findings and conventional radiographic findings. As a general rule, CT and MRI should not be performed without first obtaining conventional radiographic films.

Magnetic Resonance Imaging

Principle

MRI generates sectional images of the body by utilizing the principle of nuclear magnetic resonance (Purcell and Bloch 1946). Thus this modality does not involve the use of ionizing radiation. The MRI of biological tissue was first performed in 1973 (Lauterbur, Mansfield, Grannell).

Technique

Atomic nuclei with an odd number of protons or neutrons have an angular momentum (nuclear spin) that is analogous to a spinning top. The angular momentum generates a magnetic moment that is directed along the rotational axis (dipole). This property is possessed by hydrogen nuclei, which are present in the human body in very high concentrations. Normally the rotational axes of the hydrogen nuclei in the human body are randomly distributed, so that the average of all the nuclear moments is equal to zero. But when the hydrogen nuclei are acted upon by a constant, strong external magnetic field, they will align themselves along the magnetic field lines because of their magnetic impulse and will acquire a measurable net magnetic moment. The aligned hydrogen nuclei "precess" in a spinning motion about the external magnetic field. The frequency of this spinning motion, called the Larmor frequency, is proportional to the strength of the external magnetic field and a nucleus-specific constant (gamma). When a high-frequency (HF) magnetic field is now ap-

plied perpendicular to the first magnetic field, the hydrogen nuclei will align perpendicular to the second HF field in an attempt to escape the applied force, and their rotational axes will move on a conical surface around the field lines of the initial magnetic field. All the hydrogen nuclei will undergo a synchronous precession immediately after the excitation pulse is applied, that is, they are in phase (phase coherence). If the frequency of the second HF magnetic field is equal to the specific precession frequency (resonance) induced by the initial constant magnetic field, the rotational axes of the hydrogen atoms can be deflected from their alignment by the low HF field strengths. (The resonance is specific for each type of nucleus.) If the second HF magnetic field is then turned off, the angle between the field lines of the outer magnetic field and the rotational axes will decrease, the longitudinal magnetization along the outer magnetic field increasing with the time constant T1 (longitudinal relaxation, spin-grid alternation), and energy will be emitted to the surroundings. At the same time, the phase coherence of the hydrogen atoms will decline steadily after the second magnetic field has been switched off. The hydrogen atoms' precession is out of phase (dephasing), and the transverse magnetization component decreases until the magnetic resonance signal completely disappears. This time constant, called T2 relaxation, is caused by the reciprocal action of individual magnetic hydrogen atoms on one another (spin-spin interaction). In addition, dephasing is influenced by inhomogeneities in the external magnetic field (MR scanner, patient body, surroundings) so that the transverse relaxation does not decrease with the actual time constant T2 but decays more rapidly with the time constant T2*. The relaxation times describe the proton spins' return to alignment parallel to the magnetic field due to their interactions with one another and their surroundings.

Since the external magnetic field is shielded to varying degrees by the electron clouds of the atoms and molecules in the chemical compounds, there are slight differences in the resonant frequencies (chemical shift) which depend on the body region being examined. By analyzing the frequencies (spectroscopy), the molecular structure can be evaluated, thus providing a mechanism for tissue discrimination. The greater the magnitude of the MR signal, the more protons are present in the ROI. In addition, the atomic nuclei return to their original positions at different rates, depending on their molecular structures (relaxation time).

The images produced by MRI reflect the density of the hydrogen atoms in the body and their temporal behavior when excited by electromagnetic radiation. "Gradient fields" are used for position encoding. These are additional magnetic fields that are superimposed over the constant external magnetic field in the three cardinal spatial directions.

Owing to the amplitude and duration of their voltage pulses, the HF magnetic fields used in MRI, known as radiofrequency fields, cause the hydrogen atoms to tilt from their initial alignment by 90° or 180°. Pulse sequences commonly used in MRI are spin-echo, inversion-recovery, and saturation-recovery sequences. Sequences with smaller flip angles, such as fast low-angle shot (FLASH) sequences, shorten the acquisition time. Faster sequences simultaneously register the entire signal from a relatively large body region and use a Fourier analysis to perform separation and spatial encoding of the frequency mix (2D and 3D Fourier image acquisition; Köchli and Marincek 1998, Laubenberger and Laubenberger 1999, Vahlensieck and Reiser 2002).

Contrast agents: Complexes that contain the chemical element gadolinium (Gd) are most commonly used as MRI contrast agents. Owing to its high number (seven) of unpaired electrons, Gd has a strong paramagnetic effect. In conventional doses (standard dose = 0.1–0.3 mmol/kg body weight), tissues with increased blood flow causing increased extravasation of Gd complexes show increased signal intensity due to shortening of the T1 relaxation time in the presence of the Gd contrast agent. Because Gd is toxic in its free-ion form, it is made into a complex by chelation, which yields a nontoxic, water-soluble Gd complex. The high stability of this complex ensures that free Gd ions are not released into the body in potentially toxic amounts. Patients with severe renal failure should undergo dialysis within 24 hours to prevent dissociation of the complexes. The effect of the chelate complexes on MRI signal characteristics is determined largely by the paramagnetic Gd, while the pharmacokinetic characteristics of the complex depend on the chelate-forming agents that are used. The pharmacokinetic behavior of extracellular Gd contrast agents is characterized by a rapid rise of plasma level after IV administration followed by a distribution phase in the extracellular fluid compartment that lasts only a few minutes. The fall in the plasma level (half-life of approximately 90 minutes) is determined by the renal excretion rate. The agents are excreted by glomerular filtration in a chemically unchanged form (Köchli and Marincek 1998, Laubenberger and Laubenberger 1999, Vahlensieck and Reiser 2002).

Interpretation

MRI is distinguished by its exceptional soft-tissue contrast and its sensitive detection of inflammatory changes. Images can be acquired in arbitrary planes of section. Active inflammatory processes can be distinguished from chronic processes on images acquired after IV contrast administration.

Indications

MRI is the modality of choice for imaging inflammatory changes in bones and soft tissues. High-resolution images can define the bone marrow, cortical bone, periosteal changes, and surrounding soft tissues.

Bone-marrow and soft-tissue inflammation are most reliably detected by unenhanced, water-sensitive (T2-weighted) sequences with or without fat suppression. Inflammatory changes show definite contrast enhancement in fat-suppressed T1-weighted sequences after IV Gd administration (Bohndorf and Imhof 2001, Vahlensieck and Reiser 2002).

Indications for MRI:
- Visualization of inflammatory changes in bone marrow, cortical bone, and surrounding soft tissues
- Visualization of periosteal reactions
- Visualization of inflammatory changes in bones and soft tissues
- Detection of circumscribed abscesses

Contraindications to MRI:
- Cardiac pacemaker (strong magnetic field)
- Relative: metal implants (intramedullary nails, total replacements)
- Relative: pregnancy
- Relative: prosthetic heart valves
- Relative: claustrophobia (patient may be sedated if necessary)
- Relative: severe obesity (Köchli and Marinek 1998, Laubenberger and Laubenberger 1999)

Quality Control

MRI should employ a high-field system with a magnetic field intensity of one Tesla or more. Sequences with frequency-selective fat saturation are best for imaging inflammatory changes (German Medical Association 2000).

Special Imaging Procedures

Fistulography

Principle

A radiographic contrast medium is injected to expand the fistulous tract and check for communication with surrounding structures.

Technique

Preparation: The procedure is performed under local anesthesia. Diagnostic preparations should include conventional skeletal radiographs and CT or MRI of the fistula region.

Fistula catheterization: A catheter is introduced into the fistula under sterile conditions, and an undiluted iodinated contrast medium is injected. The flow of the contrast medium is documented by fluoroscopy, and spot radiographs are taken in several different planes, preferably perpendicular to one another. The lumen of an adjacent hollow viscus can also be opacified with contrast medium if desired (Kauffmann and Rau 2001).

Interpretation

The entire fistulous tract should be evaluated from skin level to its termination. In certain cases, interpretation of the fistulograms should be aided by CT or MRI.

Indications

Preoperative fistulography is used for the investigation of inflammatory processes involving bones, joints, and soft tissues.

Contraindications

- Immunocompromised patient
- No therapeutic implications
- Contrast extravasation into blood vessels
- Contrast allergy

Interference Factors

Problems may arise due to superficial contrast leakage from the fistula opening, incomplete contrast filling of the fistulous tract, or the inoculation of infectious organisms into deeper tissues.

Quality Control

Mark the fistula opening with a safety pin. At least two radiographs are taken in mutually perpendicular projections. Superficial contrast leakage may lead to errors of interpretation.

Diagnostic and Interventional Angiography

Principle

The current preferred technique of diagnostic catheter-based angiography is intra-arterial digital subtraction angiography (DSA). Radiographic contrast medium is injected into the vascular ROI by selective or nonselective catheterization, depending on the indication.

Technique

Preparations include taking a history geared toward the planned intervention, securing informed consent, and excluding possible contraindications. Preliminary tests depend on the ROI and may include Doppler pressure measurement, duplex scans of the limbs, and CT or MR angiography (CTA, MRA).

Antegrade puncture of the common femoral artery is performed if a simultaneous interventional procedure is planned. This requires initial MRA or CTA evaluation of the corresponding vascular region. If a stenosis is found that can be treated interventionally, this can be done in the same sitting (Kandarpa 1996, Castaneda-Zuniga 1997).

Indications

Angiography is particularly rewarding in patients with delayed wound or bone healing that have been selected for plastic reconstructive surgery. The vascular status of the affected region should first be investigated to confirm adequate blood flow.

Indications for DSA include primary vascular diseases such as arterial occlusive disease, arteriovenous malformations, aneurysms, arteriovenous fistulas, traumatic vascular injuries, vasospasm, and segmental vascular diseases. Other indications are the diagnosis of secondary vascular diseases such as vascular compression or infiltration, postoperative or postinterventional complications, and the assessment of preoperative or preinterventional vascular anatomy. If a vascular stenosis is suspected or has been confirmed, preparations should be made for an interventional procedure and DSA should be combined with percutaneous transluminal angioplasty (PTA), stent insertion, and thrombolysis.

Contraindications

Absolute contraindications to DSA include unstable patients who require preliminary treatment elsewhere, uncorrected organ failure, and indeterminate tumor masses before exclusion of an iodine-storing thyroid carcinoma.

Relative contraindications include severe previous contrast reactions, impaired renal function, equivocal thyroid function, recent myocardial infarction, severe arrhythmia, severe heart failure, coagulopathy with a markedly increased bleeding risk, limited ability to assume a recumbent position, and cardiopulmonary diseases.

General contraindications to radiographic examinations include pregnancy, superimposed oral barium contrast medium, and previous abdominal CT, upper GI series, or contrast enema (Günther and Thelen 1996, Kandarpa 1996).

Precautions in Specific Diseases

Possible precautionary measures include hydration, thyroid blockade, and sedation.

Diabetes: In consultation with the physician in charge, the insulin dose can be reduced by 50% and the examination scheduled for late morning. Antidiabetic medication with metformin should be discontinued 2–3 days before the administration of iodinated contrast media. The patient should be adequately hydrated due to the increased risk of tubular necrosis.

Thrombocytopenia: The current value should exceed 75 000 platelets/mL. Check blood count and coagulation status before the intervention.

Anticoagulated patients: Coumarins should be discontinued several days before the examination (Quick > 50%), and heparin may be substituted as required. In an emergency, give the patient fresh-frozen plasma or vitamin K (25–50 mg) at least 4 hours before the procedure.

Heparinized patients: Discontinue heparin at least 3–4 hours before the examination (PTT values < 1.25–1.5 times control values). Heparin can be resumed 6–8 hours after the examination or earlier in selected cases, although this will increase the bleeding risk.

Impaired renal function: Known risk factors for developing renal failure after contrast administration are patient age, hypertension, administered contrast dose, and preexisting proteinemia. Serum creatinine levels generally return to normal within 5–10 days after contrast administration.

Pheochromocytoma: Up to 8% of pheochromocytoma patients experience a hypertensive crisis during the procedure.

Polycytemia vera and sickle-cell anemia: Thromboembolic complications may occur after contrast administration.

Agitation and nervousness: Sedate unusually anxious patients for the examination (Günther and Thelen 1996, Kandarpa 1996).

Quality Control

On completion of the examination, place compression on the arterial puncture site for 8–10 minutes. Then apply a pressure dressing and place a sandbag over the groin for at least 2 hours. If intravascular heparin has been administered, it may be necessary to remove the sheath in two stages, and bed rest should be maintained.

Angiographic examinations via a femoral approach have a reported complication rate of 1.73%; 0.4% of which are vascular injuries and 0.26% are postprocedure bleeding (Kandarpa 1996).

Ambulatory Angiography

Ambulatory examinations can be scheduled for all cooperative patients who are able to recognize complications after completion of the procedure. **Prerequisite:** Another adult must be available to watch the patient.

Exclusion criteria: a history of severe allergies or a severe prior contrast reaction, heart failure, renal failure, poorly controlled hypertension, anticoagulant therapy in patients with a coagulopathy or electrolyte disorder.

The patient should be monitored for at least 2 hours after the examination, and fluid intake should be sufficient to ensure rapid elimination of the contrast medium (Günther and Thelen 1996, Kandarpa 1996).

Percutaneous Drainage of Joints, Bones, and Abscesses

Principle

Percutaneous aspiration of fluid collections, tumors, or abscesses is performed under CT or ultrasound guidance for diagnosis (e.g., bacteriology, histopathology) or treatment (external drainage).

Technique

Preparations: The procedure is performed under local anesthesia or under IV sedation if required. Diagnostic preparations include ultrasound, CT, or MRI of the affected skeletal region for accurate localization.

Puncture: Deep local anesthesia may be administered along the proposed needle track, depending on the location. Special coaxial needles or other biopsy needles can be used to retrieve tissue samples. Stellate biopsies can be repeatedly taken through an outer guide sheath to avoid cell dissemination along the puncture track. When dealing with an abscess or predominantly fluid lesion, first take material for bacteriologic or cytologic analysis and then introduce a 5F to 8F ring or pigtail catheter over a guidewire to drain the contents.

Interpretation

An adequate amount of biopsy material can be sampled in 80%–95% of cases. It is best to biopsy the periphery of large lesions because central portions may already be necrotic. The percutaneous drainage of abdominal abscesses is successful in 70%–90% of cases, eliminating the need for operative treatment. Comparable data are not available for skeletal interventions (Günther and Thelen 1996, Kandarpa 1996).

Indications

Indications include the drainage of uninfected fluid collections such as pseudocysts and lymphoceles, the drainage of abscesses, the sampling of bacteriologic material, and biopsies to confirm the diagnosis of primary or secondary tumors.

Contraindications

Untreated coagulopathy and technical obstacles in cases where the tumor is not accessible.

Interference Factors

Complications arise in 5%–10% of all imaging-guided biopsies and abscess-drainage procedures, depending on the institution. Complications may include infection, sepsis, bleeding, pneumothorax, and local infection at the puncture site.

Less than 2% of diagnostic aspirations and biopsies are complicated by infection, bleeding, organ injury, pneumothorax, or pancreatitis. The seeding of malignant cells along the needle track has been described in case reports but is generally regarded as extremely rare (<0.01%; Günther and Thelen 1996).

Quality Control

Laboratory values: platelets > 75 000, Quick ≥ 60%, PTT at least 1.5 times the control value. Supplement local anesthesia by analgesia in certain procedures, especially when the efficacy of local anesthesia is compromised in the infected area. Rigorous asepsis should be practiced during biopsy or drainage. An adequate diagnostic work up (MRI, CT, ultrasound) is essential. Easily accessible lesions can be biopsied or drained at bedside under ultrasound guidance. Dressings should be regularly changed and drains irrigated with 3 × 5–10 mL of sterile saline solution. Drains may be left indwelling for 2–7 days. If drainage suddenly stops, check the drain placement and take samples for bacteriologic testing before removing the drain.

Imaging Findings in Specific Disorders

M. Kroetz, U. Linsenmaier, M. Reiser

Acute and Chronic Bone Infections

Classification of Osteomyelitis

Acute Hematogenous Osteomyelitis

Sites of Occurrence and Clinical Features

Acute hematogenous osteomyelitis occurs predominantly in early childhood (see **Table 3.1** for classification of different forms of osteomyelitis). The incidence rises again after 50 years of age. Infantile hematogenous osteomyelitis is distinguished from acute juvenile osteomyelitis and acute adult osteomyelitis (Heuck 1997, Bohndorf and Imhof 2001, Resnick 2002, Vahlensieck and Reiser 2002).

Infantile osteomyelitis (up to age 12 months) is an acutely progressive disease that often shows multicentric and articular involvement. Sites of predilection are the femoral metaphyses, hips, and humerus. The diaphyseal, metaphyseal and epiphyseal blood vessels create potential pathways for epiphyseal and subpe-

Table 3.1 Classification of different forms of osteomyelitis (modified from Bohndorf)

Acute osteo-myelitis	Chronic osteo-myelitis	Special forms
Hematog-enous	Endogenous/ primary hema-togenous	Brodie abscess
		Tuberculous osteomyelitis
	Recurrent multifocal	Plasma cell osteomyelitis
		Salmonella, fungal infections
	Exogenous/ secondary	Others

riosteal spread (**Fig. 3.1**). The main causative organisms are streptococci. Males and females are affected equally (Cohen et al. 1990, Heuck 1997, Resnick 2002).

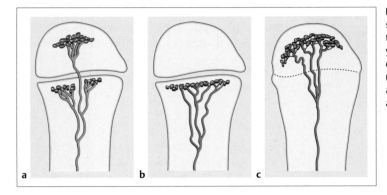

Fig. 3.1a–c Metaphyseal and epiphyseal blood supply. During the first year of life, the vessels cross the epiphyseal plate (**a**). From approximately 2 to 16 years of age, the vessels become obliterated and the epiphysis forms a barrier to hematogenous spread (**b**). By skeletal maturity, however, blood vessels again establish a connection between the epiphysis and metaphysis (**c**).

Juvenile osteomyelitis (12 months or older) is characterized by an acute onset of symptoms that are poorly localized initially. The metaphyses of the long tubular bones are most commonly affected. Usually the infection does not spread to the epiphysis due to physiologic occlusion of the meta- and epiphyseal vessels. Intra-articular spread may occur only if the joint capsule encloses portions of the metaphysis (hip, knee). Subperiosteal spread may also occur. The main causative organisms are staphylococci, and males are predominantly affected (Cohen et al. 1990, Heuck 1997, Resnick 2002).

Acute adult osteomyelitis: This is a rare disease that often takes an insidious clinical course. Sites of predilection are the axial skeleton and long tubular bones, and the diaphysis, metaphysis, and epiphysis may be involved. Articular involvement is common. Subperiosteal involvement is rare due to the thick cortex and firm periosteal attachment in adults. If subperiosteal spread does occur, it often leads to fistula formation and soft-tissue involvement. Males are predominantly affected (Heuck 1997, Bohndorf and Imhof 2001, Resnick 2002, Vahlensieck and Reiser 2002).

Chronic Hematogenous Osteomyelitis

If acute hematogenous osteomyelitis does not resolve, it may pass through a subacute stage before progressing to chronic hematogenous osteomyelitis, which is sometimes multifocal (Resnick and Petterson 1992, Heuck 1997, Bohndorf and Imhof 2001, Resnick 2002). Key imaging goals are the early detection of a reactivated, florid inflammatory process and the detection or exclusion of new inflammatory foci. This is most effectively accomplished by MRI.

Differential diagnosis of hematogenous osteomyelitis:
- Eosinophilic granuloma
- Malignant tumors: Ewing sarcoma, osteosarcoma, reticular cell sarcoma

- Necrotic tumors, posttraumatic seromas
- Abscesses due to other causes
- Periostitis due to other causes
- Noninfectious osteomyelitis (psoriasis, Reiter syndrome)

Imaging of Acute and Chronic Hematogenous Osteomyelitis

Projection Radiography

Hematogenous osteomyelitis produces radiographically detectable bone changes by 7–14 days at the earliest. Trabecular bones at that time may show ill-defined margins with a geographic, moth-eaten or permeative pattern of bone destruction. The lesion margins are indistinct. The cortex is initially eroded from the inside before varying degrees of cortical destruction can be seen. Note that destructive changes are more difficult to detect in trabecular bone than in compact bone. The infection may spread outward through the cortical bone, elevating the periosteum and causing radiographically detectable periosteal new bone formation. If the spread of infection deprives bony areas of their blood supply, these areas will become necrotic and will eventually appear on radiographs as sequestra. Reactive new bone formation may completely isolate the sequestrum from surrounding bone (involucrum). Marked associated soft-tissue swelling, especially about joints, will often develop within 3–5 days in infants and small children.

> **NOTE**
>
> Conventional radiographs initially show obliteration of fat planes and increased soft-tissue density due to edema of the paraosseous soft tissues.

The bony changes that occur during the reparative stage and in chronic hematogenous osteomyelitis depend on the virulence of the causative organism, host immune status, and treatment. Endosteal, cortical, and periosteal new bone formation produce a mixed lytic and sclerotic pattern. The initial sign of healing is centripetal sclerosis

(Gold et al. 1991, Heuck 1997, Bohndorf and Imhof 2001, Resnick 2002).

Key radiographic features of hematogenous osteomyelitis:

- Detectable soft-tissue swelling during the first 3 days
- Bony changes no earlier than 7–14 days
- Trabecular bone destruction (geographic, moth-eaten, permeative)
- Ill-defined lesion margins with convex cortical thinning
- Periosteal new bone formation
- Detectable sequestrum or involucrum (rare)
- Mixed lytic and sclerotic changes in the reparative stage

Ultrasound

The value of ultrasound in acute osteomyelitis is inversely proportional to patient age. In infants, the early phase of osteomyelitis is initially marked by edematous swelling of the deeper soft tissues. This is followed later by the appearance of a thin, echo-free subperiosteal fluid collection that visibly elevates the periosteum. The significance of ultrasound findings should not be overstated, however. The changes described above are nonspecific, and there is a substantial incidence of false-positive findings and (in up to 40% of cases) false-negative findings (Kaiser and Rosenborg 1994).

Ultrasound scans in adults can detect only associated soft-tissue involvement. Abscesses and hematomas appear as echo-free or hypoechoic masses. Diffuse soft-tissue edema leads to inhomogeneous, hyperechoic thickening of the subcutaneous tissue. Ultrasound is very accurate in the detection of joint effusions (anechoic intra-articular fluid). Usually it cannot be determined whether a bland or suppurative effusion is present.

Computed Tomography

MRI is superior to CT owing to its good soft-tissue contrast and high accuracy, especially in infants and children due to the scant fat planes in that population.

CT scanning in adults can accurately detect the destruction of trabecular and cortical bone, periosteal ossification, sclerosis, and sequestration. Bone density is increased, the density difference being most pronounced in the diaphysis (fat marrow). Gas inclusions and fat–fluid levels in the medullary cavity are relatively specific for osteomyelitis. Paraosseous abscesses can be identified by their fluid attenuation and enhancing abscess membrane. Surrounding soft tissues show an obliteration of interposed fat planes due to edema. CT findings and conventional x-ray findings coincide during the repair stage and in chronic hematogenous osteomyelitis. Both modalities show osteolytic lesions coexisting with sclerotic changes (Gold et al. 1991, Bohndorf and Imhof 2001, Reiser et al. 2001, Resnick 2002).

Magnetic Resonance Imaging

Frequency-selective and T-weighted MRI pulse sequences (STIR = short true inversion recovery) combined with fat suppression can detect inflammatory changes with high sensitivity, although they tend to overestimate the spatial extent of the inflammation. Decreased signal intensity is seen in the bone marrow and fatty tissue in T1-weighted sequences. This technique also provides detailed anatomical visualization. T2-weighted images without fat saturation show little or no contrast between inflammatory changes and normal bone marrow or fat, especially when fast (turbo) spin-echo sequences are used. Inflammation and edema in muscles appear hyperintense in T2-weighted images. The same is true for contrast-enhanced T1-weighted sequences. Contrast-enhanced T1-weighted sequences with fat suppression are particularly rewarding. Inflammatory areas in the bone marrow and in paraosseous soft tissues are delineated by their high signal intensity. An abscess membrane surrounding a fluid-filled abscess cavity can easily be identified. Sequestra are also nonenhancing but, like abscesses, are hypointense in the STIR sequence and may show little if any peripheral enhancement. If the inflammatory process spreads to the cortex, increased signal intensity is visible in the compact bone, which is normally devoid of signal. Periosteal reactions can also be identified. Fistulous tracts have fluid-equivalent signal intensity in T2-weighted and STIR

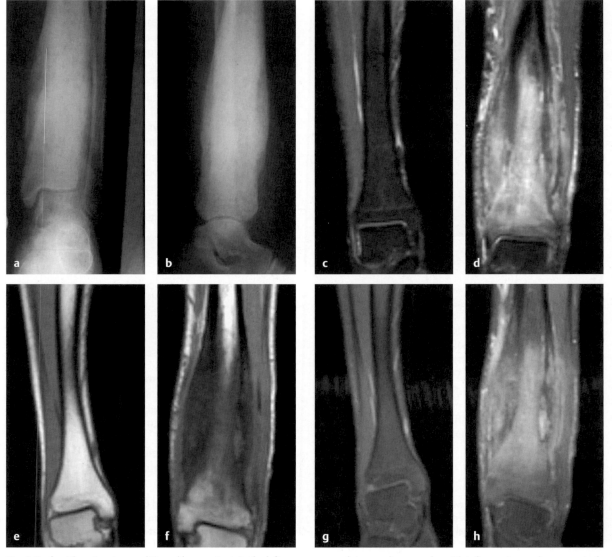

Fig. 3.3a–h Chronic osteomyelitis and hyperostosis in the left tibia of a 19-year-old male. Radiographs show massive cortical expansion in the mid- and distal tibia with increased sclerosis of the bone marrow (**a, b**). MRI (**d, f, h** left distal tibia; **c, e, g** healthy distal right tibia for comparison) shows definite fusiform cortical expansion with marked edematous imbibation of the bone mar-row and surrounding muscles with inflammatory enhancement of the entire bone and the soft tissues in this region (**c, d** = STIR se-quence, **e, f** = unenhanced T1-weighted image, **g, h** = fat-saturated T1-weighted image after contrast administration). Note the inclu-sion of the epiphysis in the meta- and epiphyseal blood supply.

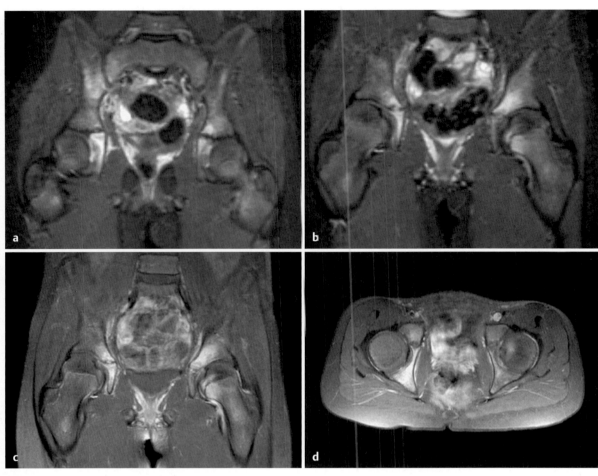

Fig. 3.4a–d CRMO in a 10-year-old girl. MRI shows involvement of the right ilium, both acetabula, and the left femoral head with pronounced bone marrow edema in STIR sequences (**a, b**). The cortex is still intact, and the synovium shows edematous imbibi-tion. Fat-saturated T1-weighted sequences after contrast adminis-tration (**c, d**) show inflammatory enhancement of the bone mar-row and synovium.

Chronic Posttraumatic Exogenous Osteomyelitis

Etiology, Sites of Occurrence, and Clinical Features

This is a primarily local bone inflammation (osteomyeli-tis), whose spread depends on the host immune status, the virulence of the causative organism, the extent of soft-tissue damage, the introduction of foreign tissue, the degree of circulatory compromise in the bone, and the stage of fracture healing. The soft-tissue infection spreads through the adjacent periosteum and compact bone into the medullary cavity. Causes are posttraumatic and post-operative infections and chronic ulcers, as in diabetes mellitus. Various organisms, often including a combina-tion of aerobes and anaerobes, may be causative. Patients present clinically with increasing local pain and signs of inflammation. Draining sinus tracts may develop in cases

that take a protracted course. Sepsis or septic arthritis may develop in untreated or poorly managed cases as a result of lymphogenous or hematogenous spread (Gold et al. 1991, Greenspan 1999, Bohndorf and Imhof 2001, Resnick 2002).

Imaging of Chronic Posttraumatic Exogenous Osteomyelitis

Projection Radiography

Soft-tissue swelling is manifested by the obliteration of fat planes in the surrounding soft tissues. Periosteal spread of the disease leads to elevation of the periosteum and incipient periosteal new bone formation (often the earli-est radiographic sign). The further course is marked by subperiosteal bone resorption and cortical destruction. If the inflammation spreads to the medullary cavity, radio-graphs show evidence of trabecular destruction. The further course of the disease is the same as in hematogenous osteomyelitis (Resnick and Petterson 1992, Greenspan 1999, Bohndorf and Imhof 2001, Resnick 2002).

> **NOTE**
>
> When postoperative infection develops after the internal fixation of a fracture, radiographs are difficult to interpret for some time. It is important to compare the radiographs with immediate postoperative films. Bony consolidation of the fracture site is delayed, and osteolytic lesions coexist with areas of new bone formation. Callus formation may be the dominant finding in more protracted cases.

Key radiographic findings in chronic posttraumatic osteomyelitis:

- Soft-tissue swelling, obliterated fat planes
- Subperiosteal bone resorption and new bone formation
- Osteolytic lesions in the medullary cavity
- Reparative stage as in hematogenous osteomyelitis
- Postoperative radiographs are difficult to interpret and should be compared with preoperative films

Fistulography

When a draining fistula is catheterized and radiographic contrast medium is injected, spot radiographs can demonstrate the communication between the bone and fistula. This will also reveal the presence of any sequestrum (**Fig. 3.5**).

Ultrasound

Ultrasound can detect inflammatory soft-tissue edema indicating an infectious focus and can identify circumscribed fluid collections due to abscess formation.

Computed Tomography

The main role of CT in chronic posttraumatic osteomyelitis is to detect a devitalized sequestrum that has become separated from the surrounding bone. The fragment is hyperdense and rimmed by fluid (Heuck 1997, Bohndorf and Imhof 2001, Reiser et al. 2001, Resnick 2002).

Magnetic Resonance Imaging

The MR signal and enhancement characteristics of the lesions in chronic exogenous osteomyelitis closely resemble those in hematogenous osteomyelitis.

> **NOTE**
>
> MRI during the first 3–6 postoperative months cannot positively distinguish surgery-related bone marrow edema from inflammatory involvement of the medullary cavity.

Fluid-sensitive sequences (STIR, T2-weighted) show greatly increased signal intensity in the bone marrow, which also shows contrast enhancement in fat-suppressed T1-weighted sequences.

> **NOTE**
>
> Abscess formation in the medullary cavity or paraosseous soft tissues, showing central fluid-equivalent signal intensity and peripheral enhancement of the abscess membrane (best appreciated in fat-saturated T1-weighted sequences), confirms the presence of a postoperative infection.

Circumscribed postoperative fluid collections, unlike inflammatory fluid collections, do not exhibit perifocal edema. MRI in chronic cases shows an inhomogeneous pattern with a combination of endosteal and periosteal new bone formation and osteolytic changes. Fistulas are best demonstrated by unenhanced fat-suppressed, fluid-sensitive sequences (STIR) and by thin-slice, fat-suppressed T1-weighted sequences after IV contrast administration (Gold et al. 1991, Vahlensieck and Reiser 1992, Bohndorf and Imhof 2001, Resnick 2002, Vahensieck and Reiser 2002; **Fig. 3.6**).

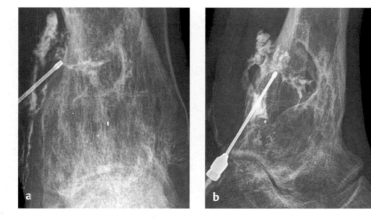

Fig. 3.5a, b Fistulograms in chronic posttraumatic osteomyelitis. Inverted fluoroscopic images in the AP (**a**) and lateral projection (**b**) show an arborizing system of fistulous tracts in the soft tissue extending into a large, trough-shaped defect in the distal tibia. Note the pronounced, inhomogeneous bone marrow sclerosis at the site of the tibial defect.

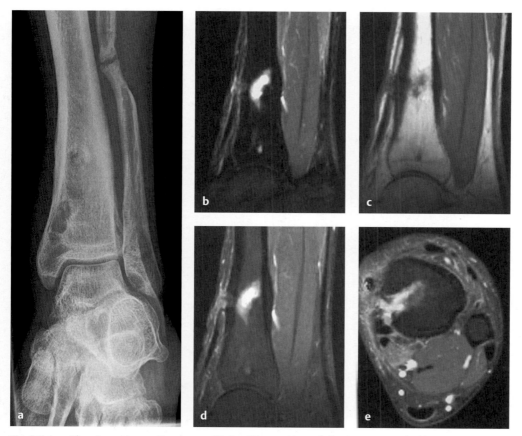

Fig. 3.6a–e Chronic posttraumatic osteomyelitis in a 22-year-old man following an open tibial fracture. Radiograph shows eccentric, irregular dia-, meta-, and epiphyseal areas of increased lucency with marginal sclerosis and cortical thickening in the distal tibia (**a**). MRI of this region (**b–e**) shows a fluid-filled defect in the bone marrow with spindle-shaped cortical expansion and fistulas tracking anteriorly (**b–d**) and medially (**e**) into the surrounding soft tissue.

Infectious Spondylitis and Spondylodiskitis

Etiology, Sites of Occurrence, and Clinical Features

Males are predominantly affected in approximately 2%–4% of all cases. Incidence shows an initial peak in infancy and childhood and a second peak in the fifth and sixth decades. Previous infections and interventional procedures or operations are predisposing factors. The infectious organisms mainly spread hematogenously via the vertebral arteries to the anterior portions of the vertebral bodies bordering the disk space (spondylitis). From there the inflammation spreads secondarily across the vertebral end plate into the disk space and avascular disk (spondylodiskitis). Generally this is followed by extension to adjacent vertebral bodies. Primary infection of the vascularized disk may occur in children. Only one vertebral segment is affected in most cases, but involvement of multiple segments may occur. The lumbar spine is most commonly affected followed by the lower thoracic spine. Involvement of the entire spinal column may occur.

The acute form of the disease is characterized by dull, localized spinal pain (occurring mainly at night), antalgic posturing, fever, and general malaise. Inflammatory markers are elevated when these symptoms are present. The chronic form causes little or no local pain, and inflammatory markers are normal or only slightly elevated, often causing a delay in diagnosis. The main causative organisms are staphylococci, Gram-negative bacteria, and *Mycobacterium tuberculosis* (Dihlmann 1987, Freyschmidt 1997, Heuck 1997, Bohndorf and Imhof 2001, Resnick 2002).

Differential diagnosis of infectious spondylitis:
- Erosive osteochondrosis
- Rheumatoid arthritis
- Tuberculous spondylitis
- Seronegative spondylarthritis
- Pseudogout
- Sarcoidosis
- Tumor metastasis

Imaging of Infectious Spondylitis

Projection Radiography

Radiographic abnormalities first appear from 1 to 3 weeks after the onset of clinical symptoms. Soft-tissue swelling may be noted during the first 2–3 weeks (psoas shadow, shifting of the paravertebral line). This is followed by a loss of intervertebral disk height and blurring of adjacent vertebral body end plates. Further progression is marked by increasing unsharpness, irregular margins, and defects in adjacent end plates ranging to marked destruction of the vertebral bodies and disk (kyphoscoliosis, gibbus). The reparative phase is characterized by a smoothing of contour defects in the vertebral body end plates, focal sclerosis of the cancellous bone, osteophyte formation, and even partial interbody fusion (Dihlmann 1987, Heuck 1997, Bohndorf and Imhof 2001, Stäbler and Reiser 2001, Resnick 2002).

Key radiographic findings in infectious spondylitis:
- Soft-tissue swelling
- Decreased height of the intervertebral disk space
- Indistinct vertebral body end plates, contour defects
- Destruction of the vertebral bodies and disk, kyphoscoliosis
- Reparative phase: smoothing of contour defects, sclerosis, osteophytes, block vertebrae

Fistulography

Fistulography can define the communication between the fistula and bone or may reveal a sequestrum or abscess cavity. MRI can also detect fistulas and define their extent after the injection of water or Gd into the fistulous opening.

Ultrasound

Paravertebral fluid collections and abscesses can be identified with ultrasound. If necessary, they can be aspirated under ultrasound guidance to obtain samples for bacteriologic analysis.

Computed Tomography

CT shows the same changes as conventional radiographs. Acquiring thin slices ensures that high-quality MPRs can be performed. Soft-tissue processes lead to the obliteration of normal fat planes, decreased density in relation to normal muscles, and occasionally to increased contrast enhancement. Abscesses have central fluid-equivalent attenuation, although somewhat higher densities may be seen depending on the blood, cellular and protein content of the abscess. Usually the hypervascularized abscess membrane is clearly delineated on postcontrast images owing to its increased contrast uptake. Infection of the bone marrow leads to increased density even in the absence of visible bone destruction. The higher the fat content of the bone marrow, the greater the density increase in the medullary cavity. Rarely, fat–fluid levels or gas inclusions may be found in the medullary cavity. Defects in the vertebral end plates are seen more clearly in CT scans than in plain radiographs—especially when only a small portion of the end plate is affected. The junction of the vertebral end plate and disk can be more precisely evaluated in sagittal and coronal reconstructions than in primary axial sections. Trabecular and cortical bone destruction, sclerosis, and sequestra are demonstrated better by CT than conventional radiographs. If epidural spread of spondylitis is suspected, CT myelography will provide a more detailed view than standard contrast-enhanced CT.

> **NOTE**
>
> CT is better than any other modality for directing percutaneous biopsies and drainage.

The infecting organism can be identified in approximately 50% of cases by the analysis of biopsy material (Heuck 1997, Bohndorf and Imhof 2001, Stäbler and Reiser 2001, Reiser et al. 2001, Resnick 2002).

Magnetic Resonance Imaging

> **NOTE**
>
> MRI is particularly useful for detecting inflammatory changes in the vertebral bodies, disks, and adjacent soft tissues. It combines high sensitivity with accurate and detailed morphologic definition.

T1-weighted images show a decrease in bone marrow signal intensity while T2-weighted spin-echo images show increased signal intensity. Inflammatory changes in the bone marrow are detected sensitively and with excellent contrast in STIR and fat-saturated T2-weighted images. Contrast-enhanced T1-weighted images with fat saturation permit the detection of abscesses in vertebral body bone marrow and disks and are essential in diagnosing chronic spondylodiskitis and detecting its reactivation. This technique can also detect epidural abscess spread in spondylitis. MRI is also very accurate in detecting the periosteal and paravertebral spread of spondylitis. The lesions do not always consist of fluid-filled abscess cavities, and enhancing paravertebral granulomatous structures may be found in nonspecific bacterial spondylitis.

T2-weighted MRI shows high, fluid-equivalent signal intensities in the intervertebral disk space. This finding aids differentiation from erosive osteochondrosis, which may closely resemble spondylitis. Another differentiating feature is the spread of bone marrow edema into the adjacent vertebral body: infectious spondylitis usually involves more than half of the vertebral body, whereas erosive osteochondrosis shows a bandlike arrangement bordering the disk space. Moreover, the T1-weighted imaging of infectious spondylitis shows at least one site where the continuity of the vertebral end plates is disrupted, whereas end-plate continuity is preserved in erosive osteochondrosis (Stäbler et al. 1998, Bohndorf and Imhof 2001, Stäbler and Reiser 2001, Resnick 2002, Vahlensieck and Reiser 2002; **Figs. 3.7 and 3.8**).

Complications of infectious spondylitis or spondylodiskitis:

- Soft-tissue abscess
- Mediastinitis
- Empyema
- Pericarditis, peritonitis, meningitis
- Cord compression by an epidural abscess
- Kyphosis
- Atlantoaxial dislocation

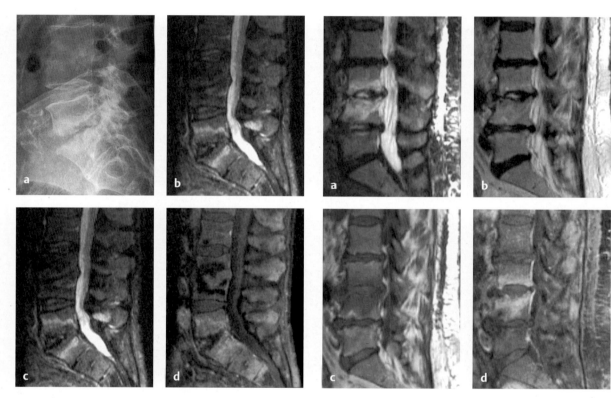

Fig. 3.7a–d Active spondylodiskitis at L5/S1 and previous spondylodiskitis at L4/L5 with the complete fusion of adjacent vertebral bodies (block vertebrae). Lateral radiograph (**a**) shows predominantly posterior osteochondrosis at L5/S1 with complete destruction of the associated end plates and increased vertebral body sclerosis. MRI at the L5/S1 level shows findings typical of active spondylodiskitis with fluid-equivalent signal intensity of the intervertebral disk and bone marrow edema in the adjacent vertebral bodies in the STIR sequence (**b**). The end plates are no longer delineated in the unenhanced T1-weighted image (**c**). The fat-saturated T1-weighted sequence shows marked enhancement of the bone marrow in the two adjacent vertebral bodies involving more than one-half the vertebral body height (**d**). MRI at L4/5 shows complete vertebral blocking with a large, nonenhancing fluid-filled defect and absence of bone marrow edema (**b–d**).

Fig. 3.8a–d Sagittal MR images (**a** = STIR image, **b** = T2-weighted image, **c** = unenhanced T1-weighted image, **d** = fat-saturated T1-weighted image after contrast administration) show changes typical of acute infectious spondylodiskitis at L3/4.

Special Forms of Osteomyelitis

Brodie Abscess

Etiology, Sites of Occurrence, and Clinical Features

The Brodie abscess is a subacute and chronic form of osteomyelitis that is caused by an organism of low virulence or develops in a patient with a good immune status. The abscess cavity measures 1–4 cm in diameter and is walled off by inflammatory granulation tissue. The interior is filled with pus. A Brodie abscess does not lead to fistula formation. It occurs predominantly in adolescents and most commonly involves the metaphyses of the tibia, distal femur, and radius. Boys are affected more frequently than girls. The Brodie abscess usually takes an insidious clinical course with no systemic manifestations or pain, often delaying diagnosis by years. The main causative organism is *Staphylococcus aureus* (Chandnani et al. 1990, Heuck 1997, Bohndorf and Imhof 2001, Resnick 2002).

Differential diagnosis of the Brodie abscess:
- Fibrous dysplasia
- Osteoblastoma
- Osteoid osteoma
- Cysts

Diagnostic Imaging

Projection Radiography

The Brodie abscess typically appears as a round-to-oval lucent zone located at the center of the metaphysis and surrounded by a sclerotic rim of variable width. Canalicular extension toward the epiphysis is occasionally seen. Periosteal reactions may occur (Heuck 1997, Bohndorf and Imhof 2001, Resnick 2002; **Fig. 3.9**).

Computed Tomography

CT scans show a pus-filled abscess cavity (HU > 20) surrounded by a sclerotic rim (Chandnani et al. 1990).

Magnetic Resonance Imaging

STIR images show a hyperintense abscess cavity surrounded by a hypointense border. The bone marrow surrounding a Brodie abscess often shows ill-defined edema of variable extent (**Fig. 3.10**). The abscess membrane enhances markedly after contrast administration (Unger et al. 1988, Mason et al. 1989, Chandnani et al. 1990, Resnick 2002, Vahlensieck and Reiser 2002).

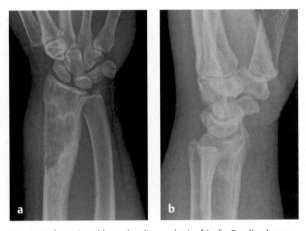

Fig. 3.9a, b   AP and lateral radiographs (**a, b**) of a Brodie abscess in the distal radius show a slightly eccentric dia- and metaphyseal lucent zone with marginal sclerosis and cortical thinning on the radial and volar sides. Pronounced soft-tissue swelling is also present over the radial and posterior sides of the distal radius.

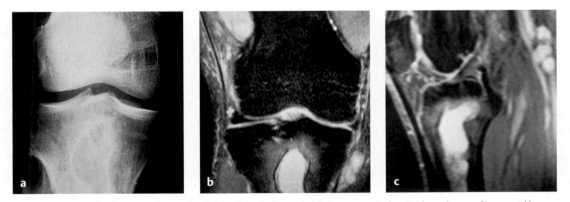

Fig. 3.10a–c   Brodie abscess in the proximal right tibia. Radiograph (**a**) shows a central metaphyseal zone of increased lucency surrounded by sclerosis. Coronal (**b**) and sagittal (**c**) STIR images show a very hyperintense abscess cavity with a hypointense rim surrounded by an extensive, ill-defined area of bone marrow edema.

Key findings in a Brodie abscess:

- Radiograph: metaphyseal osteolysis with a sclerotic rim
- CT: abscess cavity with a faintly enhancing sclerotic rim
- No evidence of fistula formation

Tuberculous Osteomyelitis

Etiology, Sites of Occurrence, and Clinical Features

Today this form of osteomyelitis occurs mainly in drug addicts, alcoholics, immunosuppressed patients, Human immunodeficiency virus (HIV)-infected patients, and immigrants from endemic regions, regardless of age or gender. Skeletal involvement by tuberculosis is almost always preceded by an oligosymptomatic primary infection in the lung or urogenital tract, for example. Hematogenous spread leads to medullary cavity involvement with the destruction of normal bone. A productive form of tuberculous osteomyelitis (granulation tissue, bone resorption) is distinguished from an exudative form (caseating necrosis, necrotic bony trabeculae). The spinal column is involved in 25%–60% of cases. Bone inflammation without articular involvement occurs in 10%–15% of cases, and there is a 10% incidence of multifocal involvement. Sites of predilection are the metaphyses of the long tubular bones and the bones of the hands and feet. In adults the infection often spreads to the adjacent joint. Growth-plate involvement may occur in children. The disease takes an insidious course characterized by debilitation (weight loss, subfibrile temperatures), pain, and local swelling without skin redness. Inflammatory markers are elevated. The main causative organism is *Mycobacterium tuberculosis* (Heuck 1997, Bohndorf and Imhof 2001, Resnick 2002).

Differential diagnosis of tuberculous osteomyelitis:

- Chronic form of another type of osteomyelitis
- Metastases
- Plasmacytoma
- Eosinophilic granuloma
- Fungal infection

Diagnostic Imaging

Projection Radiography

Radiographs in adult patients show elliptical osteolytic areas with marginal sclerosis located predominantly in the axial skeleton, calvarium, shoulder, or pelvis. Sequestra may be found in cases that take a protracted course. Children often show symmetrical involvement of the pe-

ripheral skeleton with metaphyseal osteolytic zones of varying size without marginal sclerosis. Tuberculous dactylitis is a special form affecting children but is rarely seen today. It involves the short tubular bones of the hands and feet and is characterized by soft-tissue swelling, demineralization, cortical destruction, and a lamellated periosteal reaction (Spina ventosa; Haygood and Williamson 1994, Heuck 1997, Bohndorf and Imhof 2001, Resnick 2002).

Magnetic Resonance Imaging

The MRI findings may closely resemble those of acute hematogenous osteomyelitis (zones of caseating necrosis). They may also present as soft-tissue tumors, however. Fluid-sensitive sequences (STIR, T2-weighted) show variable, inhomogeneous hyperintensity while T1-weighted images show low signal intensity before contrast administration (tuberculous granulomas) and variable irregular enhancement after contrast administration (**Fig. 3.11**; David et al. 1987, Quinn et al. 1988, Unger et al. 1988, Erdmann et al. 1991, Morrison et al. 1993, Resnick 2002).

Key findings in tuberculous osteomyelitis:

- Osteolytic areas with marginal sclerosis
- Frequent symmetrical involvement of the peripheral skeleton in children
- Tuberculous dactylitis (special form in children)
- Variable lesion appearance on MRI

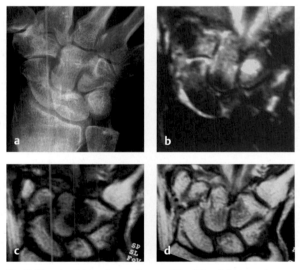

Fig. 3.11a–d Tuberculous osteomyelitis of the right hamate bone of the right hand. Radiograph (**a**) shows an elliptical area of hamate osteolysis at the insertion of the ligament between the capitate and hamate bones. STIR sequence (**b**) shows fluid-equivalent signal intensity at this site accompanied by pronounced bone marrow edema in the capitate and trapezoid bones. Unenhanced T1-weighted image (**c**) shows low signal intensity of the osteolytic area, while the postGd T1-weighted image (**d**) shows slight enhancement (with kind permission of A. Stäbler, MD).

Rare Forms of Osteomyelitis

Syphilitic Osteomyelitis

This is a chronic inflammation caused by *Treponema pallidum*. A congenital form with early or late onset is distinguished from an acquired form. The congenital form leads to syphilitic osteochondritis, diaphyseal osteomyelitis, and periostitis with periosteal reactions. The acquired form is characterized by permeative or moth-eaten osteolytic lesions, signs of periostitis, cortical sequestra, and minimal sclerosis (Heuck 1997, Bohndorf and Imhof 2001, Resnick 2002).

Fungal Osteomyelitis

Fungal osteomyelitis is a very rare condition that occurs chiefly in immunocompromised patients. Actinomycoses, cryptococcoses, blastomycoses, and histoplasmoses are the most common forms. These infections cause painless ulcerations, fistulation with soft-tissue swelling, and chronic osteomyelitis with a mixed osteolytic and sclerotic pattern (Heuck 1997, Bohndorf and Imhof 2001, Resnick 2002).

Parasitic Osteomyelitis

Soft-tissue infection in **toxoplasmosis** may spread to the bone leading to osteomyelitis. Findings include soft-tissue swelling, cystic osteolytic lesions, and circumscribed demineralization.

In 1%–2% of patients with **echinococciasis**, osteomyelitis develops in the setting of the primary infection. Hematogenous spread from the liver or lung may also occur. Sites of predilection are the spine, pelvis, long tubular bones, and skull. Radiographs show multiple small, thin-walled osteolytic lesions (histology: cysts) in which individual trabeculae may remain intact. Additional findings are cortical thinning and general expansion of the affected bone. The dominant MRI findings are cysts, which appear hyperintense in STIR and T2-weighted sequences (Heuck 1997, Bohndorf and Imhof 2001, Resnick 2002).

Joint Infections

Hematogenous Septic Arthritis

Etiology

Manifestations depend on the causative organism, the course (acute or chronic), the precipitating infection, and the site of involvement in the skeletal system. Early diagnosis is necessary to prevent joint infections and their often serious complications. This calls for the early initiation of sensitive imaging procedures.

> **NOTE**
>
> Joint infections have a variable clinical presentation and may be challenging in their diagnosis and differential diagnosis.

The infecting organisms invade the synovial tissue by hematogenous spread from a local or distant focus of infection. The organisms then spread from the synovial membrane to the synovial fluid (Dihlmann 1987, Dihlmann and Bandick 1995, Greenspan 1999, Bohndorf and Imhof 2001).

> **NOTE**
>
> Septic arthritis is particularly common in immunosuppressed patients, elderly patients, patients with chronic diseases, IV drug abusers, and moribund patients.

The development of infection depends on general and local host defenses and on the virulence and number of infecting organisms. The inflammatory process may remain confined to the synovium and joint capsule or may spread to involve the intra-articular structures and bone. Lysosomal enzymes released by bacterial phagocytosis lead to the destruction of cartilage, while the accompanying joint effusion raises the intra-articular pressure. The synovium becomes hypertrophic and forms a fibrous granulation tissue called pannus, which may infiltrate the cartilage and bone causing further destruction. The inflammatory synovial reaction also incites the release of collagenases and the infiltration of leukocytes into the synovial fluid, leading to the progression of joint destruction (Soren 1993, Fassbender 1994).

Sites of Occurrence

The knee, shoulder, and hip joints are commonly affected in adults, and involvement is usually localized to one joint (monoarthritis). Infections of the hip and knee joints are more common in children, although polyarticular disease may occur.

> **NOTE**
>
> Involvement of the sacroiliac joints, symphysis, and sterno-clavicular joints has been reported in immunocompromised patients and IV drug users.

In other less frequent cases, septic arthritis predominantly involves the hand, elbow, and ankle joint (Dihlmann 1987, Dihlmann and Bandick 1995, Greenspan 1999, Bohndorf and Imhof 2001).

Clinical Features

Swelling, local warmth, and redness are accompanied by a painful limitation of motion. Systemic manifestations include low-grade fever and malaise. Other systemic signs such as fever, chills, and sepsis may occur as the disease progresses (Soren 1993, Fassbender 1994).

Differential diagnosis of joint pain (Reeder 1993):
- Infectious arthritis
- Hematogenous septic arthritis
- Nonhematogenous arthritis
- Special forms of infectious arthritis:
  - Lyme borreliosis
  - Viral arthritis
  - Tuberculous arthritis
  - Parasitic or fungal arthritis
  - HIV-associated arthritis
  - Syphilitic arthritis
  - Leprosy-associated arthritis
- Sympathetic forms of arthritis
- Adjacent bone tumors
- Adjacent osteomyelitic foci
- Rheumatoid arthritis
- Ankylosing spondylitis
- Rheumatic polymyalgia
- Acute rheumatic fever
- Enteropathic arthropathies (mainly Crohn disease)

- Connective-tissue diseases (Reiter syndrome, systemic lupus erythematosus, scleroderma, CREST syndrome)
- Psoriatic arthropathy
- Neuropathic (diabetic) osteoarthropathy
- Hemophilic arthropathy
- Osteoarthritis
- Gout
- CPPD (calcium pyrophosphate disease)

Diagnostic Imaging

Projection Radiography

Early cases show joint-space widening due to intra-articular effusion. The effusion and associated soft-tissue swelling lead to the development of inflammatory soft-tissue signs.

These signs are variable depending on the affected joint. Fusiform soft-tissue swelling develops around the interphalangeal joints. Lateral soft-tissue swelling may be seen on the first and fifth metacarpophalangeal joints. The direct or indirect detection of joint effusion may prove difficult in certain joints, depending on the volume of the effusion: the wrist (absent pronator quadratus sign), the distal radioulnar joint, the elbow joint (*fat-pad sign*, or apparent absence of the anterior fat pad with a demonstrable posterior fat pad), the knee joint (clouding of the suprapatellar bursa), and the ankle joint (distended joint capsule). Increased fluid volumes may be seen in the acromioclavicular joint, and displacement of the humeral or femoral head may indicate a joint effusion in children.

Periarticular osteopenia develops with further progression due to inactivity and hyperemia of the affected bony area, blurring the trabecular markings of the cancellous bone (collateral sign).

> **NOTE**
>
> The onset of articular cartilage destruction is marked by radiographically detectable joint-space narrowing, which shows a more concentric pattern than in osteoarthritis.

Erosive lesions may be caused by the ingrowth of fibrous pannus tissue into the bone. Marginal erosions are most commonly found at the attachment of the joint capsule (the *bare area*). It takes at least 1 week for these changes to appear on radiographs.

The further progression of joint destruction may lead to joint deformities and ankylosis. Late stages may show a reactive sclerosis of the affected bony regions (Dihlmann 1987, Tumeh and Tomeh 1991, Soren 1993, Fassbender 1994, Reiser and Peters 1995, Freyschmidt 1997; **Fig. 3.12**).

Key radiographic findings in septic arthritis (Reeder 1993, Reiser and Peters 1995):
- Early changes:
  - Soft-tissue signs (joint effusion, capsule swelling)

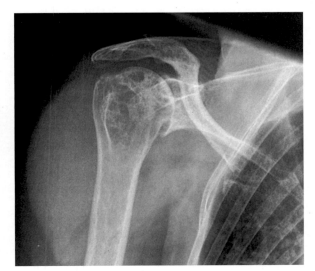

Fig. 3.12 AP radiograph of the right shoulder joint shows pronounced, concentric narrowing of the joint space. Multiple subchondral cysts are projected onto the humeral head and, to a lesser degree, onto the glenoid. Trabecular markings in the humeral head are blurred, and the position of the humeral head is slightly elevated in relation to the glenoid. A conspicuous, spindle-shaped area of soft-tissue proliferation is projected onto the deltoid muscle lateral to the right shoulder joint. In summary, this finding is typical of hematogenous septic arthritis of the right shoulder joint with suspicion of synovitis and pronounced concomitant soft-tissue proliferation.

- – Widening of the joint space
- – Periarticular osteopenia
- – Osteomyelitis due to concomitant involvement of adjacent bone
- Progression:
  - – Narrowing of the joint space (due to cartilage destruction)
  - – Erosive changes in adjacent bone (ingrowth of synovium or pannus)
  - – Joint deformity and destruction
  - – Residual damage (ankylosis, osteosclerosis)

Differential diagnosis of septic arthritis:
- Noninfectious forms of arthritis
- Rheumatoid arthritis (**Fig. 3.13**)
- Ankylosing spondylitis
- Neuropathic (diabetic) osteoarthropathy
- Synovial chondromatosis
- Pigmented villonodular synovitis (PVNS)

Fistulography

Fistulography is useful for the visualization of fistulous tracts extending from the skin surface to a joint or articular compartment and to the adjacent bone.

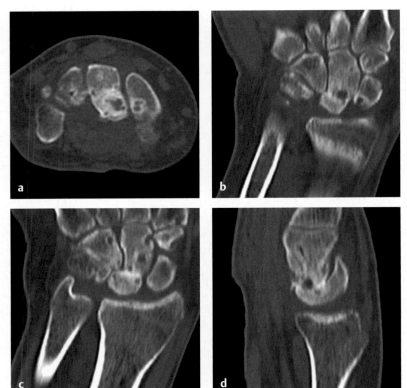

Fig. 3.13a–d Involvement of the right wrist by rheumatoid arthritis. Primary axial CT scan (**a**) and coronal (**b**, **c**) and sagittal MPRs (**d**) show multiple subchondral cysts in the carpal bones, narrowing of the intercarpal joint spaces and radiocarpal joint, and incipient fusion of the lunate and capitate bones (carpal bone formation).

Ultrasound

Ultrasound is useful for directing arthrocentesis and visualizing soft-tissue and capsular swelling and joint effusions. The internal echo pattern of the effusion yields information on the cellularity or fibrin content of the fluid. Periarticular fluid collections, synovial outpouchings (Baker cysts), fluid-filled bursae and tendons can also be visualized with ultrasound (Tumeh et al. 1987, Shiv et al. 1990, Soren 1993, Resnick 2002).

Computed Tomography

CT is used to exclude bony involvement by abscesses, diagnose advanced joint destruction, detect intra-articular fragments after trauma, define the extent of bone destruction, and detect radiopaque foreign bodies. It is also used in the preoperative planning of joint debridement.

> **NOTE**
>
> Conventional tomography and arthrography have been largely superseded by CT and MRI (**Fig. 3.13**).

> **NOTE**
>
> MRI is the most sensitive modality for detecting the early changes of septic arthritis. T2- and T1-weighted fat-suppressed sequences in at least two planes are acquired before and after Gd administration.

Magnetic Resonance Imaging

Joint effusions show markedly increased signal intensity on T2-weighted images and variable hypointensity on T1-weighted images, depending on their protein content. Intense enhancement of the synovium and proliferative synovial changes is a characteristic finding. Cartilage destruction can be detected in specific cartilage-weighted pulse sequences.

Bone erosions appear as tissue defects that show high signal intensity on T2-weighted images and low signal intensity on T1-weighted images. Heavily T2-weighted sequences can distinguish fluid (high T2 signal) from pannus (lower T2 signal). Pannus also shows intense contrast enhancement.

Inflammatory involvement of the adjacent bone can be detected in approximately 90% of cases based on increased T2-weighted signal intensity in the medullary cavity (bone marrow edema). T1-weighted images after contrast administration show increased signal intensity in the corresponding areas. These latter findings, like the presence of periosteal reactions, are not specific for septic arthritis and may also be seen in noninfectious forms of arthritis and after trauma. Frequently, however, these findings are more pronounced in septic arthritis than in noninfectious forms. MRI usually permits the confident detection of inflammatory bone involvement (Vahlensieck and Reiser 2002).

> **NOTE**
>
> The advantages of MRI over bone scintigraphy are better morphologic definition, better spatial orientation, and the more accurate differentiation of internal findings and their anatomical localization.

Differentiation is aided by detecting hemosiderin deposits in the joint space, which have low signal intensity on T2-weighted images. These deposits may be found in PVNS and hemophilic arthropathy. They require differentiation from the ossified intra-articular foreign bodies (*rice bodies*) in synovial chondromatosis, which are also hypointense or appear as signal voids. When synovitis has become chronic, fatty inclusions (lipoma arborescens) may appear in the synovium and bursa (Murphey et al. 1991, Sharif 1992, Sandrasegaran et al. 1994, Karpos et al. 1995, Rand et al. 1998, Yoshioka et al. 2000, Bohndorf and Imhof 2001, Vahlensieck and Reiser 2002; **Figs. 3.14, 3.15, 3.16**).

Complications

Joint destruction may lead to osteoarthritis, growth disturbance due to epiphyseal plate destruction, osteomyelitis of the adjacent bone, soft-tissue infections, and the rupture of tendons and capsules. Synovial cysts may also form in the bone. Epiphyseal necrosis occasionally develops in children. Late stages may be marked by postinfectious ankylosis (Dihlmann 1987, Reiser and Peters 1995, Freyschmidt 1997).

Nonhematogenous Septic Arthritis

Etiology

Nonhematogenous arthritis may be caused by the direct inoculation of infectious organisms. It may also develop as a postoperative complication, or it may result from a local inflammatory focus in bone or soft tissues spreading to involve the joint space.

Diagnostic Imaging

Radiographic signs: Early signs are periarticular soft-tissue changes, soft-tissue swelling, and gas inclusions arising from extra-articular inflammatory foci. Later stages exhibit signs of septic arthritis.

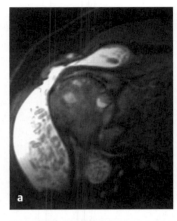

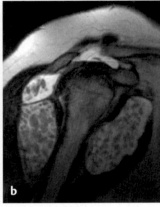

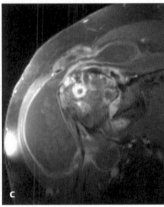

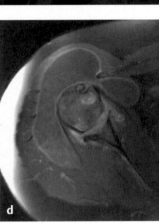

Fig. 3.14a–d Hematogenous septic arthritis of the right shoulder joint. The T2-weighted images (**a** = coronal STIR, **b** = sagittal T2-weighted) show massive expansion with effusion in the subacromial and subdeltoid bursae and axillary recess. Scans also show patchy bone marrow edema in the humeral head with multiple subchondral cysts. Fat-saturated T1-weighted images after contrast administration (**c** = coronal, **d** = axial) show pronounced enhancement of the bursae (peripheral), the entire synovium, and in the medullary cavity of the humeral head. Overall findings are typical of advanced arthritis with osteomyelitis of the humeral head, synovitis, and bursitis.

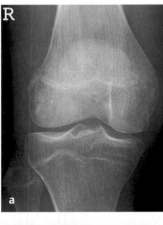

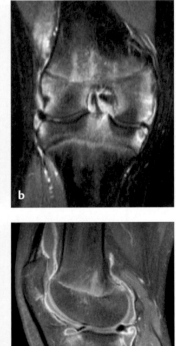

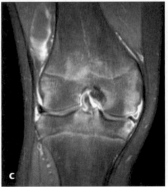

Fig. 3.15a–d Septic arthritis of the right knee joint in a 16-year-old boy. AP radiograph (**a**) shows slight medial soft-tissue swelling and no bony abnormalities. Coronal STIR image (**b**) shows definite epi- and metaphyseal bone marrow edema (hyperintense bone marrow), edematous imbibation of the synovium, and effusion in the knee joint. Fat-saturated T1-weighted images after contrast administration (**c, d**) show intense enhancement of the epi- and metaphyseal medullary cavity and synovium indicating osteomyelitis with concomitant synovitis and effusion in the suprapatellar pouch (**d**).

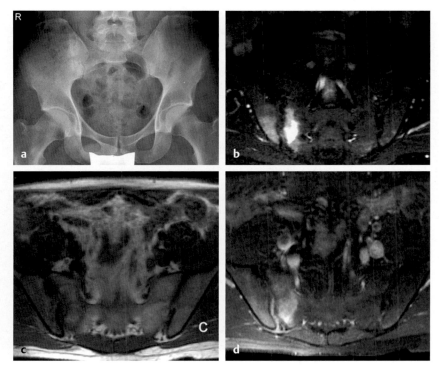

Fig. 3.16a–d Acute exacerbation of right sacroiliac arthritis in a 32-year-old man. Conventional radiograph (**a**) shows increased sclerosis of the subchondral articular surface of the right ilium and, to a lesser degree, of the right lateral mass. Paracoronal STIR image (**b**) and unenhanced axial T1-weighted image (**c**) show pronounced bone marrow edema predominantly affecting the juxta-articular portions of the ilium. Axial T1-weighted image after contrast administration shows intense inflammatory enhancement of the subchondral articular surfaces.

Postoperative Arthritis

Postoperative arthritis may develop in up to 10% of patients who undergo major joint surgery. It is generally caused by the direct inoculation of infectious organisms into the joint space or the spread of an inflammatory process into the joint.

Arthritis Caused by Direct Inoculation

Infectious organisms are frequently introduced by bite injuries, penetrating stab or gunshot wounds, or by iatrogenic inoculation in diagnostic or therapeutic arthrocentesis.

Contiguous Arthritis

Contiguous arthritis develops when a communication is established between the joint space and an adjacent inflammatory focus. This may result from enteroarticular fistulas, severe trauma, or the spread of an adjacent soft-tissue infection. Another route is by the spread of osteomyelitis into an adjacent joint. This is particularly common in infants when infectious organisms spread across the cartilage from the metaphysis to the epiphysis and then into the joint. In adults, the organisms may invade the joint directly from the metaphysis.

Blood vessels may cross the epiphyseal plate during the first year of life, creating a potential route for the spread of infection. From approximately 2 to 16 years of age, however, the epiphysis forms a barrier to the hematogenous spread of infectious organisms. When skeletal maturity is reached, a vascular connection is reestablished between the epiphysis and metaphysis (Resnick 2002).

When the growth plate is intra-articular as in the elbow, shoulder, and hip, infection can spread from the metaphysis into the joint space without involving the growth plate and may precipitate arthritis. This is a typical route for hip-joint infections in infants and small children. In rare cases of tendon infection (e.g., biceps tendon) an infectious focus may invade the joint space by spreading along the tendons (Reiser and Peters 1995, Freyschmidt 1997, Heuck 1997).

Septic Arthritis of the Hip Joint

Early radiographs are usually unrewarding, and ultrasound or MRI may be indicated as an alternative. Capsular and soft-tissue swelling may produce an "obturator sign." Intra-articular effusion may cause joint-space widening or even subluxation of the articular surfaces. The correct diagnosis is often suggested by signs of concomitant osteomyelitis in the femoral metaphysis.

Possible complications include coxarthritis, growth disturbances, angular limb deformity, destruction of the femoral head or coxa magna (enlarged and deformed femoral head), complete lysis of the femoral head, and osteonecrosis of the femoral head following an epiphyseal or metaphyseal infection (presumably due to increased pressure on the blood vessels).

Tuberculous Arthritis

Etiology

This is a chronic, destructive form of septic arthritis caused by *M. tuberculosis*. The infection often arises from a bony osteomyelitic focus, but may also spread to the joint by the hematogenous or lymphogenous route. Up to 1% of all patients with pulmonary tuberculosis also suffer from tuberculous arthritis, which generally is confined to one joint. Peak age incidence is in the fifth and sixth decades. Predisposing factors are immunosuppression, IV drug use, alcoholism, and local weakening of host defenses due to steroid injections or other causes. Large joints such as the ankle, knee, and hip are predominantly affected. The joints of the hands and feet are less frequently involved (Thijn and Steensma 1989, Haygood and Williamson 1994).

Clinical Features

Patients present with mild pain and limitation of motion. A history of tuberculosis and bacterial cultures of the joint effusion suggest the correct diagnosis and are positive in 70%–80% of cases.

Projection Radiography

Early changes such as periarticular osteopenia, slowly progressive joint-space narrowing, and marginal bone erosions (especially in weight-bearing joints) are suggestive of tuberculous arthritis. Soft-tissue swelling is nonspecific. Radiographs may also show subchondral bone destruction affecting the subchondral plate.

Further progression is marked by tuberculous synovitis, periosteal new bone formation in the setting of periostitis, subchondral sclerosis, and possible opposing areas of necrosis (*kissing* sequestra; Thijn and Steensma 1989, Haygood and Williamson 1994).

Complications

Potential complications are fistula formation, soft-tissue abscesses, intra-articular loose bodies, growth disturbance, and ankylosis.

Differential diagnosis of polyarticular joint diseases (Burgener and Kormano 1991, Reiser and Peters 1995):

Frequent causes:
- Rheumatoid arthritis
- Primary or secondary osteoarthritis
- Juvenile chronic arthritis (JCA)
- Ankylosing spondylitis
- Gout
- Pseudogout (chondrocalcinosis)
- Psoriatic arthropathy

Rare causes:
- Lyme disease
- HIV-associated arthritis
- Enteropathic arthritis
- Hematochromatosis
- Hemophilia
- Jaccoud arthritis
- Acromegaly
- Amyloidosis
- Connective-tissue diseases (mixed connective-tissue disease, Reiter syndrome, Sjögren syndrome)
- Sarcoidosis
- Viral synovitis (mumps, rubella, smallpox, hepatitis)
- Wilson disease

Differential diagnosis of monoarticular joint diseases (Burgener and Kormano 1991, Reeder 1993):

Frequent causes:
- Infectious arthritis
- Avascular arthritis
- Gout
- Secondary osteoarthritis (trauma, mechanical overload)

Rare causes:
- Neuropathic osteoarthropathy
- Pseudogout (chondrocalcinosis)
- PVNS
- Rheumatoid monoarthritis
- Amyloidosis
- Reiter syndrome
- Synovial neoplasms (synovial cysts such as Baker cysts, synovial hypertrophy due to infection, synovial osteochondromatosis, villonodular synovitis)
- Joint effusion (adjacent neoplasms in the bone)

Other Forms of Infectious Arthritis

Arthritis in Lyme Disease

Etiology, Sites of Occurrence, and Clinical Features

Lyme disease is caused by Borrelia organisms (spirochetes) transmitted by tick bites. Flulike symptoms and erythema migrans appear after an incubation period of up to 4 weeks. Involvement of the nervous system, heart, eye, and musculoskeletal system follows after a period of weeks or months. Untreated infection leads to arthralgia or frank arthritis in approximately 60% of cases.

Patients complain of intermittent mono- or oligoarticular arthritis predominantly affecting the large joints. The knees are most commonly affected, but symmetrical polyarthritis of the small joints is also observed. Individual episodes last from weeks to months and may recur over a period of years. Chronic erosive arthritis may develop in up to 10% of untreated patients. Rarely the causative organism can be cultured from joint effusion (Bohndorf and Imhof 2001, Resnick 2002).

Projection Radiography

Radiographic findings include soft-tissue signs and collateral signs, joint-space narrowing, subchondral cysts, marginal erosions, osteophytes, and occasional chondrocalcinosis.

Differential Diagnosis

The differential diagnosis includes rheumatic fever, JCA, gonococcal arthritis, Reiter syndrome, and tuberculous arthritis (Bohndorf and Imhof 2001, Resnick 2002).

Mycotic Arthritis

Etiology

Fungal infections of the joint generally occur only in immunosuppressed patients and are usually confined to one joint. Osteomyelitis occurs rarely due to histoplasmosis or cryptococcal infection. More common is a reactive immune response to fungal antigens leading to joint effusion and synovitis. Causative organisms are actinomycetes, coccidioidomycetes, and blastomycetes, which occur mainly in North America.

Projection Radiography

Radiographs show mild osteopenia and changes similar to those in tuberculous arthritis (Bohndorf and Imhof 2001, Resnick 2002).

Viral Arthritis

Etiology, Sites of Occurrence, and Clinical Features

Viral arthritis usually presents with symmetrical involvement of the metacarpophalangeal and proximal interphalangeal joints of the hands. Viral arthritis develops in up to 20% of hepatitis B infections, up to 75% of parvovirus infections, and up to 30% of rubella infections in adults.

Infectious mononucleosis, adenovirus infections, varicella, and echovirus infections may occasionally incite articular complaints.

Projection Radiography

Radiographs show nonerosive polyarticular arthritis that is usually confined to the lower limb. Rubella and parvovirus infections may cause radiographic joint-space narrowing; this may be followed by osteoarthritis. Hepatitis B usually causes a nonerosive arthritis of the finger, ankle, and knee joints. Up to 35% of HIV-infected patients may develop arthralgia predominantly affecting the elbow, shoulder, and knee joints.

Syphilitic Arthritis

Etiology

Articular involvement by syphilis has been described in 2%–3% of patients but is rarely encountered today.

Projection Radiography

Osteopenia, joint-space narrowing, erosion, sclerosis, and ankylosis have been described (Bohndorf and Imhof 2001, Resnick 2002).

Arthritis in Leprosy

This form presents clinically with severe joint pain and swelling and massive joint effusion chiefly involving the ankle, knee, hand, finger, and elbow. Differentiation is required from neuropathic osteoarthropathy in leprosy.

Arthritis Caused by Nonpyrogenic Organisms

Etiology, Sites of Occurrence, and Clinical Features

Up to 1 in 5000 persons inoculated with the BCG vaccine complain of arthritis or osteomyelitis. Reactive arthritis occurs in approximately 1% of patients. Arthritis caused by atypical mycobacteria mainly affects the peripheral joints.

Projection Radiography

Radiographic features resemble those of tuberculosis. Tendosynovitis can often be identified.

Parasitic Arthritis

Helminthiasis may cause arthritis and arthralgia in sporadic cases. Mono- or oligoarticular arthritis, especially of the hand and ankle joints, may occasionally occur in toxoplasmosis (Reiser and Peters 1995, Freyschmidt 1997, Heuck 1997, Bohndorf and Imhof 2001, Vahlensieck and Reiser 2002).

Radiologic differential diagnosis of joint-space narrowing (Reeder 1993, Bohndorf and Imhof 2001, Resnick 2002):

Frequent causes:
- Osteoarthritis
- Hematogenous septic arthritis
- Ankylosing spondylitis
- Osteoarthritis secondary to avascular necrosis
- Rheumatoid arthritis
- Psoriatic arthropathy
- Other chronic forms of arthritis in advanced stages (gout, JCA, enteropathic arthritis, neuropathic arthritis, arthritis in connective-tissue diseases)

Rare causes:
- Hemophilic arthropathy
- PVNS
- Pseudogout
- Reiter syndrome
- Hemophilic arthropathy

- Stickler syndrome (autosomal dominant connective-tissue disorder with cataracts, myopia, hyperextensible joints, and arthritis)
- Winchester syndrome (very rare, only 12 cases known worldwide; presents in first year of life with arthritis of small joints, facial dysmorphia, skin thickening, and contractures)

Radiologic differential diagnosis of joint space widening (Reeder 1993, Bohndorf and Imhof 2001, Resnick 2002):

Frequent causes:
- Early stage of hematogenous septic arthritis
- Hemarthrosis due to acute intra-articular hemorrhage (e. g., caused by trauma or hemophilia)
- Serous joint effusion (rheumatoid arthritis, connective tissue diseases)
- Posttraumatic dislocation or subluxation, widening of the joint capsule
- Perthes disease

Rare causes:
- Inflammatory synovial thickening
- Rheumatoid arthritis, gout, tuberculosis, fungal arthritis
- Winchester syndrome
- Faber lipogranulomatosis
- PVNS
- Interposed cartilage fragments after trauma
- Neuropathic osteoarthropathy
- Synovial neoplasms

Radiologic differential diagnosis of arthritis with osteopenia (Reeder 1993, Bohndorf and Imhof 2001, Resnick 2002):

Frequent causes:
- Hematogenous septic arthritis, tuberculosis
- Rheumatoid arthritis

Rare causes:
- HIV-associated arthritis
- Enteropathic arthritis
- Fungal arthritis
- JCA
- Lupus erythematosus
- Lyme disease
- Connective-tissue diseases (Sjögren syndrome)
- Transient osteoporosis
- Scleroderma
- Reflex sympathetic dystrophy

Radiologic differential diagnosis of arthritis with little or no osteoporosis (Reeder 1993, Bohndorf and Imhof 2001, Resnick 2002):
- Osteoarthritis (degenerative, posttraumatic, erosive)

- Ankylosing spondylitis
- Gout
- Neuropathic osteoarthropathy
- Pseudogout
- Psoriatic arthropathy

Pustulotic Arthro-Osteomyelitis, SAPHO Syndrome

Etiology, Sites of Occurrence, and Clinical Features

Pustulotic arthro-osteomyelitis occurs in middle age with no gender predilection. Up to 10% of patients with plantopalmar pustulosis develop destructive inflammatory, proliferative hyperostotic changes in their bones and joints. Osteoarticular involvement is particularly common in the sternoclavicular joint. The term SAPHO describes a syndrome consisting of **s**ynovitis, **a**cne, **p**ustulosis, **h**yperostosis, and **o**steomyelitis. Eighty percent of patients present initially with painful, bilateral swelling of the sternoclavicular joints and limited motion (fibroostitis of the costoclavicular ligament). Fifty percent of patients have primary involvement of the axial skeleton, and up to 30% have erosive or nonerosive arthritis of the extremities. The clinical course is marked by alternating exacerbations and remissions for years. A chronic persistent course is rarely observed. The etiology of pustulotic

arthro-osteomyelitis is uncertain, but bacterial and viral infections, autoimmune processes, and reactive arthro-osteomyelitis have been proposed (Heuck 1997, Resnick 1998, Heyem et al. 1999, Bohndorf and Imhof 2001, Resnick 2002).

Differential diagnosis of pustulotic arthro-osteomyelitis:

- Degenerative changes in the sternoclavicular joints
- Infectious arthritis and spondylodiskitis
- Metastases
- Diffuse idiopathic skeletal hyperostosis

Diagnostic Imaging

Projection Radiography

The sternoclavicular joints often show symmetrical erosive destruction of the articular surfaces with partially irregular joint-space widening. The medial portions of the clavicles are expanded and show increased sclerosis. As the disease progresses, there is ossification of the costoclavicular ligaments with bony ankylosis of the sternoclavicular joints. The spinal column shows diffuse sclerosis of single or multiple vertebrae (ivory vertebrae), syndesmophytes, osteophytes, and calcification of the anterior longitudinal ligament. Erosive bone destruction of the costovertebral joints may occur at an early stage. A mixed pattern of increased sclerosis and circumscribed

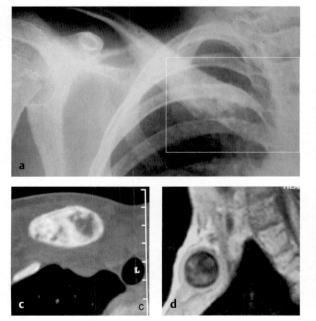

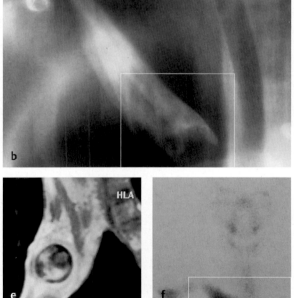

Fig. 3.17a–f SAPHO syndrome with involvement of the right sternoclavicular joint. Conventional radiograph (**a**), conventional coronal tomogram (**b**), and axial CT (**c**) show expansion and increased sclerosis of the medial clavicle with destruction of the medial articular surface. Sagittal T2-weighted MRI (**d**) and T1-weighted MRI after contrast administration (**e**) show concentric

hypertrophy of the clavicle with increased sclerosis, destruction of the medial articular surface, bone marrow edema, and moderate irregular enhancement. Two-phase bone scintigraphy (**f**) shows markedly increased uptake in the right sternoclavicular joint (with kind permission of A. Stäbler, MD).

osteolytic areas with periosteal reactions develops in the sacroiliac joints, the long tubular bones, and the flat bones (**Fig. 3.17**). Soft-tissue swelling may occur at retrosternal, paravertebral, and paraosseous sites in addition to soft-tissue calcification (Hayem et al. 1999, Heuck 1997, Bohnhof and Imhof 1998, Boutin and Resnick 1998, Resnick 2002).

Bone Scintigraphy

Bone scintigraphy is a very rewarding study in SAPHO syndrome. A "steerhorn" pattern of uptake may be seen in the sternoclavicular joints. Bone scintigraphy is also excellent for detecting the frequent multifocal occurrence of skeletal lesions.

Computed Tomography

CT is generally unnecessary in SAPHO syndrome. It may be useful in selected cases, however, such as excluding an osteoplastic tumor when severe sclerosis is present. High-resolution CT can provide detailed, nonsuperimposed views of bone destruction and sclerotic changes. The findings coincide with those of conventional radiographs, but CT is superior to radiographs for the accurate localization of findings (Heuck 1997, Boutin and Resnick 1998, Hayem et al. 1999, Bohndorf and Imhof 2001, Resnick 2002).

Magnetic Resonance Imaging

Pustulotic arthro-osteomyelitis can generally be diagnosed on the basis of clinical findings combined with plain radiographs. MRI is useful only for distinguishing inflammatory skeletal changes from reactive changes. MRI can detect multifocal involvement owing to its large field of view (STIR sequences, HASTE [half-Fourier acquisition single-shot turbo spin-echo] sequences; Heuck 1997, Boutin and Resnik 1998, Hayem et al. 1999, Bohndorf and Imhof 2001, Resnick 2002; **Fig. 3.18**).

Key findings in pustulotic arthro-osteomyelitis:

- Sternoclavicular hyperostosis
- Multifocal hyperostotic bone involvement (ivory vertebrae)
- Erosive destruction of the costovertebral joints
- Inflammatory enthesopathies with new bone formation
- Signs of peripheral or axial arthritis
- Hyperostotic changes in long tubular bones
- Spinal changes that resemble ankylosing spondylitis
- Soft-tissue involvement

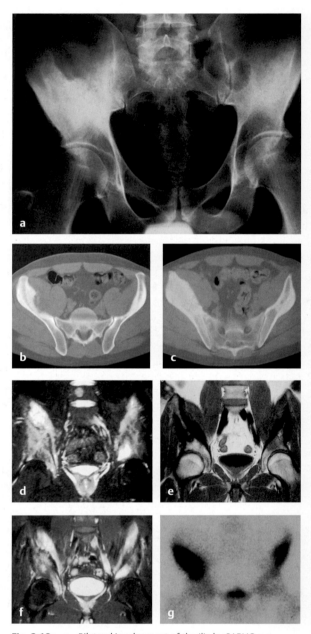

Fig. 3.18a–g Bilateral involvement of the ilia by SAPHO syndrome. Pelvic radiograph (**a**) shows bilateral increased sclerosis of the ilium, more pronounced on the right side and extending to the right sacroiliac joint. Axial CT scans (**b, c**) show bilateral fusiform expansion of the cortical bone, more pronounced on the right side, with marked sclerosis of the medullary cavity in that region. The anterior portion of the right sacroiliac joint is also affected. MRI STIR sequence (**d**) shows pronounced, bilateral bone marrow edema in the hypertrophic ilium with patchy, edematous imbibation of the surrounding soft tissue. Unenhanced coronal T1-weighted image (**e**) defines the extent of bilateral fusiform ilial sclerosis. Fat-saturated T1-weighted image after contrast administration (**f**) shows marked enhancement of the sclerotic bones with minimal enhancement of surrounding soft tissues. Two-phase bone scintigraphy (**g**) shows markedly increased uptake in the ilia, particularly on the right side (with kind permission of A. Stäbler, MD).

Implant Complications

Prosthetic Loosening and Infection

Biplane radiographs are usually sufficient to investigate suspected prosthetic loosening, which is confirmed if an implant fracture or periprosthetic fracture is detected. The migration of prosthetic components in follow-up examinations is another sign of prosthetic loosening.

> **NOTE**
>
> Prosthetic loosening is confirmed by comparing current radiographs with prior films. In the case of cemented implants, a cement fracture and a lucent zone between the cement and metal are definite signs of prosthetic loosening.
>
> With an uncemented prosthesis, increased sclerosis of the cancellous bone under the tip of the implant (total hip replacement) and periosteal reactions about the tip of the implant stem (shoulder, hip) are signs of prosthetic loosening.

If DSA shows that the prosthesis or cement is rimmed by contrast medium, prosthetic loosening is confirmed. If prosthetic loosening is questionable, the arthroplasty can be imaged fluoroscopically to check for relative motion between the implant and bone. Wear debris from a polyethylene acetabular component may incite foreign-body granulomas leading to the destruction of acetabular bone. Radiographs may show circumscribed bone destruction, which should not be confused with bone resorption around a loose prosthesis (Greenspan 1999, Freiberg 2001).

Definite signs of prosthetic loosening:
- Resorption zone between the prosthesis and cortex
- Periprosthetic fracture
- Prosthetic fracture
- Cement fracture
- Prosthetic migration or displacement

With a periprosthetic infection, radiographs show circumscribed osteolytic zones of increased lucency bordering the prosthesis. Soft-tissue swelling may also be noted as an incidental finding, but soft-tissue ultrasound is more accurate for this application and can detect even small amounts of joint effusion or fluid resulting from an infected prosthesis. In rare cases a chronic periprosthetic infection may incite a periosteal reaction adjacent to the implant (Greenspan 1999, Reiberg 2001).

> **NOTE**
>
> Generally, however, it is impossible to distinguish between prosthetic loosening and periprosthetic infection on radiographs.

If doubt exists and a correct diagnosis would have therapeutic implications, arthrography should be performed. Articular fluid should be aspirated if possible to provide material for microbiologic examination, which could confirm possible infection of the prosthesis. If the prosthesis is loose, arthrography (preferably using the DSA technique) will show a contrast rim of variable width surrounding the prosthesis.

Diabetic Osteoarthropathy

Etiology, Sites of Occurrence, and Clinical Features

Diabetic foot syndrome (DFS) is one of the most frequent complications of diabetes mellitus. The principal causes are peripheral polyneuropathy, macroangiopathy, and also microangiopathy, which is common in diabetes mellitus.

When a diabetic foot is caused by **polyneuropathy,** sensation is absent or diminished. Pedal pulses are not diminished. The skin is warm and dry, pes cavus is frequently present, and often only one foot is affected initially. Decreased sensation leads to unphysiologic weight bearing and planar ulcers, which are most pronounced at the metatarsal level. The ulcers are painless, have a livid base are surrounded by a hyperkeratotic zone, and bleed easily.

Cases with a **vascular** cause are generally bilateral and the femoral, tibial, and peroneal vessels are most commonly affected. Sensation is preserved, but pedal pulses are absent and the skin is shiny, cold, atrophic, and hairless. Further progression is marked by ulceration and gangrene. Ischemic ulcers are painful, have a fibrotic base, and do not bleed.

The pathogenesis of diabetic foot may involve either one of the above causes or may involve a combination of both factors.

Regardless of its pathogenesis, DFS may lead to diabetic osteoarthropathy with an increased susceptibility to infections. Diabetic osteoarthropathy occurs in approximately 2%–4% of patients with long-standing diabetes mellitus (Freyschmidt 1997). The midfoot and forefoot are most commonly affected. Typical findings are cortical bone destruction, periosteal reactions, osteoporotic changes, subluxations, and eventual fragmentation and necrosis of bone and cartilage with joint-space obliteration by debris. Angiopathy is often manifested by pronounced calcification of blood vessels in the foot and lower leg.

A special form of diabetic osteoarthropathy caused by diabetic polyneuropathy is the "Charcot joint." Characterized by painless bone destruction developing over a period of 1–2 years, this condition has been classified into three stages by Eichenholtz (1966). Stage I is characterized by aseptic bone inflammation with hyperemia, fragmentation, and dislocations. The surrounding soft tissue may be painless, red, and swollen. Stage II is characterized by new bone formation, and stage III by consolidation and resolution.

Infections develop either through fissures in the dry, poorly vascularized skin between the toes or secondarily after tiny injuries in polyneuropathic DFS. Infections spread in the soft tissue along muscle compartments, giving rise to abscess formation and cellulitis. The most severe form of soft-tissue infection is necrotizing fasciitis. A subcutaneous facia becomes infected, leading to necrosis and gangrene of the skin above the lesion. Soft-tissue infections may also spread to the bone and incite a severe osteomyelitis that is difficult to treat. In contrast to Charcot osteoarthropathy, these infections are extremely painful and invariably involve the surrounding soft tissues.

Differential diagnosis of diabetic osteoarthropathy:

The section below focuses on the evaluation of bones and soft tissues in osteoarthropathy. Angiologic procedures, which are usually at the forefront of diagnostic procedures in DFS, will not be covered in this chapter.

Diagnostic Imaging

Projection Radiography

The minimum requirements for a conventional radiographic work up of diabetic osteoarthropathy are an AP view, lateral view, and a lateral weight-bearing view of the foot. Only the lateral weight-bearing view is useful for evaluating the arch and pressure points, which are usually abnormal in diabetics.

"Debris" refers to the pronounced fragmentation and destruction of bones and cartilage leading to loss of the physiologic anatomy of the bony structures and obliteration of the joint space by tiny, quartzlike bone fragments (Dihlmann 1987, Freyschmidt 1997). This bone destruction, which may lead to the complete loss of normal anat-

omy, requires strict differentiation from bone destruction due to osteomyelitis. Osteomyelitis is secondary to a preexisting soft-tissue infection and may be confined to individual bones. Debris, on the other hand, is characterized by extensive, noninflammatory destruction of metatarsal anatomy that generally does not involve the soft tissues (Dihlmann 1987, Freyschmidt 1997, Heuck 1997).

The increasing destruction of cartilage and bone, usually painless in the neuropathic joint, often leads to subluxations and occasional dislocations in diabetic osteoarthropathy. The metacarpal joints are predominantly affected, but subluxation and dislocation may also occur in the metatarsal and interphalangeal joints (Dihlmann 1987, Freyschmidt 1997, Heuck 1997, Bohndorf and Imhof 2001).

Long-standing DFS is characterized by increasing subchondral sclerosis and periosteal new bone formation with osteophytic spurring. This leads to a combination of bone destruction (debris) and periosteal new bone formation (Dihlmann 1987, Freyschmidt 1997, Heuck 1997, Bohndorf and Imhof 2001).

Key findings in diabetic osteoarthropathy:
- Debris: fragmentation and necrosis of cartilage and bones, which fill in the former joint space
- Subluxations, especially in the metatarsophalangeal joints
- Destruction of the articular surface
- Subchondral sclerosis
- Periosteal new bone formation
- Massive soft-tissue swelling
- Vascular calcifications

Computed Tomography

CT is usually an adjunctive study in DFS. Bone destruction is so pronounced in most cases that adding CT scans has no therapeutic implications.

CT is most commonly used to direct preoperative planning. Thin slices are acquired and MPRs should always be obtained. CT should also be performed if an intra-articular loose body is suspected or if subluxations coexist with an intra-articular fracture (Reiser and Peters 1995, Greenspan 1999, Bohndorf and Imhof 2001).

Magnetic Resonance Imaging

MRI is used in DFS to evaluate the extent of soft-tissue involvement. It can sensitively detect bone marrow edema and bone infection, though it may be difficult or impossible in some cases to differentiate noninfectious bone marrow edema from osteomyelitis.

In cases with diffuse soft-tissue inflammation, MRI shows more or less pronounced, diffuse enhancement in T2-weighted or STIR sequences. Unenhanced T1-weighted sequences show diffuse hypointensity. T1-weighted contrast-enhanced images show marked enhancement in the inflamed soft tissue. This enhancement is most pronounced in fat-saturated sequences. Often, however, it is not possible to distinguish reactive soft-tissue inflammation from cellulitis.

On the other hand, the presence of a soft-tissue abscess combined with an ulcer or fistula confirms a soft-tissue infection. The abscess contents show high fluid-equivalent signal intensity on T2-weighted SE and STIR images. The abscess is hypointense on T1-weighted images, and its membrane shows intense peripheral enhancement after contrast administration.

Bone marrow edema may develop in DFS as a result of bone destruction and associated unphysiologic weight bearing on affected bones, or it may result from florid osteomyelitis. This produces increased signal intensity in T2-weighted and STIR sequences and decreased signal intensity in unenhanced T1-weighted sequences. Bone marrow edema due to unphysiologic weight bearing continues to show relatively low signal intensity after IV contrast administration. Florid osteomyelitis, on the other hand, shows definite enhancement. Enhancement may also occur in bone marrow edema secondary to unphysiologic weight bearing. The likelihood of osteomyelitis increases in cases where an ulcer is accompanied by a soft-tissue defect (Craig et al. 1997). This is not found when bone marrow edema results from unphysiologic loads.

The Charcot joint in stage I is a special case: Because it is an aseptic bone inflammation and therefore an active process, it is characterized by bone marrow edema and contrast enhancement, making it difficult to distinguish from osteomyelitis. When osteomyelitis is present, it should show markedly higher T2-weighted signal intensity than bone marrow edema in Charcot arthropathy. An indirect differentiating feature is that florid osteomyelitis is always associated with pronounced soft-tissue inflammation, whereas a stage I Charcot joint is usually confined to bony structures. On the other hand, cases where a stage I Charcot joint does show soft-tissue involvement may be indistinguishable from osteomyelitis by MRI. Another differentiating criterion that suggests osteomyelitis is the presence of cortical destruction. In a stage II or III Charcot joint, the bone marrow shows low signal intensity in all MRI sequences (Craig et al. 1997, Freyschmidt 1997, Bohndorf and Imhof 2001, Vahlensieck and Reiser 2002; **Fig. 3.19.**)

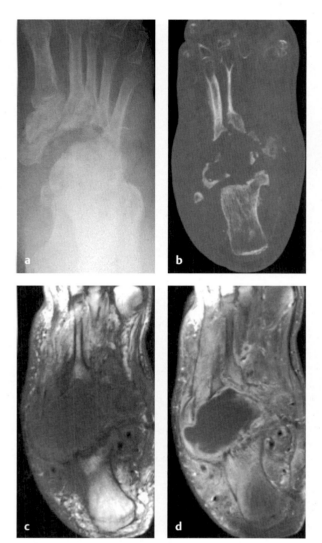

Fig. 3.19a–d A 64-year-old man with a long history of type-2 diabetes. AP radiograph (**a**) of the right foot shows complete destruction of the metatarsus with a large central defect, remaining portions of the navicular and the medial and intermediate cuneiform bones, shortening of the foot, and pronounced soft-tissue swelling. Axial CT (**b**) accurately defines the extent of bone destruction and the condition of the metatarsal joints. MRI in axial T1-weighted sequences before (**c**) and after (**d**, fat-saturated) contrast administration shows a fluid collection of several centimeters in the lateral metatarsal area with pronounced marginal contrast enhancement. Enhancement is also seen at the bases of the metatarsal bones, in the remnants of the metatarsals, and in the surrounding soft tissues. The overall findings are consistent with very advanced diabetic arthropathy with osteomyelitis and abscess formation and nearly complete destruction of the metatarsus and edematous, inflammatory imbibition of the surrounding soft tissue.

Delayed Union, Bone Defect, and Nonunion

Etiology

Undisplaced fractures and anatomically immobilized fractures will undergo primary healing when the fracture surfaces are approximated with adequate compression. In this case the fracture line will fuse by endosteal callus formation.

Displaced or dehiscent fractures will undergo secondary healing, in which the fracture site is bridged predominantly by periosteal callus (Greenspan 1999).

Diagnostic Imaging

Projection Radiography

Periosteal callus formation often cannot be visualized if the fracture site is devoid of periosteum, as in the intra-articular portion of the femoral neck. Likewise, endosteal callus cannot be seen until calcification has occurred. The initially radiolucent callus is transformed into laminar bone by enchondral ossification, and this bone is clearly visible on radiographs.

CT scans with MPRs should be added in cases where bones are covered by dressings or splints, positioning problems arise, the progression of ossification or bony union is unclear, or internal fixation devices are still present in the ROI (Greenspan 1999, Bohndorf and Imhof 2001).

Complications

Delayed union is present if the bone ends have not fused by 16 to 18 weeks, depending on the fracture site and patient age. Nonunion is present if fusion still fails to occur after that period. Radiographs show rounded bone fragments with sclerotic ends that are separated by a definite gap. Fluoroscopy demonstrates relative motion of the fragments.

Pseudarthrosis is a variant of nonunion in which a synovialike capsule forms at the fracture site and creates a false joint space by approximately 6–8 months after the fracture. Several types of nonunion are described below.

Nonunions

Atrophic, Nonreactive Nonunion

There is no bony reaction whatsoever at the fragment ends. There is scant vascularity, and scintigraphy shows little or no radionuclide uptake. Surgical treatment consists of intensive decortication and, if necessary, autologous bone grafting.

Reactive (Hypertrophic) Nonunion

A reactive nonunion is characterized by hypertrophic bone formation and increased sclerosis of the bone ends, possibly leading to deformity of the bone ends or of the affected limb. Generally the bone is well vascularized, and increased tracer uptake is found at scintigraphy. Surgical treatment consists of internal fixation (Greenspan 1999, Bohndorf and Imhof 2001).

Infected Nonunion

The radiographic appearance of an infected nonunion depends on the activity of the inflammatory process. Older, inactive infectious foci display irregular margins, cortical thickening, uniform periosteal thickening, and increased sclerosis of the bony callus.

Actively infected nonunions are characterized by soft-tissue swelling, the destruction of cortical bone and callus, and periosteal reactions (Greenspan 1999, Bohndorf and Imhof 2001).

Diagnostic Imaging

Three stages of nonunion can be distinguished on radiographs: the resorption stage with a gaping fracture line (I), the formation of bone-resorption zones and cysts (II), and progressive sclerosis of the fracture ends with an absence of bony fusion (III).

The nonunion site shows increased signal intensity in T2-weighted MRI sequences. The adjacent bone shows a variable degree of bone marrow edema, depending on the activity of the process. Bony sclerosis typically leads to progressive hypointensity in all sequences. Contrast agents (Gd chelates) can provide information on bone

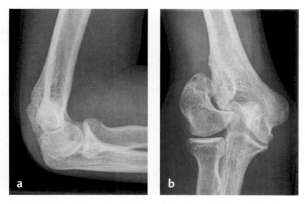

Fig. 3.20a, b Nonunion of the radial epicondyle 9 months after a fracture of the distal humerus. Biplane radiographs show a broad fracture line extending into the intercondylar notch with no evidence of endosteal or periosteal callus formation. A small sclerotic strip is visible at the fracture ends. AP radiograph (**a**) does not show malalignment of the distal fragment. Lateral radiograph (**b**) shows anterior tilting of the distal fragment by at least 15°. Despite the nonunion, there are no visible abnormalities in the humeroradial joint. There is no evidence of effusion in the right elbow joint.

viability and possible associated infections (Vahlensieck and Reiser 2002; **Fig. 3.20**).

Risk factors for fracture nonunion:

- Inadequate blood supply caused, for example, by vascular damage, extensive soft-tissue injuries, periosteal injuries, extensive internal fixation, or osteonecrosis
- Incomplete immobilization, loosening of an internal fixation device, or distraction of the fracture fragments
- Infection, osteomyelitis
- Loss of bony substance, bone sequestrum, osteolysis, dehiscent bone fragments
- Gaping of the fragments due to adjacent osteonecrosis of the bone ends
- Soft tissue interposed between the fragments

Bibliography

Bloch F, Hansen WW, Packard M. Nuclear Induction. Phys Rev 1946;69:127

Bohndorf K, Imhof H. Musculoskeletal Imaging. Stuttgart: Thieme; 2001

Boutin RD, Resnick D. The SAPHO syndrome: an evolving concept for unifying several idiopathic disorders of bone and skin. AJR Am J Roentgenol 1998;170(3):585–591

Bundesärztekammer. Leitlinien der Bundesärztekammer zur Qualitätssicherung in der Röntgendiagnostik. Dtsch Arztebl 1995;92(34/35):A2272–A2285

Bundesärztekammer. Leitlinien der Bundesärztekammer zur Qualitätssicherung in der Magnet-Resononz-Tomographie. Dtsch Arztebl 2000;97(39):A2557–A2568

Burgener FA, Kormano M. Differential Diagnosis in Conventional Radiology. Stuttgart: Thieme; 1991

Castaneda-Zuniga WR. Interventional Radiology. New York: Williams & Wilkins; 1997

Chandnani VP, Beltran JD, Morris CS, et al. Acute experimental osteomyelitis and abscesses: detection with MR imaging versus CT. Radiology 1990;174(1):233–236

Cohen MD, Cory DA, Kleiman M, Smith JA, Broderick NJ. Magnetic resonance differentiation of acute and chronic osteomyelitis in children. Clin Radiol 1990;41(1):53–56

Craig JG, Amin MB, Wu K, et al. Osteomyelitis of the diabetic foot: MR imaging-pathologic correlation. Radiology 1997;203(3):849–855

David R, Barron BJ, Madewell JE. Osteomyelitis, acute and chronic. Radiol Clin North Am 1987;25(6):1171–1201

Dihlmann W. Gelenke-Wirbel-Verbindungen. Stuttgart: Thieme; 1987

Dihlmann W, Bandick J. Die Gelenksilhouette. Das Informationspotential der Röntgenstrahlen. Berlin: Springer; 1995

Eichenholtz PN. Charcot Joints. Springfield, IL: CC Thomas; 1966

Erdman WA, Tamburro F, Jayson HT, Weatherall PT, Ferry KB, Peshock RM. Osteomyelitis: characteristics and pitfalls of diagnosis with MR imaging. Radiology 1991;180(2):533–539

Fassbender HG. Inflammatory reactions in arthritis. In: Davies M, Dingle JT, Page C, eds. Immunopharmacology of Joints and Connective Tissue. London: Academic Press; 1994

Freiberg AA. The Radiology of Orthopaedic Implants. St. Louis: Mosby; 2001

Freyschmidt J. Skeletterkrankungen: Klinisch-radiologische Diagnose und Differentialdiagnose. Berlin: Springer; 1997

Gold RH, Hawkins RA, Katz RD. Bacterial osteomyelitis: findings on plain radiography, CT, MR, and scintigraphy. AJR Am J Roentgenol 1991;157(2):365–370

Greenspan A. Orthopedic Radiology. Philadelphia: Lippincott Williams & Wilkins; 1999

Günther RW, Thelen M. Interventionelle Radiologie. Stutttgart: Thieme; 1996

Hayem G, Bouchaud-Chabot A, Benali K, et al. SAPHO syndrome: a long-term follow-up study of 120 cases. Semin Arthritis Rheum 1999;29(3):159–171

Haygood TM, Williamson SL. Radiographic findings of extremity tuberculosis in childhood: back to the future? Radiographics 1994;14(3):561–570

Heuck A. Skelettradiologie. Stuttgart: Thieme; 1997

Jones KM, Unger EC, Granstrom P, Seeger JF, Carmody RF, Yoshino M. Bone marrow imaging using STIR at 0.5 and 1.5 T. Magn Reson Imaging 1992;10(2):169–176

Jurik AG, Egund N. MRI in chronic recurrent multifocal osteomyelitis. Skeletal Radiol 1997;26(4):230–238

Kaiser S, Rosenborg M. Early detection of subperiosteal abscesses by ultrasonography. A means for further successful treatment in pediatric osteomyelitis. Pediatr Radiol 1994 24(5):336–339

Kandarpa A. Handbook of Interventional Radiologic Procedures. Boston, Ma: Little, Brown & Co.; 1996

Karpos PA, Spindler KP, Pierce MA, Shull HJJ Jr. Osteomyelitis of the pubic symphysis in athletes: a case report and literature review. Med Sci Sports Exerc 1995;27(4):473–479

Kauffmann GW. Röntgenfibel – Praktische Anleitung für Eingriffe in der Röntgendiagnostik. Heidelberg: Springer; 2001

Köchli VD, Marincek B. Wie funktioniert MRT? Berlin: Springer; 1998

Laubenberger T, Laubenberger J. Technik der medizinischen Radiologie. Cologne: Deutscher Ärzteverlag; 1999

Link TM, Berning W, Scherf S, et al. CT of metal implants: reduction of artifacts using an extended CT scale technique. J Comput Assist Tomogr 2000;24(1):165–172

Linsenmaier U, Rieger J, Pfeifer KJ. Konventionelle Strahl-endiagnostik. In: Scriba PC, Pforte A, eds. Taschenbuch der medizinisch-klinischen Diagnostik. Berlin: Springer; 2000:290–303

Mason MD, Zlatkin MB, Esterhai JL, Dalinka MK, Velchik MG, Kressel HY. Chronic complicated osteomyelitis of the lower extremity: evaluation with MR imaging. Radiology 1989;173(2):355–359

Morrison WB, Schweitzer ME, Bock GW, et al. Diagnosis of osteomyelitis: utility of fat-suppressed contrast-enhanced MR imaging. Radiology 1993;189(1):251–257

Murphey MD, Wetzel LH, Bramble JM, Levine E, Simpson KM, Lindsley HB. Sacroiliitis: MR imaging findings. Radiology 1991;180(1):239–244

Purcell EM, Tarrey HC, Pound RV. Resonance absorption by nuclear magnetic moments in a solid. Phys Rev 1946;69:37

Quinn SF, Murray W, Clark RA, Cochran C. MR imaging of chronic osteomyelitis. J Comput Assist Tomogr 1988;12(1):113–117

Rand T, Schweitzer M, Rafii M, Nguyen K, Garcia M, Resnick D. Condensing osteitis of the clavicle: MRI. J Comput Assist Tomogr 1998;22(4):621–624

Reeder MM. Gamnuts in Bone, Joint and Spine Radiology. New York: Springer; 1993

Reiser M, Peters PE. Radiologische Differentialdiagnose der Skeletterkrankungen. Stuttgart: Thieme; 1995

Reiser MF, Takahashi M, Modic M, Bruening R. Multislice CT. Berlin: Springer; 2001

Resnick D. Diagnosis of Bone and Joint Disorders. Philadelphia: Saunders; 2002

Resnick D, Petterson H. Skeletal Radiology. London: Merit Communications; 1992

Sandrasegaran K, Saifuddin A, Coral A, Butt WP. Magnetic resonance imaging of septic sacroiliitis. Skeletal Radiol 1994;23(4):289–292

Sharif HS. Role of MR imaging in the management of spinal infections. AJR Am J Roentgenol 1992;158(6):1333–1345

Shiv VK, Jain AK, Taneja K, Bhargava SK. Sonography of hip joint in infective arthritis. Can Assoc Radiol J 1990;41(2):76–78

Soren A. Arthritis and Related Affections. Clinic, Pathology and Treatment. Berlin: Springer; 1993

Stäbler A, Baur A, Krüger A, Weiss M, Helmberger T, Reiser M. Differential diagnosis of erosive osteochondrosis and bacterial spondylitis: magnetic resonance tomography (MRT). [Article in German] Rofo 1998;168(5):421–428

Stäbler A, Reiser MF. Imaging of spinal infection. Radiol Clin North Am 2001;39(1):115–135

Sundaram M, McDonald D, Engel E, Rotman M, Siegfried EC. Chronic recurrent multifocal osteomyelitis: an evolving clinical and radiological spectrum. Skeletal Radiol 1996;25(4):333–336

Thijn CJP, Steensma JT. Tuberculosis of the Skeleton with Accent on Radiology. Berlin: Springer; 1989

Tumeh SS, Aliabadi P, Weissman BN, McNeil BJ. Disease activity in osteomyelitis: role of radiography. Radiology 1987;165(3):781–784

Tumeh SS, Tohmeh AG. Nuclear medicine techniques in septic arthritis and osteomyelitis. Rheum Dis Clin North Am 1991;17(3):559–583

Unger EC, Moldofsky P, Gatenby R, Hartz W, Broder G. Diagnosis of osteomyelitis by MR imaging. AJR Am J Roentgenol 1988;150(3):605–610

Vahlensieck M, Reiser M. Bone marrow edema in MRT. [Article in German] Radiologe. 1992;10:509–515

Vahlensieck M, Reiser M. MRT des Bewegungsapparats. Stuttgart: Thieme; 2002

Yoshioka H, Nakano T, Kandatsu S, Koga M, Itai Y, Tsujii H. MR imaging of radiation osteitis in the sacroiliac joints. Magn Reson Imaging 2000;18(2):125–128

Zynamon A, Jung T, Hodler J, Bischof T, von Schulthess GK. The magnetic resonance procedure in the diagnosis of osteomyelitis. Its value and comparison with skeletal scintigraphy. [Article in German] Rofo 1991;155(6):513–518

Nuclear Medicine Imaging of Bone Inflammations

S. Adams, G. Hoer

Introduction

In contrast to morphologically based imaging modalities, the agents used in nuclear medicine imaging (**radiopharmaceuticals**) are formulated in such a way that they are incorporated into metabolic processes (**indicator method**) without altering them. Once they have been incorporated into the body, radiopharmaceuticals are subject to the same transport, metabolic, and excretory processes as other substances. The radioactive isotopes emit radiation, which enables them to be tracked both qualitatively and quantitatively within the body. In many cases nuclear medicine imaging can detect pathology before any radiographic abnormalities are seen.

Inflammations in bone cause a change in regional blood flow. Inflammatory hyperemia is associated with an increase in vascular permeability due to gap formation in the endothelium. Additionally, regional edema may develop due to the exudation of plasma proteins. Changes in the basement membrane allow inflammatory cells (e.g., granulocytes, monocytes) to actively migrate into the interstitium. Because the cortex in osteomyelitis does not provide an outlet for increased pressure within the bone, pus is extruded into the medullary spaces of the cortex at an early stage, causing the cortex to become perforated beneath the periosteum. Compression of the nutrient vessels leads to early intraosseous necrosis. Penetration of the cortex causes periosteal elevation with subperiosteal abscess formation. Only then can the classic signs of inflammation—pain, heat, redness, swelling, and loss of function—be identified.

The goal of imaging in bone inflammations is to detect the inflammation early and prevent the development of chronic disease with associated complications. Inflammatory scintigraphic methods can demonstrate the pathophysiologic processes, often providing a specific diagnosis of the inflammatory process (Dams et al. 2000, Forstorm et al. 2000, Ruscowski et al. 2000, Van der Laken et al. 2000, Gallowitsch et al. 2002, McCarthy et al. 2002; **Tables 3.2 and 3.3**). Depending on the radiotracers used, there is a trend toward the use of molecular PET (positron emission tomography) for imaging the "molecular messengers" of tumor proliferation (with ^{18}F-thymidine), demonstrating molecular genetic processes, and differentiating them from inflammatory reactions (Shields et al. 1998; **Table 3.4**). Infectious processes meet their energy requirements through aerobic or anaerobic glycolysis. Activated leukocytes and macrophages may show an increase in both oxygen and glucose utilization.

NOTE

Imaging with 18F-FDG (fluorodeoxyglucose = glucose analogue) and PET makes it possible to perform metabolic studies (*glucose scan*) with a previously unattainable information yield on bone tumors (local extension, distant metastases), periprosthetic inflammations (occult periprosthetic inflammatory foci), and the viability of posttraumatic bone grafts.

Table 3.3 Pathophysiologic principles of inflammatory scintigraphy in bone

Radiopharmaceutical (experimental)	Pathophysiologic basis
^{99m}Tc-ciprofloxacin	Antibiotic
^{18}F-leucocytes	Diapedesis, chemotaxis
^{131}I-interleukin-8	Mediator
^{99m}Tc-PEG liposomes	
^{99m}Tc-neutrophile elastase inhibitors	Inhibitor
^{18}F-cox1/cox2 inhibitors	Inhibitor

Table 3.2 Pathophysiologic principles of inflammatory scintigraphy in bone

Radiopharmaceutical (clinically established and applied)	Pathophysiologic basis
Bone scintigraphy	Perfusion, mineralization
Radiolabeled (^{111}In-oxine, ^{99m}Tc-HMPAO)	Diapedesis, chemotaxis
Leukocyte scans	
Radiolabeled (^{111}In-oxin, ^{99m}Tc, ^{123}I) immunoglobulins	Exudation, chemotaxis = antibodies against a granulocyte antigen
^{67}Gallium citrate	Exudation, transferrin receptor binding
^{99m}Tc-nano-HSA (particle size < 1 µm) (= human serum albumin)	Diapedesis
^{18}F-FDG (fluorodeoxyglucose)	Perfusion, increased tissue permeability = intracellular uptake in activated leukocytes via glucose transporters

Table 3.4 PET imaging in trauma surgery and orthopedics

Radio-nuclide	Indication	Application
^{18}F-FDG	Malignant bone tumors or metastases	Differential diagnosis
	Inflammatory or septic processes	Septic prosthetic loosening
	Bone implants	Viability assessment
Research		
^{18}F-fluoride	Bone metastases	
^{18}FDG with ^{18}F-fluoride	Search for metastases and malignant tumors	Differentiating bone from soft-tissue metastases
^{124}I-FIAU	Gene or genomic function	For example, p53-mediated gene induction

Leukocyte Scintigraphy

Principle

Localization of inflammatory processes using autologous white blood cells radiolabeled with ^{99m}Tc-HMPAO or ^{111}In-oxine.

Technique

Patients do not require special preparations before scanning with ^{111}In-oxine-labeled leukocytes. When ^{99m}Tc-HMPAO-labeled autologous leukocytes are used, children should be fasted for up to 4 hours before the examination to reduce hepatobiliary excretion and intestinal transit. The patient should be fully informed about the principle and conduct of the examination before injecting the radiopharmaceutical. Clinical information about previous tests, current laboratory values (inflammatory markers), and previous surgery and other trauma is important for interpreting the scintigraphies. Indwelling catheters, stomas (e.g., ileal conduit, colostomy), tracheostomies, and skin or soft-tissue infections or injuries must be identified or excluded to avoid false-positive findings. For inflammatory imaging, leukocytes are isolated from venous blood and labeled with the appropriate radiopharmaceutical. The autologous leukocytes are then reinjected in the dose prescribed by DGN guidelines.

The intestinal excretion of HMPAO cleavage products requires early imaging of the abdomen or pelvis within 3 hours. Regional scans of the limbs can be acquired at 4–8 hours. Images with ^{111}In-labeled leukocytes are acquired at 1–4 and 16–30 hours. The scan duration is much longer than with ^{99m}Tc-labeled leukocytes due to the lower tracer activity. SPECT provide nonsuperimposed, 3D high-contrast images of individual skeletal regions (e.g., pelvis, spine). High-resolution multi-head gamma camera systems (high-resolution SPECT) and the coincidence SPECT acquisition of positron emitters broaden the indications for imaging trauma-surgery and orthopedic cases at PET centers and satellite PET units (Gericke et al. 1998, Santiago et al. 1999, Kälicke et al. 2000).

Application

^{111}In-labeled leukocytes provide stable labeling with no detectable tracer elution from the white blood cells. ^{111}Indium has a much longer physical half-life (67.5 hours) than ^{99}technetium (6 hours), leading to a higher level of patient radiation exposure. ^{111}Indium is a cyclotron product (unlike ^{99m}technetium, which is a generator product) and is not always available. ^{111}Indium compounds are also more costly to produce (**Table 3.6**).

Table 3.6 Indications for scanning with radiolabeled autologous leukocytes

^{111}In-oxine-labeled leukocytes	^{99m}Tc-labeled leukocytes
Chronic osteomyelitis	Musculoskeletal infections
Urinary tract infections (no renal uptake)	Septic arthritis, osteomyelitis
Chronic inflammatory bowel diseases	Localization of acute inflammatory foci in patients with fever (with or without local symptoms)
	Inflammatory or ischemic bowel diseases

Interpretation

Intravascular activity is high immediately after the injection. Late static scans show physiologic uptake in the liver, spleen, bone marrow, and large blood vessels (with decreasing intensity). The biodistribution corresponds roughly to that of the reticuloendothelial system (RES). Unlike ^{99m}Tc-labeled leukocytes, ^{111}indium-oxine-labeled leukocytes do not show activity in the kidneys, bowel, or bladder.

False-positive findings are caused by granulation tissue, which is typically located at skin level in patients with intestinal or urinary stomas. The use of indwelling peripheral cannulas or central catheters for reinjecting the labeled leukocytes may lead to false-positive soft-tissue or central vascular uptake. Other areas of increased leukocyte uptake, some reactive, are found in recent myocardial infarctions, necrotic tumors, and inflammatory reactions to foreign bodies or prosthetic material.

Inflammatory bone marrow diseases at a central location (e.g., in the spine) are difficult to detect due to high tracer uptake in the liver, spleen, and bone marrow. Leukocyte scintigraphy can detect active inflammatory bone processes as hot spots with a sensitivity of 80%–92%, its sensitivity increasing from the center of the body toward the periphery (Streule et al. 1988, Becker 1994). Note that bone marrow expansion may hinder the detection of a peripheral inflammatory focus.

False-negative findings are caused by chronic inflammatory foci (e.g., chronic osteomyelitis), which may represent lymphocyte-mediated infections and are sometimes encapsulated.

over, it is extremely likely that the injected antibodies will undergo complexing by the reticuloendothelial system, rendering them useless for the diagnosis of inflammatory processes. Thus, imaging should be preceded by a HAMA test as well as a detailed patient history (protein allergy, previous nuclear medicine imaging). The history should include information about trauma or fractures, inflammatory diseases, and any history of drain or catheter insertion after surgery. [99mTc]-labeled Fab fragments should not cause induction of HAMA (Becker et al. 1996). Ensure that the patient is fully informed about the principle and conduct of scintigraphy before injecting the radiopharmaceutical (allergy risk!).

Both complete antibodies and Fab fragments are available for granulocyte scintigraphy (DGN guidelines, Hansen et al. 1993, Fratz et al 1998, Gratz et al. 1998; **Table 3.7**).

Inflammatory Imaging with [99mTc]-Labeled Antibodies

Principle

When administered intravenously, [99mTc]-labeled antibodies bind to granulocytes in the blood stream and bone marrow (including their precursors such as myelocytes and promyelocytes). Thus, granulocyte scintigraphy with radiolabeled antibodies can be used not only for inflammatory imaging but also for bone-marrow scintigraphy (e.g., for the detection of metastases).

Application

Technique

When complete antibodies are used for granulocyte scintigraphy, immunoscintigraphy can lead to the induction of human antimouse antibodies (HAMA), which may evoke allergic reactions in repeated examinations. More-

Interpretation

With a normal scintigraphic distribution of MABs, scans demonstrate the hematopoietic bone marrow in the pelvis, spinal column, ribs, sternum, skull, and proximal diaphyses of the long tubular bones. Children show an

Table 3.7 Inflammatory imaging with [99mTc]-labeled antigranulocyte antibodies

	Complete antibodies	Fab fragment
Administered activity	370–555 MBq	740–925 MBq
Antigen	NCA-95 antigen	NCA-90 antigen
Cell binding	50%	10%
Biodistribution	Bone marrow, spleen, liver, kidney, and bladder (due to excretion)	Bone marrow, liver, spleen, intense uptake in the kidneys, nonspecific intestinal activity (4–6 h p.i.)
Scans	Whole-body scans at 2–4 or 16–24 h	Whole-body scans at least 1 h p.i. Late scans at 6–8 h
	SPECT of the trunk at 16–20 h p.i. (lower background activity)	SPECT of the trunk at 16–20 h p.i. (lower background activity)

age-related distribution of hematopoiesis with physiologic extension into the distal portions of the humerus and femur. Both children and adults show an accumulation of MABs in the liver and spleen. The renal uptake of Fab fragments is much higher than that of complete antibodies due to accumulation in the renal tubules. Inflammatory foci in central skeletal regions may be difficult to interpret (false-negative findings) due to intense physiologic uptake in the hematopoietic system. Administration of antibiotics may also reduce the diagnostic accuracy of immunoscintigraphy (antibiotics should be discontinued 3 days before scanning if clinically feasible). As with autologous leucocytes, pay particular attention to possible cold lesions (photopenic defects) in the spinal column.

Inflammatory processes are generally dynamic in that they show increasing radiopharmaceutical uptake over time (compare the intensity in the early phase with delayed scans). Bone marrow islands, which may occur in long tubular bones following replacement arthroplasty, show a constant uptake pattern that distinguishes them from peripheral bone inflammations. Immunoscintigraphy can detect peripheral inflammatory bone diseases with a sensitivity between 77% and 86% (Gratz et al. 1998, Devillers et al. 2000, Kaim et al. 2000).

NOTE

Scintigraphy with MABs appears to be more accurate than MRI in differentiating postoperative scars from reactive inflammatory bone processes. By comparison, MRI can detect low-grade infections with higher sensitivity than bone scans and immunoscintigraphy combined (Kaim et al. 2000).

Remove indwelling cannulas no earlier than 30 minutes after the antibody injection to allow for the immediate treatment of any allergic reactions.

Before immunoscintigraphy is repeated, blood should be drawn to check for a possible elevated HAMA titer.

TIPS AND TRICKS

The radiopharmaceutical must undergo quality control before the monoclonal antibody is injected. If binding is inadequate, free 99mtechnicium will significantly degrade image quality due to nonspecific uptake in organs (e.g., thyroid gland, stomach) and hepatobiliary and renal excretion (artifacts!).

The anatomical correlation of findings can be improved by performing skeletal scintigraphy and by comparison with coregistered radiographs (SPECT can be used for better localization if necessary). In the future, multimodal fusion images (which are already obtained routinely in oncology) will probably be used more frequently in skeletal examinations and may include combined PET/CT imaging.

67Galium Citrate Scintigraphy

Principle

The radiopharmaceutical 67galium citrate is an iron analogue that accumulates in inflammatory tissue by three pathophysiologic mechanisms:

- Binding to transferrin receptors (90%)
- Binding to lactoferrin (macrophages phagocytize this complex in inflammatory tissue)
- Direct radiotracer uptake by microorganisms (binding to bacterial proteins)

Technique

DGN guidelines recommend 100–220 MBq of administered activity in adults. As with other radiopharmaceuticals, the dose in children is adjusted for body weight and surface area and ranges from 1.5 to 2.6 MBq (maximum activity: 9–19 MBq; DGN guidelines).

Approximately 20% of the administered activity is eliminated by renal excretion within the first 24 hours and then chiefly by hepatobiliary excretion to the bowel. This could lead to errors of interpretation, especially in evaluating retroperitoneal lymph nodes. Administration of a laxative before scanning is recommended. Physiologic excretion into the bowel is unlikely to occur during the first 4–6 hours after injection. Whole-body or partial-body scintigraphies (plus SPECT if necessary) are acquired 24–72 hours after administration of the radiopharmaceutical. Delayed scans > 96 hours p.i. may be advisable owing to the long half-life of 78 hours.

NOTE

The long physiologic half-life and kinetics of the radiopharmaceutical lead to increased radiation exposure and thus require rigorous patient selection criteria, especially in children!

Pregnancy and lactation are relative contraindications according to DGN guidelines and require special consideration.

The scanning speed is 6–10 cm/min, which may result in scan times of at least 30 minutes for whole-body scintigraphy. To avoid motion artifacts, inform the patient of the duration of the examination in advance and position him or her comfortably on the examination table. 67Galium citrate is useful for the localization of inflammatory diseases as well as tumor detection. For this reason, the history should not only include information on inflammations (clinical presentation, laboratory findings, treatment, tests) but should also cover oncologic aspects (histology, surgeries, chemotherapy, radiotherapy, etc.). Given its similarity to iron, blood transfusion or hemolysis may adversely affect the distribution of the radiopharmaceutical.

Application

Gallium scintigraphy is used for the localization of inflammatory diseases, especially in the trunk and spinal column. It is also used to search for foci of chronic osteomyelitis, for example, when more informative tests (PET) are not available. Gallium scanning is also useful for the diagnosis and follow-up of inflammatory lung diseases (e.g., tuberculosis, sarcoidosis), especially in immunocompromised patients (e.g., AIDS [acquired immunodeficiency syndrome]) and patients with FUO.

Interpretation

A normal gallium scan demonstrates uptake in the liver, spleen, bones, and bone marrow. Physiologic uptake is additionally found in the bowel, nasopharynx, lacrimal and salivary glands, and in the female breast. Glandular tissue shows symmetrical uptake in the corresponding regions. Asymmetrical uptake, especially in inflammatory foci, may lead to false-positive findings.

Positive findings have been described in malignant melanoma, lung cancer, and in Hodgkin and non-Hodgkin lymphomas. A normal gallium scan shows little pulmonary uptake compared with other radionuclides, with the result that interstitial and opportunistic lung diseases, as in immunocompromised patients, can be readily detected (Harwood et al. 1987, Moser et al. 1990, Karkavitsas et al. 1997, Cortes-Blanco et al. 1999). Panpulmonary contrast activity in the lungs is the scintigraphic correlate of AIDS pneumonia. Pulmonary imaging has good sensitivity, but the low specificity is a disadvantage (Karkavitsas et al. 1997). Other causes of diffusely increased pulmonary uptake include idiopathic pulmonary fibrosis, pneumoconiosis, asbestosis, and drug toxicity (interstitial pneumonitis after chemotherapy). Iron preparations, multiple blood transfusions, or hemolysis may saturate the transferrin receptors with associated decreased uptake in the liver, spleen, bones, and bone marrow (Palestro 1994). A combination of three-phase bone scintigraphy, leucocyte scintigraphy, and gallium scintigraphy may be helpful in distinguishing between acute and chronic osteomyelitis (Etchebehere et al. 1998). A review of the literature shows that inflammatory changes in bones and joints can be detected with a sensitivity of 70%–98% (Abramovici and Robinstein 1988, Sordahl et al. 1993, Love et al. 2000, Sapienza et al. 2000). SPECT is superior to planar gallium scintigraphy, especially in the spinal column (Vorne et al. 1989).

The selection of radiopharmaceuticals for inflammatory imaging is influenced by clinical findings, the physiologic distribution of the agents, their availability, and the radiation exposure associated with their use (Kühnel et al. 2000; **Table 3.8**). On the basis of the whole-body format and rapid availability of technetium-labeled agents for the localization of inflammatory bone processes, [67]gallium citrate is not widely used in Germany but is commonly used in the U.S.

> **NOTE**
>
> Scintigraphy with the cyclotron product [67]gallium citrate involves a relatively high radiation exposure, and radiogallium is not always available.
>
> To avoid false-positive findings (especially in the abdomen), the patient should empty the bowel before the start of the examination.
>
> The patient should be informed of the long acquisition times and the need for imaging on multiple days.
>
> The result of the examination will be available no earlier than 48 hours p.i.
>
> Do not institute antibiotic therapy prior to scanning.

Table 3.8 Physiologic distribution and radiation exposure from radiopharmaceuticals commonly used for inflammatory imaging

Radiopharmaceutical	Radiation exposure (half-life, equivalent dose)	Physiologic distribution	Availability
[99m]Tc-diphosphonate	Physical half-life = 6 h; 4.4 mSv at 555 MBq	Vessels and soft tissues (early phase), bones (late phase)	Always available; tracer is generator product
[67]Gallium citrate	Physical half-life = 78 h; 27 mSv at 220 MBq	Liver, spleen, kidney, bowel, bones, bone marrow, lacrimal and salivary glands, nasopharynx	Not immediately available; tracer is cyclotron product
[99m]Tc-labeled antigranulocyte antibodies	Physical half-life = 6 h; 3.9 mSv at 370 MBq	Liver, spleen, bone marrow, lung; some hepatobiliary excretion to the bowel	Always available; tracer is generator product
[111]In-labeled leukocytes	Physical half-life = 67.5 h; 15 mSv at 25 MBq	Liver, spleen, lung	Time-consuming preparation, not immediately available; tracer is cyclotron product

Inflammatory Imaging with 99mTc-Labeled Nanocolloids

Principle

Nanometer-sized 99mtechnetium-labeled colloidal particles derived from human serum albumin leave the intravascular space through intercellular leaks in the endothelium and basement membrane (= **diapedesis**) at the site of the inflammation. Local radiopharmaceutical uptake depends on the activity of the inflammatory focus (De Schrijver et al. 1987). Besides diapedesis, IV injection is followed by an active metabolic uptake of the protein particles by phagocytic cells of the reticuloendothelial system in the bone marrow, liver, and spleen.

Technique

No patient preparation is required. The referring physician should provide the nuclear-medicine physician with all information noted in the previous sections. The adult dose is approximately 500 MBq of the 99mTc-labeled agent administered by IV injection. The activity dose in children is based on the table of the Pediatric Task Group of the EANM (European Association of Nuclear Medicine). Anterior and posterior whole-body images are acquired 1 hour after injection and may be supplemented if necessary by regional scans or SPECT in coronal, axial, and sagittal planes.

Application

The most common indication for inflammatory imaging with 99mTc-labeled nanocolloids is the search for inflammatory foci (especially in the knee and hip joints) and the investigation of FUO.

Interpretation

Scintigraphy normally shows intense radiotracer uptake in the RES of the liver, spleen, and bone marrow.

Nanocolloid scintigraphy detects bone inflammation with a reported sensitivity of approximately 90% (specificity = 85%) (DGN guidelines, Streule et al. 1988, Van Dalen et al. 1988, Al Attia et al. 2001). Direct comparison of leukocyte scans with the 99mTc-labeled tracer shows that both methods yield identical results, the nanocolloid scan providing a slightly better depiction of chronic inflammatory foci. Leukocyte scanning appears to be better than scanning with human serum albumin particles for characterizing the intensity of an inflammatory focus by semiquantitative analysis (region-of-interest technique = ROI technique) (Streule et al. 1988, Papos et al. 1998).

Hyperemia, which is common in inflammatory reactions, leads to increased radiopharmaceutical uptake in the affected region during the perfusion and blood-pool phases of three-phase bone scintigraphy. This uptake is nonspecific, however, and may also result from increased blood flow due to malignant tumors and other causes. According to studies by Höflin et al., colloid scintigraphy shows increased uptake only when hyperemia is caused by an inflammatory process—not when increased blood flow is due to other causes (Höflin 1988). This phenomenon may be advantageous in inflammatory imaging with nanocolloids. Other advantages of 99mTc-nanocolloid scintigraphy compared with 111In-leukocyte scintigraphy are the simple technique, availability, low radiation exposure, and the prompt reporting of results.

The sensitivity of nanocolloid scans for detecting foci of bone inflammation decreases from the periphery toward the center of the body due to intense hyperphagocytosis of the radiopharmaceutical in the reticuloendothelial system.

> **NOTE**
>
> 99mTc-nanocolloid scintigraphy is a simple screening method for inflammatory foci. The IV cannula should be left indwelling for at least 30 minutes after the injection, and the patient should be observed for possible protein allergies.
>
> Bone scans and current radiographs should be available for anatomical localization.
>
> The sensitivity of 99mTc-nanocolloid scintigraphy in the detection of bony inflammatory foci decreases from the periphery toward the center (due to intense uptake in the RES).

Inflammatory Imaging with 18F-FDG Positron Emission Tomography

Principle

Activated leukocytes (macrophages, neutrophilic granulocytes) are strongly dependent on anaerobic glycolysis in inflammatory processes. This increased glucose metabolism of inflammatory cells can be detected by positron-emission tomography (PET) with 18fluorine-labeled deoxyglucose (18F-FDG).

Technique

The patient should be fasted for at least 4–6 hours before the 18F-FDG PET examination but is allowed unsweetened beverages such as mineral water. Determine the current blood glucose level and body weight before administering the FDG. The blood glucose level should not exceed 120 mg%, because hyperglycemia can reduce FDG uptake in tumors and other tissues. In patients with a poorly regulated blood sugar level, postpone FDG PET until it can be performed under stable conditions (normoglycemia) with the patient on standard medication. Again, it is necessary to take a detailed history that covers inflammatory diseases, trauma, previous operations or biopsies, and previous radiotherapy or chemotherapy.

Whole-body scans are acquired 40–60 minutes after the injection of approximately 5 MBq/kg body weight ^{18}F-FDG (total activity approximately 250–500 MBq). The activity administered in children should conform to the table of the Pediatric Task Group of the EANM. Dynamic scans can be acquired to quantify the glucose metabolism of inflammatory or neoplastic processes (e.g., using the Patlak analysis or simple standard uptake values [SUVs]; Dimitrakopoulou-Strauss et al. 2002). Diazepam should be used in anxious patients to suppress neuroadrenergic stimulation, which results from the activation of paravertebral ganglia, for example, and causes diffuse tracer uptake in the neck muscles (*lobster sign*).

Because of the potential for tracer uptake in muscles, the patient is not allowed to move or speak (laryngeal and lingual muscles!) before or after the injection and should be positioned comfortably during the examination. Reduce bladder activity (superimposed artifacts) by having the patient void before scanning.

Patient preparations for ^{18}F-FDG PET:
- Fasted for 4–6 hours
- Current blood glucose level (<120 mg%)
- History (inflammatory diseases, operations, radiation, or chemotherapy?)
- Avoid muscular artifacts by positioning the patient comfortably and telling him/her not to move and speak as little as possible before and after the injection
- Void before the examination

Application

The most frequent indications for FDG PET are oncologic investigations as described by the Third Consensus Conference in 2000 (Reske and Kotzerke 2000). Other indications (not yet confirmed in larger studies) may be the investigation of FUO and evaluation for chronic osteomyelitis in the peripheral skeleton or spinal column. ^{18}F-FDG PET imaging already has an adjunctive role in assessing the viability of bone grafts (Piert et al. 1999).

Interpretation

Following IV administration, the glucose analogue ^{18}F-FDG enters the cells via glucose transporters and is incorporated into the glucose metabolic pathway. In the first step, ^{18}F-FDG is phosphorylated to ^{18}F-FDG-6-phosphate by the enzyme hexokinase. Because of this chemical change (desoxy substitution), ^{18}F-FDG-6-phosphate is not metabolized further within the cell and is retained there (*metabolic trapping*). The rate of accumulation of the metabolic tracer in the tissue reflects both intracellular

transport and the hexokinase activity of the corresponding cells. Uptake of the glucose analogue is nonspecific because glucose metabolism is increased not just in tumor cells but also in inflammatory processes (activated leukocytes).

Physiologically increased uptake is found in the brain, myocardium, liver, bowel, and also in the kidneys and bladder due to urinary excretion. Uptake also occurs in bone marrow and muscles, depending on their degree of activation (Yao et al. 1995). The salivary glands, throat, nose, pharynx, and eye muscles also show moderate ^{18}F-FDG utilization. Thus, it may be difficult to detect tumors located in tissues that show intense physiologic tracer uptake (low lesion-to-background ratio!). Interpretation errors may also result from uptake in benign lesions (e.g., thyroid adenomas) and in postoperative changes (e.g., seroma) (Kubota et al. 1992, Yamada et al. 1995). Scan acquisitions at different times may aid in differentiating malignant from benign (e.g., inflammatory) lesions (Gupta et al. 1998, Zhuang et al. 2001b).

The possible clinical applications of FDG PET in inflammatory imaging are determined by the tracer distribution patterns described above. One advantage of FDG over radiopharmaceuticals previously used for inflammatory imaging is its superior spatial resolution. In one comparative study, FDG PET could positively distinguish between osteomyelitis and inflammatory reactions in the surrounding soft tissues. Furthermore, FDG PET is better for detecting chronic osteomyelitic foci in the truncal skeleton (Zhuang et al. 2001b; **Table 3.9**) than immunoscintigraphy with antigranulocyte antibodies, which frequently detects nonspecific cold lesions (intense antibody uptake in the liver, spleen, and bone marrow = low lesion-to-background ratio) (Guhlmann et al. 1998a).

> **NOTE**
>
> ^{18}F-FDG PET is increasingly used to explore possible inflammatory causes of prosthetic loosening after knee and hip replacements (Zhuang et al. 2001b; **Table 3.9**).

Metal artifacts apparently do not hamper the interpretation of ^{18}F-FDG PET findings, as they do in MRT and CT for example (Guhlmann et al. 1998b, Kälicke et al. 2000). Another advantage is the ability to quantify different de-

Table 3.9 Detection of inflammatory prosthetic loosening by ^{18}F-FDG PET

	Sensitivity (%)	Specificity (%)	Accuracy (%)
Overall	90.5	81.1	–
Knee	90.9	72.0	77.8
Hip	90.0	89.3	89.5

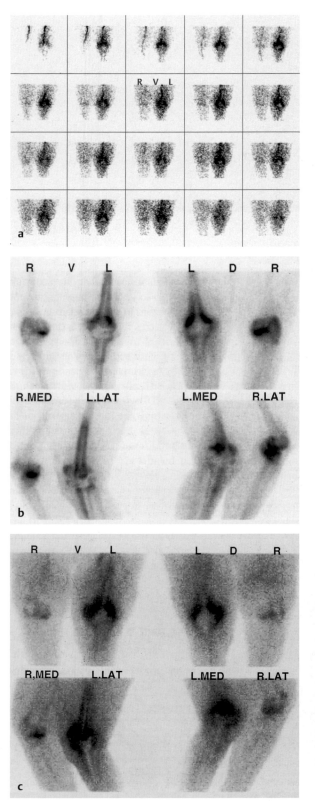

Fig. 3.23a–c See text

Case 3:

A 67-year-old woman presented with signs of inflammation in the left knee joint following a total knee replacement. Septic prosthetic loosening was suspected.

Three-phase sequential scintigraphy of the knee joints with ⁹⁹ᵐTc-diphosphonate showed definite hyperperfusion in the left knee joint (**Fig. 3.23a**). Increased hyperemia was noted about the femoral condyles in the soft-tissue phase (**Fig. 3.23b**). The mineralization phase showed intense bone hypermetabolism in the femoral condyles bordering the femoral component on the left side (**Fig. 3.23c**). Bone metabolism showed little if any increase along the tibial component (with kind permission of Prof. Dr. V. Nicolas, Department of Radiology and Nuclear Medicine, Bergmannsheil University Hospital, Ruhr University Bochum, Germany).

Diagnosis: Florid inflammation of the left knee joint (predominantly on the femoral side) by *S. aureus* with no evidence of prosthetic loosening.

Case 4:

A 55-year-old man presented with FUO up to 38.5° after undergoing chemotherapy for an embryonic testicular carcinoma. Morphologic imaging showed no evidence of an infectious focus.

Whole-body scintigraphy with ⁶⁷gallium citrate at 72 hours p.i. showed focal tracer uptake projected over the right side of the mandible (paramedian) and a bilateral increase in pulmonary uptake (**Fig. 3.24**).

Diagnosis: Acute dental root infection (culture: *S. aureus*) accompanied by a toxic reaction in the lungs to bleomycin administration.

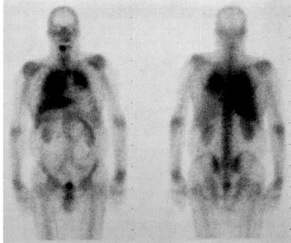

Fig. 3.24 See text

Case 5:

A 45-year-old woman presented with known rheumatoid arthritis. She had an approximately 3-week history of unexplained febrile episodes to 39.5° and pain in the lower extremities. She underwent a total left hip replacement in October, 2001. She was not taking antibiotics at the time immunoscintigraphy was performed.

Antigranulocyte scintigraphy with a [99m]-labeled antibody was performed. Whole-body scintigraphy (**Fig. 3.25a**) and a regional scan (**Fig. 3.25b**) of the lower leg at 4 hours p.i. (image washout) showed patchy antibody uptake projected over the distal portions of both lower legs consistent with acute inflammatory foci (arrows).

Diagnosis: Acute bilateral tibial osteomyelitis (biopsy: *S. aureus*).

Case 6:

A 35-year-old man presented with a suspected fracture of the right scaphoid bone after an athletic injury. The right side of the wrist was tender to pressure. Conventional radiographs showed no abnormalities.

Two-phase scintigraphy showed markedly increased metabolic activity in the right scaphoid bone (**Fig. 3.26a**) with moderately increased perifocal hyperemia (**Fig. 3.26b**). Other whole-body scintigraphic findings were normal for age (**Fig. 3.26c**).

> **NOTE**
>
> Fractures can be diagnosed on the basis of increased bone metabolism within 2–10 days in patients less than 60 years of age. Scintigraphy can detect peripheral fractures (e.g., of the limbs) earlier than central fractures (e.g., of the spine).

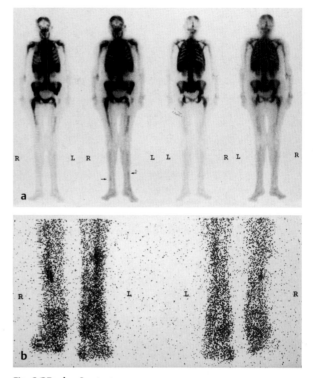

Fig. 3.25a, b   See text

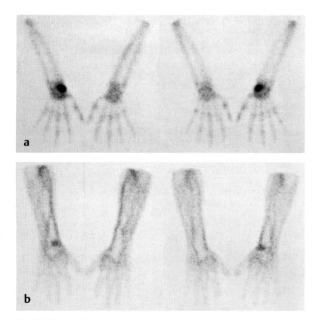

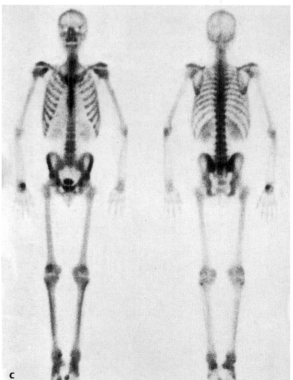

Fig. 3.26a–c   See text

Bibliography

Abramovici J, Rubinstein M. Tc-99m-Nanocolloids: An alternative approach to diagnosis of inflammatory lesions of bones and joints. Eur J Nucl Med 1988;14:244

Al Attia HM, Al Haider ZY, Khadim RA, El Higrisy M, Adams BK. The role of scintigraphy with technetium-99m nanocolloid in patients with peripheral joint pain. Clin Rheumatol 2001;20(4):255–258

Becker W. Entzündungen. In: Büll U, Schicha H, Biersack H-J, Knapp W, Reiners C, Schober O, eds. Nuklearmedizin. Stuttgart: Thieme; 1994:404–418

Becker W. The contribution of nuclear medicine to the patient with infection. Eur J Nucl Med 1995;22(10):1195–1211

Becker W, Palestro CJ, Winship J, et al. Rapid imaging of infections with a monoclonal antibody fragment (LeukoScan). Clin Orthop Relat Res 1996;329(329):263–272

Collier BD. Orthopaedic applications of single photon emission computed tomographic bone scanning. In: Fogelman I, ed. Bone Scanning in Clinical Practice. Berlin: Springer; 1987:175–187

Cortés Blanco A, Sáez Lavilla C, Martínez Lázaro R, Arazo Garcés P, Borraz López MV, Ascaso Bandrés A. Human immunodeficiency virus (HIV) infection. The effectiveness of different diagnostic sequences in suspected pulmonary infection. [Article in Spanish] Med Interna 1999;16(1):15–20

Dams ETM, Oyen WJG, Boerman OC, et al. 99mTc-PEG liposomes for the scintigraphic detection of infection and inflammation: clinical evaluation. J Nucl Med 2000;41(4):622–630

De Schrijver M, Streule K, Senekowitsch R, Fridrich R. Scintigraphy of inflammation with nanometer-sized colloidal tracers. Nucl Med Commun 1987;8(11):895–908

Devillers A, Garin E, Polard JL, et al. Comparison of Tc-99m-labelled antileukocyte fragment Fab' and Tc-99m-HMPAO leukocyte scintigraphy in the diagnosis of bone and joint infections: a prospective study. Nucl Med Commun 2000;21(8):747–753

DGN-Leitlinien. www.nuklearmedizin.de

Dimitrakopoulou-Strauss A, Strauss LG, Heichel T, et al. The role of quantitative (18)F-FDG PET studies for the differentiation of malignant and benign bone lesions. J Nucl Med 2002;43:510–518

Etchebehere EC, Etchebehere M, Gamba R, Belangero W, Camargo EE. Orthopedic pathology of the lower extremities: scintigraphic evaluation in the thigh, knee, and leg. Semin Nucl Med 1998;28(1):41–61

Fogelman I, Maisey MN, Clarke EM. An Atlas of Clinical Nuclear Medicine. Cologne: Deutscher Ärzte-Verlag; 1994

Forstrom LA, Mullan BP, Hung JC, Lowe VJ, Thorson LM. 18F-FDG labelling of human leukocytes. Nucl Med Commun 2000;21(7):691–694

Gallowitsch HJ, Heinisch M, Mikosch P, et al. Tc-99m ciprofloxacin in clinically selected patients for peripheral osteomyelitis, spondylodiscitis and fever of unknown origin—preliminary results. [Article in German] Nuklearmedizin 2002;41(1):30–36

Gericke M, Stabell U, Eckart L, et al. High resolution Knochen-SPECT mit der Prism 3000 3-Kopf-Kamera: Erste Ergebnisse bei Erkrankungen des Bewegungsapparates. Pickeractuell 1998;16:13–16

Gratz S, Behr T, Schmitt HA, et al. 99mTc-labeled antigranulocyte monoclonal antibody Fab' fragments (LeukoScan) for diagnostic imaging of bone and soft tissue infections. J Nucl Med 1998;39(Suppl.):34

Gratz S, Becker W. Bedeutung der SPECT bei der Knochenszintigraphie. Der Nuklearmediziner 2000;2:105–115

Gratz S, Dörner J, Fischer U, et al. 18F-FDG hybrid PET in patients with suspected spondylitis. Eur J Nucl Med Mol Imaging 2002;29(4):516–524

Guhlmann A, Brecht-Krauss D, Suger G, et al. Fluorine-18-FDG PET and technetium-99m antigranulocyte antibody scintigraphy in chronic osteomyelitis. J Nucl Med 1998a;39(12):2145–2152

Guhlmann A, Brecht-Krauss D, Suger G, et al. Chronic osteomyelitis: detection with FDG PET and correlation with histopathologic findings. Radiology 1998b;206(3):749–754

Gupta N, Gill H, Graeber G, Bishop H, Hurst J, Stephens T. Dynamic positron emission tomography with F-18 fluorodeoxyglucose imaging in differentiation of benign from malignant lung/mediastinal lesions. Chest 1998;114(4):1105–1111

Hahn K. Nuklearmedizinische Diagnostik der Osteomyelitis im Kindesalter. In: Feine U, Müller-Schauenburg W, eds. Skelettszintigraphie. Nürnberg: Wachholz-Verlag; 1989:107–114

Hansen HJ, Goldenberg DM, Newman ES, Grebenau R, Sharkey RM. Characterization of second-generation monoclonal antibodies against carcinoembryonic antigen. Cancer 1993;71(11):3478–3485

Harwood SJ, Carroll RG, Anderson M, et al. SPECT gallium scanning for lymphoma and infection. Clin Nucl Med 1987;12(9):694–702

Höflin F. Target activity enhancement by thermally induced hyperemia in the scintigraphy of inflammation in the extremities. Eur J Nucl Med 1988;14:244

Hör G, Frey KW, Keyl W, Hertel E. Comparison of scintigraphy and X-ray diagnosis in osteomyelitis. [Article in German] Fortschr Geb Rontgenstr Nuklearmed 1969;110(5):708–716

Hör G, Keyl W, Langhammer H, et al. Ergebnisse der Scanner- und Kameraszintigraphie im Vergleich mit Röntgendiagnostik (Nativaufnahme, Angiographie) und Thermographie bei Skeletterkrankungen. In: Pabst HW, Hör G, eds. Nuklearmedizin. Stuttgart: Schattauer; 1974:377–382

Kälicke Th, Schmitz A, Risse JH, et al. Fluorine-18 fluorodeoxyglucose PET in infectious bone diseases: results of histologically confirmed cases. Eur J Nucl Med 2000;27(5):524–528

Kaim A, Ledermann HP, Bongartz G, Messmer P, Müller-Brand J, Steinbrich W. Chronic post-traumatic osteomyelitis of the lower extremity: comparison of magnetic resonance imaging and combined bone scintigraphy/immunoscintigraphy with radiolabelled monoclonal antigranulocyte antibodies. Skeletal Radiol 2000;29(7):378–386

Karkavitsas N, Damilakis J, Tzanakis N, Xilouris A, Samiou M, Bouros D. Effectiveness of Tc-99m sestamibi compared to Ga-67 in patients with pulmonary sarcoidosis. Clin Nucl Med 1997;22(11):749–751

Kubota R, Yamada S, Kubota K, Ishiwata K, Tamahashi N, Ido T. Intratumoral distribution of fluorine-18-fluorodeoxyglucose in vivo: high accumulation in macrophages and granulation tissues studied by microautoradiography. J Nucl Med 1992;33(11):1972–1980

Kühnel G, Börner AR, Döhring J, Weckesser E, Knapp WH. 18F-FDG-Positronenemissionstomographie in der Entzündungsdiagnostik. Der Nuklearmediziner 2000;2:97–103

Love C, Patel M, Lonner BS, Tomas MB, Palestro CJ. Diagnosing spinal osteomyelitis: a comparison of bone and Ga-67 scintigraphy and magnetic resonance imaging. Clin Nucl Med 2000;25(12):963–977

McCarthy TJ, Sheriff AU, Graneto MJ, Talley JJ, Welch MJ. Radiosynthesis, in vitro validation, and in vivo evaluation of 18F-labeled COX-1 and COX-2 inhibitors. J Nucl Med 2002;43(1):117–124

Moser E, Tatsch K, Kirsch CM, Küffer G, Goebel FD. Value of 67gallium scintigraphy in primary diagnosis and follow-up of opportunistic pneumonia in patients with AIDS. Lung 1990;168(Suppl):692–703

Palestro CJ. The current role of gallium imaging in infection. Semin Nucl Med 1994;24(2):128–141

Papós M, Barát F, Nárai G, Dillmann J, Láng J, Csernay L. Tc-99m HMPAO leukocyte and Tc-99m nanocolloid scintigraphy in posttraumatic bone infection. Clin Nucl Med 1998;23(7):423–428

Piepsz A, Hahn K, Roca I, et al. Paediatric Task Group European Association Nuclear Medicine. A radiopharmaceuticals schedule for imaging in paediatrics. Eur J Nucl Med 1990;17(3-4):127–129

Piert M, Winter E, Becker GA, et al. Allogenic bone graft viability after hip revision arthroplasty assessed by dynamic [18F]fluoride ion positron emission tomography. Eur J Nucl Med 1999;26(6):615–624

Reske SN, Kotzerke J. FDG-PET for clinical use. Results of the 3rd German Interdisciplinary Consensus Conference, "Onko-PET III", 21 July and 19 September 2000. Eur J Nucl Med 2001;28(11):1707–1723

Ruscowski M, Qu T, Pullman J, et al. Inflammation and infection imaging with a 99mTc-neutrophil elastase inhibitor in monkeys. J Nucl Med 2000;41(2):363–374

Santiago JF, Jana S, Gilbert HM, et al. Role of Fluorine-18-Fluorodeoxyglucose in the Work-up of Febrile AIDS Patients. Experience with Dual Head Coincidence Imaging. Clin Positron Imaging 1999;2(6):301–309

Sapienza MT, Hironaka F, Lima AL, et al. Evaluation of inflammatory activity in chronic osteomyelitis. Contribution of scintigraphy with polyclonal antibodies. [Article in Portuguese] Rev Assoc Med Bras 2000;46(2):106–112

Schmitz A, Risse HJ, Kälicke T, Grünwald F, Schmitt O. FDG-PET for diagnosis and follow-up of inflammatory processes:

initial results from the orthopedic viewpoint. [Article in German] Z Orthop Ihre Grenzgeb 2000;138(5):407–412

Shields AF, Grierson JR, Dohmen BM, et al. Imaging proliferation in vivo with [F-18]FLT and positron emission tomography. Nat Med 1998;4(11):1334–1336

Sorsdahl OA, Goodhart GL, Williams HT, Hanna LJ, Rodriquez J. Quantitative bone gallium scintigraphy in osteomyelitis. Skeletal Radiol 1993;22(4):239–242

Streule K, de Schrijver M, Fridrich R. 99Tcm-labelled HSA-nanocolloid versus 111In oxine-labelled granulocytes in detecting skeletal septic process. Nucl Med Commun 1988;9(1):59–67

Van Dalen A, Stemfort AF, de Jonge-Bok M, De Schrijver M. Three-phase scintigraphy of Tc-99m nanocoll vs. Tc-99m MDP in orthopedics. Eur J Nucl Med 1988;14:244

van der Laken CJ, Boerman OC, Oyen WJG, van de Ven MT, van der Meer JW, Corstens FH. Radiolabeled interleukin-8: specific scintigraphic detection of infection within a few hours. J Nucl Med 2000;41(3):463–469

Vorne M, Soini I, Lantto T, Paakkinen S. Technetium-99m HM-PAO-labeled leukocytes in detection of inflammatory lesions: comparison with gallium-67 citrate. J Nucl Med 1989;30(8):1332–1336

Yamada S, Kubota K, Kubota R, Ido T, Tamahashi N. High accumulation of fluorine-18-fluorodeoxyglucose in turpentine-induced inflammatory tissue. J Nucl Med 1995;36(7):1301–1306

Yao WJ, Hoh CK, Hawkins RA, et al. Quantitative PET imaging of bone marrow glucose metabolic response to hematopoietic cytokines. J Nucl Med 1995;36(5):794–799

Zhuang HM, Cortés-Blanco A, Pourdehnad M, et al. Do high glucose levels have differential effect on FDG uptake in inflammatory and malignant disorders? Nucl Med Commun 2001a;22(10):1123–1128

Zhuang H, Pourdehnad M, Lambright ES, et al. Dual time point 18F-FDG PET imaging for differentiating malignant from inflammatory processes. J Nucl Med 2001;42(9):1412–1417

4

Antibiotic Therapy

Oral Antibiotic Therapy

H. Breithaupt

Introduction

There exist several antibiotics for the treatment of bone infections; most are administered intravenously. The antibiotic treatment of osteomyelitis raises several questions:

- Is it a hematogenous or locally spread infection?
- Which pathogens are involved?
- Are the pathogens sensitive or resistant to antibiotic treatment?
- Have the antibiotics proven successful in clinical studies?

- Does the patient have primary or concomitant diseases?
- What is the risk–benefit relationship compared with other antibiotics?
- What is the dosage and expected duration of the therapy?
- What will it cost?

Acute Diffuse Osteomyelitis

Acute diffuse osteomyelitis arises through hematogenous spread and affects patients of all ages. *Staphylococcus aureus* is the most common pathogen; other germs are less often involved.

- Newborns: β-hemolytic streptococci, *Escherichia coli*
- Children: group A streptococci, *Haemophilus influenzae*
- Adults: 60% *S. aureus*, 30% coagulase-negative staphylococci, 10% each: *E. coli*, *Serratia marcescens*, and *Pseudomonas aeruginosa*
- After injury to the sole of the foot: 90% *P. aeruginosa*
- Heroin abuse: *S. aureus*, *P. aeruginosa*, etc
- AIDS patients: candida, *Aspergillus*, atypical mycobacteria, etc

Therapy for acute, diffuse osteomyelitis should be both specific and applied in high daily doses—with bactericidal antibiotics for 6–8 weeks:

- *S. aureus*: 3 × 4 g flucloxacillin IV or 3 × 600–900 mg clindamycin IV
- *S. aureus*, streptococci: 3 × 900 mg clindamycin IV
- Streptococci, sensitive staphylococci: 3 × 10 million IU penicillin G IV

- Sensitive staphylococci and *Staphylococcus epidermidis*: 3 × 5 g fosfomycin IV or 3 × 600 mg linezolid IV or per os

Empirical antibiotic therapy for unidentified pathogens can begin after a sample of infected material has been taken:

- Unknown pathogens: 3 × 900 mg clindamycin IV
- Children: clindamycin ± cefotaxim IV (max. 50 mg/kg/day)
- Immunocompromised patients: 3 × 2 g ceftazidim IV plus 3 × 1–2 mg/kg tobramycin IV (max. 2 weeks) or 3 × 500 mg ciprofloxacin per os
- *S. epidermidis*: 2 × 1 g vancomycin IV plus 3 × 500 mg fusidinic acid per os or 2 × 300 mg rifampicin per os; alternative: 3 × 600 mg linezolid IV or per os

Oral sequential therapy can be initiated after 2–4 weeks of parenteral therapy if there has been clinical improvement and the C-reactive protein (CRP) has normalized:

- *S. aureus*: 3 × 1–2 g flucloxacillin per os
- *S. aureus*, streptococci: 3 × 600 mg clindamycin per os
- *S. aureus*, Gram-negative pathogens (also *P. aeruginosa*), *Brucella*: 3 × 500 mg ciprofloxacin per os

Chronic Osteomyelitis

Chronic osteomyelitis usually arises when pathogens are spread after a trauma, or following soft-tissue infection, or through intraoperative contamination, but also when acute infections have not been sufficiently cured. The **spectrum of pathogens** depends on the origin of the infection:

- Trauma: staphylococci, *E. coli*, *Proteus*, *P. aeruginosa* (often mixed infections)
- Postoperative: staphylococci, *E. coli*
- Diabetic gangrene: aerobic and anaerobic mixed infections
- Foreign bodies: *S. aureus*, *S. epidermidis*, *P. aeruginosa*

Surgical debridement is of decisive importance in the therapy of chronic osteomyelitis:

- Complete removal of infected, devitalized tissue (debridement, sequestrotomy, removal of infected bone substitute)
- Improvement of circulation by plastic surgery (e.g., transplantation of bones, muscles, and/or skin)
- Local application of antibiotics as adjuvant therapy (e.g., gentamicin polymethylmethacrylate [PMMA])

Antibiotic therapy is only a supportive or inflammation-suppressing measure without curative intent in chronic osteomyelitis. Usually long-term therapy (clinical symptoms, CRP) is required with the accompanying risk of developing antibiotic resistance. Antibiotics with confirmed effect which enter the bone constitute the specific treatment of chronic osteomyelitis:

- Unknown pathogens: 3 × 3 g ampicillin/sulbactam IV (rapid intervention is required)
  Alternative: 3 × 900 mg clindamycin IV plus 3 × 2 g cefotaxim IV
- *S. aureus*: 3 × 600–900 mg clindamycin IV or per os or 3 × 500 mg ciprofloxacin per os

Alternative: betalactam antibiotic plus rifampicin (or fusidinic acid)
- Methicillin-resistant *S. aureus* (MRSA): 2 × 1 g vancomycin IV ± 1 × 600 mg rifampicin per os
  Alternative: 2 × 600 mg linezolid IV or per os
- Coagulase-negative staphylococci: 2 × 1 g vancomycin
  Alternatives: 2 × 600 mg linezolid IV or per os or 3 × 500 mg fosfomycin IV plus 2 × 300 mg rifampicin per os (or 3 × 500 mg fusidinic acid per os)
- Streptococci: 3 × 600–900 mg clindamycin IV or per os
- Enterococci: 3 × 2–5 g ampicillin IV
  Alternative: 2 × 1 g vancomycin IV
- Enterobacteria: 3 × 500 mg ciprofloxacin per os or 1 × 2 g ceftriaxon IV or IM
- Salmonella: 3 × 500 mg ciprofloxacin per os or 3 × 2 g cefotaxim IV
- *P. aeruginosa*: 3 × 2 g ceftazidim IV plus 3 × 1–2 mg/kg tobramycin IV (during the first 2 weeks) or 3 × 500 mg ciprofloxacin per os ± 3 × 1–2 mg/kg tobramycin IV (during the first 2 weeks)
- Anaerobic pathogens (often mixed infections): 3 × 600–900 mg clindamycin IV or per os or 3 × 3 g ampicillin; sulbactam IV or 3 × 1 g imipenem; cilastatin IV or 1 × 400 mg moxifloxacin per os
- *Brucella*: 1 × 500 mg levofloxacin per os
- *Pasteurella multocida*: 3 × 10 million IU penicillin G IV
  Alternatives: 1 × 2 g ceftriaxon IV or intramuscular or 1 × 200 mg doxycyclin per os
- Mycobacterium tuberculosis: 5 mg/kg isoniazid plus 10 mg/kg rifampicin plus 25 mg/kg pyrazinamid per os plus 25 mg/kg ethambutol per os
- Fungal infections: 800 mg fluconazol per os
  Alternative: voriconazol 2– 3 × 200 mg per os or caspofungin 50 mg

Antibiotic Profiles

Benzylpenicillin

Penicillin G

Evaluation:
+++ strepto-, pneumo-, and meningococci
++ *Treponema*, *Borrelia*, *Leptospira*, gonococci (except β-lactamase producers), *S. aureus* (except β-lactamase

producers), *Corynebacterium diphtheriae*, *P. multocida*, Clostridia (except *Clostridium difficile*), *Bacteroides* (except *Bacteroides fragilis*), fusobacteria, peptostreptococci, actinomycetes
— enterobacteria, *Pseudomonas*, β-lactamase producers (*Haemophilus*, *Moraxella catarrhalis*, etc.) *Nocardia*, *Mycoplasma*, *Chlamydia*

Side effects: Allergies (exanthema, fever) 2%, anaphylaxis 1:40 000, neurotoxicity (myoclonia, coma, and fits with high doses)

Dosage: Up to 3 × 10 million IU/day

Penicillins Suitable for Staphylococci

Flucloxacillin: Staphylex, etc. (IV, per os)
Oxacillin: InfectoStaph (IV)
Dicloxacillin: InfectoStaph (per os)

Evaluation: Antibiotic of choice for *S. aureus* (except when methicillin-resistant), narrow-spectrum antibiotic

Side effects: Like penicillin G, hepatitis ± cholestasis (3%)

Dosage: 3 × 2–4 g/d (IV), 3 × 1–2 g/d (per os)

Obsolete combinations: Amoxicillin + flucloxacillin, mezlocillin + oxacillin

Aminopenicillins

Ampicillin: Binotal, etc. (IV)

Amoxicillin: Clamoxyl, etc. (per os)

Evaluation:
+++ enterococci, *Haemophilus*, *Listeria*
++ strepto-, pneumo-, meningococci, *Salmonella*, *Shigella*, *Proteus mirabilis*, *E. coli* (30%–50% are resistant)
− other enterobacteria, *Pseudomonas*, β-lactamase producers (e.g., *S aureus*, *M. catarrhalis*)

Side effects: Like penicillin G, ampicillin exanthema (approximately 15%, in mononucleosis 70%–100%)

Dosage: Ampicillin 3 × 2–5 g/d (IV), amoxicillin 3 × 1 g/d (per os)

Aminopenicillin + Betalactamase Inhibitors

Ampicillin/sulbactam: Unacid (IV)

Sultamicillin: Unacid PD (per os)

Amoxicillin/clavulanate: Augmentan, etc. (per os, IV)

Evaluation: Extended broad-band effectiveness against Gram-positive, Gram-negative, and anaerobic pathogens
+++ enterococci, *Haemophilus*, *Listeria*
++ *S. aureus*, streptococci, pneumococci, meningococci, *M. catarrhalis*, *E. coli*, *Klebsiella*, *P. mirabilis/vulgaris*, *Salmonella*, *Shigella*, and anaerobic bacteria (including *B. fragilis*)
− *Pseudomonas*, problematic Gram-negative pathogens, *Enterococcus faecium*, *Mycoplasma*, *Chlamydia*

Side effects: Like those of aminopenicillins (exanthemas are rarer, diarrhea is more frequent.). Clavulanate: hepatitis ± cholestasis 1:10 000

Dosage: Ampicillin/sulbactam 3 × 3 g/d (IV), amoxicillin/clavulanate 3 × 2.2 g/d (IV) or 3 × 500 mg (per os), sultamicillin 2 × 750 mg (per os)

Acylureido Penicillins

Mezlocillin: Baypen, etc.

Piperacillin: Pipril, etc.

Evaluation:
+++ Gram-negative pathogens (antibiogram!), enterococci
++ *Pseudomonas* (piperacillin)
+ Gram-positive pathogens
− β-lactamase producers (e.g., *S. aureus*, *Haemophilus*), *E. faecium*

Side effects: Like those of penicillin G, reversible neutropenia (after a cumulative dosage of >100 g)

Indications: Piperacillin/sulbactam for severe (nosocomial) infections with Gram-negative pathogens (+ aminoglycoside)

Dosage: Piperacillin 3 × 4 g/d + sulbactam 3 × 1 g/d or piperacillin + tazobactam 3 × 4/0.5g IV

Betalactamase Inhibitors

Sulbactam: Combactam

Evaluation: β-lactamase inhibitor is licensed for combination with mezlocillin, piperacillin, cefotaxim, or penicillin G
 Broadened spectrum and increased effectiveness against:

- *S. aureus*
- *E. coli*, *Proteus* species, *Klebsiella*
- *B. fragilis*

The resistances of *Pseudomonas*, enterobacteria, and *Serratia* are not influenced.

Side effects: Diarrhea

Indications: Used in combination with piperacillin for severe Gram-negative infections and severe aerobic–anaerobic mixed infections. Combined with penicillin G for diabetic gangrene or infection with actinomycosis.

Dosage: 3 × 1 g/d (IV)

Fixed combination (with a reserve penicillin): Piperacillin + tazobactam

Standard Cephalosporin

Cefazolin: Elzogram, etc.

Evaluation:
++ effective against pneumococci, streptococci, staphylococci, *E. coli*, *Klebsiella*, and *P. mirabilis*
— enterococci, *Pseudomonas*, problematic Gram-negative pathogens

Side effects: Allergies (3%, 10% cross allergies with penicillins)

Indications: Initial treatment for mild and moderately severe infections, intraoperative prophylaxis

Dosage: 3 × 2 g/d, 1 × 2 g (for a 3-hour operation)

Cephalosporins (Second Generation)

Cefuroxim: Zinacef, etc.

Cefotiam: Spizef

Evaluation:
++ effective against pneumococci, streptococci, staphylococci, *Haemophilus*, *Klebsiella*, *P. mirabilis*, *E. coli*
— enterococci, *Pseudomonas*, problematic Gram-negative pathogens

Side effects: Like those of standard cephalosporins.

Indications: Initial treatment of moderately severe infections that are probably caused by Gram-negative pathogens

Dosage: Cefuroxim 3 × 1.5 g/d, cefotiam 3 × 2 g/d

Reserve Cephalosporins

Cefotaxim: Claforan, etc.

Ceftriaxon: Rocephin, etc.

Ceftazidim: Fortum (*Pseudomonas*)
Cefepim: Maxipime (*Pseudomonas*)

Evaluation:
+++ Gram-negative pathogens (e.g., *E. coli*, *Klebsiella*, all *Proteus* species, *H. influenzae*), *P. aeruginosa* (ceftazidim, cefepim)
+ less effective against Gram-positive pathogens.
— enterococci, anaerobic pathogens, *Listeria*

Side effects: Like those of other cephalosporins

Dosage: Cefotaxim 2–3 × 2 g/d, ceftriaxon 1 × 2 g/d (1st day: 1 × 4 g), ceftazidim 3 × 2 g/d

Carbapenems

Imipenem + cilastatin: Zienam

Meropenem: Meronem
Ertapenem: Invanz

Doripenem: Doribax

Evaluation:
++ very broad spectrum against Gram-positive and Gram-negative pathogens, including *P. aeruginosa* and anaerobic bacteria
— *Stenotrophomonas maltophilia*, *Burkholderia cepacia*, *C. difficile*, and fungi
   Cilastatin inhibits the breakdown of imipenem in the kidneys.

Side effects: Diarrhea (3%), allergies (3%), cross-allergies with other β-lactams (20%), elevation of transaminases (5%), phlebitis, fits (imipenem)

Indications: Severe, therapy-resistant nosocomial infections and therapy-resistant meningitis (meropenem). Not to be used as primary therapy or on a normal ward!

Dosage: Imipenem/cilastatin 3 × 1 g/d, meropenem 3 × 1 g/d (in meningitis 3 × 2 g/d)

Aminoglycosides

Gentamicin: Refobacin, etc.
Netilmicin: Certomycin
Tobramycin: Gernebcin, etc. (*Pseudomonas*)
Amikacin: Biklin, etc. (reserve aminoglycoside)

Evaluation:
+++ Gram-negative enterobacteria
++ *S. aureus*
— streptococci, pneumococci, enterococci, anaerobic bacteria

Side effects: Oto- and nephrotoxicity, curarelike effect (respiratory paralysis) if infused too rapidly

Dosage: 1 × 3–5 mg/kg (30–60-minute infusion), for example 1 × 240–360 mg/d; amikacin 1 × 7.5–15 mg/kg

Precaution: Because of the risk of irreversible deafness:
- Adjust the dose with elevated creatinine
- Do not give for longer than 2 weeks
- 24-hour lowest level <1–2 µg/mL
- Monotherapy is obsolete (except local therapy for osteomyelitis)

Lincosamides

Clindamycin: Sobelin, etc.

Evaluation:
+++ anaerobic bacteria (including *B. fragilis*), *S. aureus*, streptococci, pneumococci
— enterobacteria, enterococci, *Haemophilus*, *Pseudomonas*

Kinetics: Bioavailability approximately 90%. No dose reduction in renal insufficiency

Side effects: Soft stools, diarrhea, colitis, hepatotoxicity, phlebitis, allergies (rare)

Dosage: 3 × 600–900 mg/d (IV), 3 × 300–600 mg/d (per os)

Glycopeptides

Vancomycin: half-life 5 hours
Teicoplanin: half-life 50 hours

Evaluation:
+++ *S. aureus* (even if methicillin resistant), coagulase-negative staphylococci, streptococci, pneumococci, enterococci, *C. difficile*
— enterobacteria, *B. fragilis*

Side effects: Allergies up to 12% (e.g., skin, fever, anaphylaxis), histamine flush (vancomycin), phlebitis, oto-and nephrotoxicity?

Dosage: Vancomycin: 2 × 1 g/d (30–60-minute infusion. Avoid infusing rapidly!)
Teicoplanin: 1 × 400 mg/d (1st day 800–1200 mg)

Monitoring: Do not go below a valley level of 15 µg/mL. Avoid peak values higher than 40 µg/mL.

Fosfomycin

Fosfomycin: Infectofos

Evaluation:
++ *S. aureus*, streptococci, pneumococci, *Haemophilus*, *E. coli*, *P. mirabilis*, *Serratia*, *Salmonella*, *Shigella*, *Citrobacter*
— enterococci, *Pseudomonas*, *Listeria*, anaerobic bacteria

Side effects: Nausea, vomiting, diarrhea (10%), headache, phlebitis, hypernatremia, hepatotoxicity, allergies (rare)

Indications: Severe infections with sensitive pathogens (antibiogram!), for example, osteomyelitis, endocarditis, and brain abscess. Combine with betalactam antibiotics.

Dosage: 3 × 3–5 g/d

Gyrase Inhibitors

Norfloxacin: Barazan, etc. (urinary-tract infections)
Enoxacin: Enoxor (per os)

Ofloxacin: Tarivid (IV, per os)

Ciprofloxacin: Ciprobay (IV, per os)
Levofloxacin: Tavanic (IV, per os)

Moxifloxacin: Avalox (IV, per os)

Evaluation:
+++ enterobacteria, *P. aeruginosa* (ciprofloxacin), *Yersinia*, *Legionella*, *Brucella Haemophilus*, *M. catarrhalis*
++ *S. aureus*, atypical mycobacteria, *Chlamydia*, *Mycoplasma*, *Rickettsia*
— streptococci, **pneumococci**, enterococci, anaerobic bacteria. **Moxifloxacin** is effective against Gram-positive and anaerobic pathogens!

Side effects: Ca. 1% central nervous system (CNS) manifestations (like sleep disturbances and restlessness), psychoses 1 : 14 000, tendopathies (0.1%), GI complaints (1%), allergies (1%, e.g., exanthemas, fever, liver damage)

Dosage:
Ofloxacin: 2 × 200 mg/d per os, up to 2 × 400 mg/d IV
Levofloxacin: 1 × 250 mg/d per os
Ciprofloxacin: 2 × 500 mg/d per os, up to 3 × 400 mg/d IV
Moxifloxacin: 1 × 400 mg/d IV, per os

Oxazolidinon

Linezolid: Zyvoxid (IV, per os)

Evaluation:
+++ Gram-positive pathogens, also penicillin-resistant pneumococci, MRSA, coagulase-negative staphylococci, glycopeptide-resistant enterococci
— *H. influenzae*, *M. catarrhalis*, *Neisseria*, enterobacteria, *Pseudomonas*

Side effects: IG complaints (vomiting in 1%–2%), mild CNS symptoms, reversible thrombo- and leukopenia, anemia, increase in blood pressure with serotoninergic or adrenergic drugs

Kinetics: Complete resorption, half-life 5–7 hours, renal elimination (30% unchanged)

Dosage: 2 × 600 mg (IV, per os). No dose restriction with hepato- or renal insufficiency.

Fusidinic Acid

Fusidinic acid: Fucidine

Evaluation:
+++ staphylococci, even penicillinase producers and some methicillin-resistant species, some *B. fragilis*
+ streptococci, pneumococci, enterococci
— enterobacteria

Side effects: GI complaints (stomach ache, vomiting, diarrhea), rarely disturbances of liver function and allergies

Kinetics: Almost complete resorption, good tissue penetration, half-life 4–6 hours (in terminal renal failure 6–8 hours), metabolic clearance 80%–90%

Dosage: 3 × 500 mg per os with meals

Comment: reserve antibiotic for severe staphylococcal infections

Ansamycin

Rifampicin: Rifa, etc.

Evaluation:
–++ *Mycobacterium tuberculosis*, *Mycobacterium leprae*, staphylococci (also MRSA), streptococci (also when penicillin C resistant), enterococci, meningococci, gonococci, *H. influenzae*, *Legionella*, *Chlamydia*
++ *Mycobacterium kansasii*, *Mycobacterium marinum*
+ *Mycobacterium avium-intracellulare*, *Mycobacterium fortuitum*, enterobacteria
— *Mycoplasma*

Side effects: Rise in transaminases (5%–20%; if above 100 IU/L ± cholestasis, discontinue treatment). Allergic reactions (exanthema, fever, eosinophilia), reversible neutropenia and thrombocytopenia (blood counts), colors saliva, tears, sweat, urine, and stools orange. Induces enzymes dependent on cytochrome P450.

Kinetics: Good bioavailability and penetration (also intracellular). Half-life: 2–5 hours. Mostly metabolic clearance.

Dosage: Up to 1 × 600 mg IV to 1 × 750 mg per os. No dose reduction with renal insufficiency.

Comment: First-choice tuberculostaticum. For combination therapy of infections that are difficult to reach (like foreign-body infections).

Further Reading

Kucers A, Crowe SM, Grayson ML, Hoy JF, eds. The Use of Antibiotics. A Clinical Review of Antibacterial, Antifungal and Antiviral Drugs. 5th ed. Oxford: Butterworth Heinemann; 1997
Kuntz P, Pieringer-Müller E, Hof H. Infektionsgefährdung durch Bißverletzungen. Dtsch Arztebl 1996;93:B765–B768
Lew DP, Waldvogel FA. Osteomyelitis. N Engl J Med 1997;336(14):999–1007

Mader JT, Calhoun J. Osteomyelitis. In: Mandell GL, Bennett JE, Dolin R, eds. Mandell, Douglas and Bennett's Principles and Practice of Infectious Diseases. 5th ed. Philadelphia: Churchill Livingstone; 2000:1182–1200

Nadal D, Zbinden R. Illnesses caused by Bartonella. Cat-scratch disease, bacillary angiomatosis, bacillary peliosis hepatis, endocarditis. [Article in German] Internist (Berl) 1996;37(9):890–894

Norden C, Gillespie WJ, Nade S, eds. Infections in Bones and Joints. Boston: Blackwell Scientific Publications; 1994

Schultheis K-H, Rehm KE, Ecke H, eds. Chirurgische Infektionen von Knochen, Gelenken und Weichteilen. Berlin: De Gruyter; 1991

Simon C, Stille W. Antibiotika-Therapie in Klinik und Praxis, 10th ed. Stuttgart: Schattauer; 1999

Smith JW, Hasan MS. Infectious arthritis. In: Mandell GL, Bennett JE, Dolin R, eds. Mandell, Douglas and Bennetts's Principles and Practice of Infectious Diseases. 5th ed. Philadelphia: Churchill Livingstone; 2000:1175–1182

Local Antibiotic Therapy

L. Frommelt

Why Use Local Antibiotics to Treat Infections of the Musculoskeletal System?

Local antibiotics for the treatment of surgical wound infections have rightly been in disfavor, because their application is difficult to control and there is always a risk that adjacent flora will develop resistance. Considering the increasing number of resistant pathogens worldwide, this is of great importance. In 2002 the first vancomycin-resistant *S. aureus* (VRSA) species in patients after very long-term treatment with vancomycin was reported in the USA. The published correlation between the use of vancomycin in the USA and the increase in clinically relevant vancomycin-resistant enterococci (VRE) by Kirst et al. in 1998 is especially impressive. Between 1984 and 1996 the use of vancomycin increased from 2000 kg to almost 12 000 kg per year. Up to 1989 there were no known enterococcal resistances to vancomycin, however thereafter the portion of resistant pathogens identified in clinical settings continually increased to almost 25%. The current skepticism concerning the uncontrolled use of local antibiotics in wound treatment is thus understandable.

Infections of the skeletal system are, however, exceptional because of their special pathogenesis, which appears to justify the local application of anti-infectious substances. The application of local antibiotics must, however, play only an adjuvant role alongside surgical debridement. These infections have a strong tendency to recur, and therapeutic success depends decisively on the thoroughness of surgical debridement. Antibiotics alone cannot control these infections. If local and systemic antibiotics are integrated into the surgical concept, they can ensure the success of the surgical intervention and its

sustainability. The key to understanding lies in the formal pathogenesis of bone infections, especially chronic forms.

Periprosthetic infections in joint prostheses represent a special situation. This foreign-body infection can serve as a model for chronic osteomyelitis and is, therefore, an ideal example of pathogenesis.

In these infections it is the foreign body which maintains the infection. In osteomyelitis there are naturally occurring foreign bodies, that is, bone sequestra, with which pathogens interact as with foreign bodies. Recurrences originate from these sequestra, and they are also the place where the pathogens withdraw and wait.

Common to all infections are the following defined stages from contamination by the potential pathogen to manifest infectious disease: contamination, adherence to a surface, colonization of the surface, invasion of the underlying tissue, and infection. The appearance of clinical symptoms accompanies the manifestation of the infectious disease, which is only terminated by the elimination of the pathogen or death of the host. The immune system, and in particular phagocytizing cells like granulocytes and macrophages, is able to eliminate bacteria. This is possible in so far as the pathogens do not multiply faster than the immune system can eliminate them. If the capacity of the cellular defenses is exhausted, the pathogens can continue to multiply, and the infection spreads. Antibiotics directly affect the ability of the bacteria to multiply and thereby shift the equilibrium to the advantage of the host's immune defenses. The immune system can then destroy the pathogens and end the infection. Antibiotics are a means to self-help, which influences the dual relationship between pathogen and host to the advantage of the host.

In the presence of a foreign body, there is a competing interaction, that is, between the foreign body and the immune system. The incorporation of bone substitute triggers a foreign-body reaction, whose goal is to remove the bone substitute. If this is not successful, a granuloma is formed. The foreign body is isolated from the internal milieu and can no longer be attacked by the immune defenses. This phenomenon can be observed with foreign bodies as well as with certain bacteria, like tuberculosis bacteria.

However, not only the host interacts with the foreign body, but also the pathogen. Bacteria that are able to produce amoeboid forms colonize foreign bodies by building a biofilm and are then irreversibly bound to the surface of the foreign body. The bacteria then transform from the planktonic form, which is characterized by rapid multiplication, rapid metabolism, and high sensitivity to antibiotics, to the amoeboid form, characterized by extremely slow multiplication, reduced metabolism, and a generally high resistance to several antibiotics. Costerson et al. (1995) observed among amoeboid forms of *P. aeruginosa* an 800-fold higher minimal inhibitory concentration (MIC) than among planktonic forms. Among staphylococci, an approximate 250-fold increase in the MIC has been reported. This means conventional systemic therapy only reaches these bacteria in concentrations which cannot influence them, or only inadequately.

A mixture of planktonic and amoeboid forms of pathogens is present in clinically manifest chronic osteomyelitis or a periprosthetic infection, whereby the clinical symptoms are mainly caused by the planktonic forms. Systemic antibiotic therapy affects almost exclusively the planktonic bacteria, influencing symptoms of the infection without eliminating the pathogen reservoir of the amoeboid forms. To clear up the infection, both the planktonic and the amoeboid forms must be eradicated. For this reason the application of local antibiotic therapy in these infections is justified.

> **NOTE**
>
> Local antibiotic therapy can achieve concentrations up to 1000 times higher than with systemic therapy alone.

In this way, both amoeboid and planktonic bacteria can be reached; local and systemic antibiotics should be combined. This therapy can only succeed together with qualified surgical debridement in which implanted foreign material (metal, synthetic material, bone cement, etc.) and infected bone tissue and sequestra, if present, should be removed.

Local Application of Antibiotics in Infections of the Skeletal System

The following text briefly characterizes the forms of local antibiotic treatment currently available.

Antibiotics and Bone Transplants

Directly after the end of WWII, when antibiotics became available, these were used for the local therapy of osteomyelitis. In 1946 Prigge instilled penicillin locally after filling bone defects stemming from chronic osteomyelitis with autogenous trabecular bone. In 1947 de Grood mixed bone grafts with penicillin and filled in osteomyelitic bone defects. Winkler (2000) has reported bone transplants loaded with tobramycin and vancomycin. He showed that bones can both bind antibiotics and release them slowly (**Table 4.1**).

Antibiotics and Plaster of Paris

Another form of application of calcium sulfate (plaster) as an antibiotic carrier is plaster of Paris (POP). Antibiotics are added to the plaster, which is used to fill in osteomyelitic bone defects and bone cysts. Kovacevic first reported the use of POP in 1953. Mackey (1982) published an investigation in which 60%–80% of the antibiotics were released immediately after implantation. This was followed by a slow release over 7–9 weeks until the POP beads dissolved. This is, then, a slightly retaining system which, like an intramuscular injection, can supply high concentrations quickly and release them into the blood stream. This is also the cause of possible toxic side effects of the administered antibiotics (**Table 4.2**).

Table 4.1 Bone transplants and antibiotic characteristics

Carrier substance	Bone grafts
Resorptive behavior	Partially resorptive, osteoconductive
Release	Delayed
Known effective antibiotics	Cephalotin, ciprofloxacin, clindamycin, dicloxacillin, penicillin, netilmycin, piperacillin, rifampicin, ticarcillin, tobramycin, vancomycin
Form of antibiotic	Liquid
Application	Presently not generally available
Comments	Procedure not generally available
	Also possible in xenotransplants (bovine or equine bones)
	Rifampicin is released over the longest time period

Table 4.2 POP and antibiotic characteristics

Carrier substance	Calcium sulfate (plaster) cylinder / beads / paste
Resorptive behavior	Completely resorbable
Release	60%–80% initially
Known effective antibiotics	Cephalozolin, fusidinic acid, gentamicin, lincomycin, penicillin, sulfonamides, teicoplanin, tobramycin, vancomycin
Form of antibiotic	Liquid
Application	Generally available
Comments	Because of its rapid initial release, there is a possible danger of undesired toxic side effects.

Antibiotics and PMMA Bone Cement

In 1970 Buchholz and Engelbrecht reported mixing antibiotics with PMMA bone cement. Buchholz used antibiotic-loaded bone cement to affix prostheses in periprosthetic infections and as prophylaxis when performing joint implantations. It was shown that several antibiotics can be released from PMMA bone cement. This does not, however, happen to the same extent in all antibiotics. Some antibiotics, like rifampicin, react with the PMMA bone cement and change the release behavior so much that the substance loses its function. Other temperature-sensitive antibiotics are irreversibly inactivated by the polymerization heat. It is, therefore, necessary to test the antibiotics for their suitability for use in PMMA bone cement before applying them.

The release behavior shows that this is a highly retaining system in which the antibiotic release correlates directly with the surface of the bone cement. Klemm used PMMA bone cement loaded with antibiotics as a substance carrier to treat osteomyelitis. He used beads placed in the osteomyelitic defects. These were later strung on a wire and implanted in the carrier as chains, which simplified removal of the beads (Klemm 1979).

As a whole, the antibiotic-loaded PMMA bone cement is a system in which high concentrations of antibiotics are initially released. Even with a large amount of bone cement, only low levels of antibiotics are found in serum, thereby making toxic side effects of the antibiotics improbable (**Table 4.3**).

Antibiotics and Collagen

Collagen sponges containing gentamicin have been commercially available since 1987. Bovine collagen is used onto which the aminoglycoside is attached. It is released by diffusion and enzymatic degradation of the collagen carrier system. This is a slightly retarded system in which the antibiotics are almost completely released within the first hours. This applies to hydrophilic, that is, easily soluble gentamicin sulfate. To slow down release, besides the gentamicin sulfate, the hydrophobic, hardly soluble gentamicin crobefat is used in one product (Septocoll, Biomet, Berlin, Germany). Gentamicin crobefat is slowly split into the effective gentamicin phosphate and a flavinoid, providing slow release of the antibiotic. Gentamicin secretion can be ensured for 48–72 hours.

Because of bovine spongiform encephalopathy (BSE), which can be transmitted to humans as the new variant of Creutzfeldt–Jacob disease (vCJD), there are now collagen fleeces which no longer use bovine collagen, but equine collagen, since up to now there is no known equine form of spongiform encephalopathy (Septocoll-E).

Other antibiotics, teicoplanin and cefotaxim, have been used experimentally, and a fairly slow release could be observed. A preparation using calf collagen has special characteristics—aside from teicoplanin, bone morphogenic proteins (BMP) are released and have a bone-building effect.

All collagen products have a good hemostatic effect, which results from thrombocyte activation on contact (**Table 4.4**).

Table 4.3 PMMA bone cement and antibiotic characteristics

Carrier substance	PMMA
Resorptive behavior	Not resorbable, bioinert (if there is no abrasion)
Release	Delayed
Known effective antibiotics	Amikacin, ampicillin, carbenicillin, cephalotin, cefazolin, cefazedon, cefotaxim, cefoperazon, cefuroxim, ciprofloxacin, clindamycin, colistin, dicloxacillin, fusidinic acid, kanamycin, lincomycin, mezlocillin, neomycin, netilmycin, ofloxacin, oxacillin, penicillin, piperacillin, polymyxin B, rifampicin, streptomycin, ticarcillin, tobramycin, vancomycin
Form of antibiotic	Crystalloid (if liquid, stability of PMMA is lost)
Application	Generally available, some pharmaceutical products available
Comments	Release of antibiotics depends on the ability to absorb water (depends on the kind of PMMA)
	Antibiotics must be tested for each different kind of PMMA
	Antibiotics must not be inactivated by heat produced during polymerization
	Antibiotics must not react with the PMMA, for example, rifampicin considerably lengthens the setting time and decreases stability

Table 4.4 Collagen and antibiotic characteristics

Carrier substance	Collagen
Resorptive behavior	Resorbable
Release	Gentamicin sulfate—only slight delay
	Gentamicin crobefat—delayed release due to poor solubility
Known effective antibiotics	Cefotaxim, gentamicin, teicoplanin
Form of antibiotic	Bound to collagen
Application	Pharmaceutical products available
Comments	Secretion characteristics are similar to those of POP, but collagen has a distinctly shorter reabsorption time.

Antibiotics and Other Carrier Substances—Prospects

The use of resorbable polymers, like those used in suture material or for resorbable bone screws, opens up new dimensions in local antibiotic therapy. Antibiotics are released from inclusions during resorption of the carrier on the degradable surface. Different synthetic polymers of glycolic acid or lactic acid are suitable for this kind of local antibiotic therapy. One speaks of so-called polylactones. In these materials the speed of release correlates directly with the speed of resorption of the biomaterial. By combining different polylactones, the dosage can be controlled on site.

A further approach is to load the bone replacement materials with antibiotics. Loading of hydroxyapatite has been relatively well tested.

Use of PMMA Bone Cement as a Carrier for Therapy and Prophylaxis

Bone cement containing antibiotics has been in clinical use for over 30 years, providing a wealth of experience in therapy and prophylaxis of skeletal infections. The local application of antibiotics in bone infections is the most widely used worldwide.

PMMA bone cement containing antibiotics serves as a carrier substance in the form of chains consisting of PMMA beads (Septopal, Biomet, Berlin, Germany). Emphasis is placed on antibiotic release, which depends directly on the surface characteristics of the carrier. The round surface is optimal for this purpose and is purely therapeutic. The chains should be removed after a suitable period of time. Biomechanical characteristics of the bone cement do not play a role in this kind of application.

If bone cement containing antibiotics is used to stabilize prostheses, it remains in place. Since any addition to the bone cement—even antibiotics—worsens its biomechanical characteristics, this must be taken into consideration when the indication is established.

> **NOTE**
> Experience has shown that no more than 10% antibiotics should be added to the bone cement.

Antibiotics added to bone cement used to stabilize prostheses serves both as therapy for periprosthetic infections and as a prophylaxis. In prophylaxis, the surface of the implant is exchanged for a surface containing antibiotics. The antibiotics hinder bacterial colonization and serve as a barrier. If a periprosthetic infection already exists, initial local antibiotic concentrations influence amoeboid forms of bacteria which remain at the operation site. In addi-

tion, the surface is protected from new colonization of the freshly implanted prosthesis, just as in prophylaxis.

> **NOTE**
> A synthesis is offered by the so-called spacer. This is an antibiotic carrier whose geometry is adapted to the anatomical features where it is to be placed, thereby releasing antibiotics less ideally than PMMA chains. However, a spacer protects the anatomical structures (ligaments, etc.) from alterations after the infected prosthesis has been removed, especially in the knee joint. The biomechanical characteristics are of secondary importance in this application, as it only serves as a temporary place-holder system. After the infection has subsided, a new prosthesis can be inserted.

The different possible uses are summarized in **Table 4.5**.

Antibiotics and PMMA Bone Cement

The release of antibiotics from PMMA bone cement occurs by diffusion according to Fick's laws. There are two phases of release:
1. Momentary release from the surface of the cement
2. Delayed (very slow) diffusion from within the bone cement to the surface

Maximum local secretion in very high concentrations takes place within the first 20 minutes after implantation of the antibiotic-containing bone cement. In the second

Table 4.5 Possible uses of PMMA bone cement containing antibiotics

	Indication	Purpose	Characteristics Stability	Geometry	Duration
Carrier	Therapy	Release of antibiotics	Not necessary	Maximal surface (bead)	Temporary
Prosthesis fixation	Prophylaxis	Barrier to colonization	Necessary	Depends on implant	Permanent
	Therapy	Release of antibiotics	Necessary	Depends on implant	Permanent
		Barrier to colonization			
Spacer	Therapy	Release of antibiotics	Relatively necessary	Depends on implant	Temporary

phase, far lower concentrations are locally secreted due to the slow transport of antibiotics from the interior of the PMMA to the surface. Depending on the antibiotic used, concentrations are reached over different time intervals that can affect at least the planktonic forms of bacteria and prevent their colonization of the cement surface.

PMMA Characteristics and Antibiotic Release

The ability of the PMMA bone cement to release antibiotics correlates directly with its ability to adsorb water. This ability depends on two material characteristics, that is, porosity and wettability by watery solutions.

> **NOTE**
>
> This means that the more hydrophilic the PMMA compound, the more suitable the bone cement for the release of antibiotics.

Both Plexiglas and bone cement consist of PMMA. This demonstrates the variability in appearance of this material and explains why the degree of hydrophilia must be taken into account in individual cases when evaluating the suitability of a PMMA bone cement. This should be experimentally confirmed for each compound.

Characteristics of Antibiotics and their Release from PMMA Cement

Not all antibiotics are equally suited for release from a PMMA matrix.

Antibiotics used for this purpose must not react chemically with PMMA or its constituents and must remain stable at higher temperatures so that they are not inactivated by heat produced during polymerization. The fact that only very small changes in a molecule can have dramatic effects is demonstrated by thiamphenicol, which only differs from chloramphenicol in one sulfur bond and can be easily released from Palacos PMMA-bone cement (Heraeus Medical, Wehrheim, Germany), whereas chloramphenicol cannot be eluted at all. An example of thermic inactivation is imipenem, which is inactivated at 60 °C. Good release from PMMA bone cement can be achieved in unrealistic conditions (a very small test object and continuous cooling with ice water during the polymerization phase). Rifampicin can be released from bone cement, but it lengthens the polymerization phase to the extent that it remains a tough, flexible mass for over 24 hours.

Since these are complex interactions, antibiotic release from the different types of bone cement must be experimentally tested.

The suitability of an antibiotic results from these data, the total release times, and the bactericidal characteristics. Lincomycin and clindamycin are exceptions. These antibiotics are purely bacteriostatic, but have proven clinically useful. Substances like vancomycin, which only have a very slow bactericidal effect and poor release characteristics, should be viewed critically. Such substances should only be administered in individual cases with special resistances and then, if possible, only be used in combination with other effective substances.

Choice and Dosage of Antibiotics in Bone Cement

In individual cases, the choice of antibiotic must be based on the pathogen and its resistance. The pharmacokinetic characteristics of the antibiotic, as well as the characteristics of the pathogen, must be taken into consideration. Local therapy must be combined with systemic therapy which is suited to the special pharmacologic conditions in the bone.

Establishing the correct dose of antibiotics in bone cement has been purely empirical. Higher dosage is limited in that adding more than 10% of the antibiotic to the PMMA bone cement severely interferes with its mechanical characteristics, which can negatively influence the length of time the artificial joints can support weight bearing.

Table 4.6 shows exemplary doses which have proven successful in clinical use.

Table 4.6 Choice of antibiotic additions to PMMA bone cement with examples of pathogens. (Only apply after individually testing the resistance of the pathogens!)

Antibiotics	Dose per 40 g PMMA bone cement	Release duration concentrations > breakpoint NCCLS in wound secretion[*]	Examples of pathogens
Clindamycin + gentamicin	1.0 g + 1.0 g	38 days 21 days (tobramycin)	Staphylococci Streptococci Propioni bacteria
Cefuroxime + gentamicin	3.0 g + 1.0 g	No information available 21 days (tobramycin)	Staphylococci Streptococci Propioni bacteria
Vancomycin + ofloxacin + gentamicin	2.0 g + 1.0 g + 1.0 g	3 days 3 days (ciprofloxacin) 21 days (tobramycin)	Staphylococci (resistant) *Corynebacterium amycolatum*
Vancomycin + gentamicin	3.0 g + 1.0 g	3 days 21 days (tobramycin)	Staphylococci (resistant) *Corynebacterium amycolatum*
Vancomycin + ampicillin + gentamicin	2.0 g + 1.0 g + 1.0 g	3 days No information available 21 days (tobramycin)	Enterococci *Listeria*
Cefotaxim + gentamicin	2.0 g + 1.5 g	No information available 21 days (tobramycin)	Enterobacteriaceae
Cefoperozon + amikacin	2.0 g + 2.0 g	No information available No information available	*P. aeruginosa*
Streptomycin	2.0 g	No information available	Mycobacterium tuberculosis

[*]The data on concentrations in wound secretions derive from animal experiments by Adams et al. (1992). Antibiotics that were not tested, but according to the author's experiments permit analogous conclusions, are in parentheses. Local antibiotic therapies for infections should be combined with systemic antibiotic therapy!
NCCLS = National Committee for Clinical Laboratory Standards

Limits to Local Antibiotic Therapy

Before applying local antibiotic therapy, radical surgical debridement of all bone necroses and removal of all foreign material is obligatory. Local antibiotic therapy is not a primary, but an adjuvant form of therapy. If this principle is not heeded, infections will certainly recur.

Local antibiotic therapy only leads to resistances in exceptional cases, for example, when pathogens survive and are exposed to low levels of antibiotics for a long time. The development of resistances like in systemic therapies, which usually occur in areas with physiologic flora, is improbable because, for example, when using clindamycin-gentamicin loaded PMMA bone cement, clindamycin is no longer traceable in the serum from the third or fourth day.

If the pathogens change, this indicates a selection of germs with resistances to the antibiotics in use.

A further rare but important cause for failure of this type of therapy is pathogens which are able to produce so-called small colony variants. These staphylococci are generally resistant to gentamicin and can survive within cells. Cases have been confirmed in which this mechanism was responsible for persisting infection. Local antibiotic therapy should no longer be applied in such cases. Despite the data in the Norwegian Prosthesis Register reporting good effects of prophylaxis with locally applied gentamicin, we must assume that this has only proven effective in rare cases.

Practical Tips for the Local Application of Antibiotics in PMMA Bone Cement

Since there are few forms of pharmaceutically produced bone cement that contain antibiotics, in practice it is often necessary to add the antibiotics by hand during the operation.

> **NOTE**
>
> It is of greatest importance to produce a homogeneous mixture of PMMA polymeric powder and pulverized antibiotics before adding the fluid monomer, which triggers the polymerization process.

Otherwise inclusions of antibiotic powder arise in the PMMA matrix, which worsens both the release properties and the stability of the bone cement.

Antibiotic powder must not be added to the fluid monomer because this causes the powder to form clumps, which become inclusions in the hardened bone cement with the above-described problems.

Watery solutions must not be mixed into artificial materials because then polymerization is not ensured and the desired material characteristics, like stability, cannot be achieved.

> **NOTE**
>
> If industrially produced bone cements containing antibiotics are available, they should be used instead of cements mixed by hand because industrial products have controlled production methods.

Tips for Mixing Antibiotics into Bone Cement by Hand

When producing the mixture consisting of PMMA polymer beads (powder) and an antibiotic powder, as homogeneous a mixture as possible must be produced before polymerization can take place. This should correspond to the rules for producing mixtures that are followed by pharmacists. The procedure is described in **Table 4.7**.

> **NOTE**
>
> Intraoperative mixing of antibiotics:
> - Mix the powders together.
> - Never use liquid antibiotics.
> - Never add more than 10% (weight) antibiotic powder.
> - If industrial products are available, use them!

Table 4.7 Procedure for mixing antibiotics to the gentamicin-PMMA bone cement

Instruments	Procedure
Suitable sterile container	1. Put the antibiotic powder into the mixing container under sterile conditions.
Sterile spatula (plastic or metal)	2. Add the same amount of PMMA polymer powder.
	3. Mix well with the spatula.
	4. Add the same amount of PMMA-polymer powder to the mixture that is already in the container.
	5. Mix well with the spatula.
	6. Continue this procedure until all the PMMA polymer powder is used up.
	7. Add PMMA monomer fluid and prepare according to producer's instructions.

Legal Aspects of Mixtures Prepared by Hand

The individual mixing of antibiotics to bone cement raises legal issues. Since neither the antibiotic nor the bone cement is being used according to regulations, that is, according to the producer's approval, this nullifies the producer's liability for the product.

> **NOTE**
>
> Legally this is considered an individual therapeutic experiment, which is fundamentally possible according to the treatment contract between patient and physician if the patient consents and it can be proved that s/he has received sufficient information about the procedure. The physician is legally liable.

For this reason also, only products should be used that are sterile and are approved as drugs by the authorities or are individually prepared according to the prescription of a medical doctor or a surgeon. Raw chemicals are never to be used, as they have neither been compounded precisely nor been subjected to toxicologic testing.

The legal assessment emphasizes the recommendation to use industrially manufactured products whenever they are available.

Bibliography

Adams K, Couch L, Cierny G, Calhoun J, Mader JT. In vitro and in vivo evaluation of antibiotic diffusion from antibiotic-impregnated polymethylmethacrylate beads. Clin Orthop Relat Res 1992;278(278):244–252

Boss JH, Shajrawi I, Mendes DG. The nature of the bone-implant interface. The lessons learned from implant retrieval and analysis in man and experimental animal. Med Prog Technol 1994;20(3-4):119–142

Brisou JF. Biofilms—Methods of Enzymatic Release of Micro Organisms. Boca Raton, FL: CRC Press; 1995

Buchholz HW, Engelbrecht H. Depot effects of various antibiotics mixed with Palacos resins. [Article in German] Chirurg 1970;41(11):511–515

Buchholz HW, Elson RA, Lodenkämper H. The infected joint implant. In: McKibbin B, ed. Recent Advances in Orthopaedics 3. New York: Churchill Livingston; 1979:139–161

Costerton JW, Lewandowski Z, Caldwell DE, Korber DR, Lappin-Scott HM. Microbial biofilms. Annu Rev Microbiol 1995;49:711–745

De Grood M. Het plomberen van restholden na osteomyelitis met bone-chips. Ned Tijdschr Geneeskd 1947;91:2192–2196

Frommelt L. Periprosthetic infection—bacteria and the interface between prosthesis and bone. In: Learmonth ID, ed. Interfaces in Total Hip Arthroplasty. London: Springer; 2000

Frommelt L, Renzig-Köhler K, Fenner T. Gentamicinhaltige Knochenzemente – In-vitro-Vergleich der Elution von Gentamicin aus unterschiedlichen Spezialitäten. Krankenhauspharmazie 2003;24:320–324

Gehrke T, von Foerster G, Frommelt L. Pharmacokinetic study of a gentamicin/clindamycin bone cement used in one-stage revision arthroplasty. In: Walenkamp GHIM, Murray DW, eds. Bone Cements and Cementing Technique. Berlin: Springer Verlag; 2001

Gristina AG. Biomaterial-centered infection: microbial adhesion versus tissue integration. Science 1987;237(4822):1588–1595

Josefsson G, Kolmert L. Prophylaxis with systematic antibiotics versus gentamicin bone cement in total hip arthroplasty. A ten-year survey of 1,688 hips. Clin Orthop Relat Res 1993;292(292):210–214

Kirst HA, Thompson DG, Nicas TI. Historical yearly usage of vancomycin. Antimicrob Agents Chemother 1998;42(5):1303–1304

Klemm K. Gentamicin-PMMA-beads in treating bone and soft tissue infections (author's transl). [Article in German] Zentralbl Chir 1979;104(14):934–942

Kovacevic B. [Problem of hematogenous osteomyelitis.]. Langenbecks Arch Klin Chir Ver Dtsch Z Chir 1953;276:432–443

Lindner B. Physikalische Analyse des Freisetzungsmechanismus von Chemotherapeutika aus dotiertem Polymethylmetacrylat. Inaugural dissertation, Kiel, 1981

Law HT, Fleming RH, Gilmore MFX, McCarthy ID, Hughes SP. In vitro measurement and computer modelling of the diffusion of antibiotic in bone cement. J Biomed Eng 1986;8(2):149–155

Mackey D, Varlet A, Debeaumont D. Antibiotic loaded plaster of Paris pellets: an in vitro study of a possible method of local antibiotic therapy in bone infection. Clin Orthop Relat Res 1982;167(167):263–268

McMaster WC. Technique for intraoperative construction of PMMA spacer in total knee revision. Am J Orthop 1995;24(2):178–180

Oxborrow NJ, Stamer J, Andrews M, Stone MH. New uses for gentamicin-impregnated polymethyl methacrylate spacers in two-stage revision hip arthroplasty. J Arthroplasty 1997;12(6):709–710

Prigge EK. The treatment of chronic osteomyelitis by use of muscle transplant or iliac graft. J Bone Joint Surg Am 1946;28:576–593

Steinbrink K, Frommelt L. Treatment of periprosthetic infection of the hip using one-stage exchange surgery. [Article in German] Orthopade 1995;24(4):335–343

Sutherland IW. Bacterial exopolysaccharides—their nature and production. In: Sutherland IW, ed. Surface carbohydrates of the prokaryotic cell. London: Academic Press; 1977

Winkler H, Janata O, Berger C, Wein W, Georgopoulos A. In vitro release of vancomycin and tobramycin from impregnated human and bovine bone grafts. J Antimicrob Chemother 2000;46(3):423–428

Zimmerli W, Lew PD, Waldvogel FA. Pathogenesis of foreign body infection. Evidence for a local granulocyte defect. J Clin Invest 1984;73(4):1191–1200

Prophylaxis and Therapy of Infections with Resistant Pathogens ____

H. Breithaupt

Introduction ___

Nosocomial infections in emergency surgery and orthopedics primarily concern wound infections and postoperative infections of the bones and joints. Errors in antibiotic therapy and hygiene can lead to an increase in infections with resistant pathogens.

Antibiotic Prophylaxis ___

The **goal** of perioperative antibiotic prophylaxis is to reduce the number of pathogens and inhibit their growth at the operation site to prevent wound infections and their complications.

Antibiotics are administered in a sufficiently high dose as a short infusion immediately before the operation begins. The antibiotic of choice is **cefazolin**, which is effective against *S. aureus* and normal enterobacteria (like *E. coli*). Broad-spectrum antibiotics are not superior to cefazolin for prophylaxis. They are considerably more expensive and lead more often to resistance.

Only intraoperative antibiotic prophylaxis is needed; postoperative prophylaxis makes no sense. Postoperative prophylaxis administered until drains are removed does not lower the incidence of infections, but promotes the development of nosocomial infections with resistant pathogens.

Prophylactic administration of antibiotics longer than 2 days leads to a selection of resistant organisms, which can then be passed on from patient to patient so that the prophylactic regime on the affected ward must repeatedly be changed due to new cases of resistance (**Table 4.8**).

General rules for antibiotic prophylaxis:
- **Begin** antibiotic administration immediately before the operation (e.g., during the beginning of anesthesia)
- Only administer antibiotics **during** the operation (if the operation lasts longer than 3 hours, give another 2 g cefazolin)
- **Do not administer postoperative prophylaxis** (except for open fractures or severely contaminated wounds)

Table 4.8 Antibiotics in emergency surgery and orthopedic surgery

Arthroscopy	No prophylaxis
Operations on the hip and other "clean" surgical interventions	2 g cefazolin
Open fractures or severely polluted wounds	3 × 2 g cefazolin + 3 × 0.6 g clindamycin or: 3 × 3 g ampicillin/sulbactam for 1–3 days
Extensive gunshot, stab, or crush injuries	Prophylaxis against gangrene with 3 × 10 mil. IU penicillin G (or 3 × 0.6 g clindamycin)

- **Relatives** may enter the room without a protective apron. They must disinfect their hands before leaving the room.
- **Transport** the patient on a rolling stretcher or in a wheelchair; wash down afterwards and change the linen. The patient, especially the mobile patient, should disinfect his/her hands before leaving the room. Accompanying personnel must know and apply hygienic measures to control multiresistant pathogens. This also applies to personnel in the department of destination, who must be informed of the arrival of a patient with multiresistant pathogens in advance. Diagnostic and therapeutic measures can, but do not have to be, scheduled at the end of the program. Patients with infected wounds should receive a fresh dressing before being transported.
- **Examining instruments**, like thermometers, blood-pressure cuffs, tourniquets, and stethoscopes, may only leave the room and be used on other patients after sufficient disinfection.

- Change **bed linen** twice a week and, of course, more often when dirty. It should be removed without releasing particles into the air if possible and put into a laundry bag placed next to the bed. According to accident-prevention regulations, laundry of patients with multiresistant pathogens does not belong in the so-called infectious laundry. Blankets and pillows are sent to the laundry at the end of the patient's stay.
- Dispose of **dressing material** and all **garbage** in the normal hospital garbage (no infectious garbage).
- Transport **instruments** to the central sterilization department without previous disinfection and put into the cleaning and disinfecting machines without any direct manipulation. If they remain on the ward for a while (weekend), the instruments should be completely covered with cleansing solution in the transport container.
- If necessary, perform **room disinfection** continuously with normal disinfectants in the usual concentration. Final disinfection should include all horizontal surfaces in the room.

Special Measures for MRSA

MRSA currently plays a prominent role in comparison to other multiresistant pathogens due to its **frequent occurrence**.

> **NOTE**
>
> MRSA could be more effectively combated with less frequent use of reserve antibiotics and good standard hygiene than by applying special isolation measures to patients colonized with MRSA.

The decisive factor in the transmission of *S. aureus* and, thereby, for MRSA is **transmission by the hands of personnel**. Airborne transmission is far less important and is probably more common in droplets than dust.

The **natural colonization with *S. aureus*** is primarily in the nose and secondarily in other moist body parts, like the perineum, groin, and armpit. Persistent nasal colonization with *S. aureus* is present in 20% of the population, and intermittent colonization has been found in 60%. Twenty percent have no adhesion molecules and therefore are never colonized by *S. aureus*. Nasal and perineal colonization need not be simultaneous.

The **worldwide spread of MRSA** is probably a result of MRSA selection during antibiotic treatment and is secondarily a result of pathogen spread due to deficient hygiene.

Patients at risk of MRSA are above all those with natural colonization by *S. aureus* who have been hospitalized for a long time and had contact with other MRSA carriers or received long-term antibiotic treatment.

Selective screening of patients at risk of MRSA when they are admitted to hospital and also during their hospital stay should help to limit the spread of MRSA on the wards. Examining personnel for MRSA should only take place if the above-described measures to control the infection prove insufficient to hinder transmission *and* if the epidemiologic correlation indicates the presence of a MRSA carrier in the surroundings, for example, more frequent postoperative infections. Only then does general screening make sense. MRSA species identified in screening should be compared with those isolated from patients by means of typing. Colonized personnel should only be treated with mupirocin if the epidemiologic correlation has been confirmed. During screening normally only the nose is examined, although transmission usually occurs through the hands of the personnel. It must also be remembered that most colonizations are transient and only last for a few days.

Decontamination of MRSA colonization applies above all to decolonization of the anterior nasal passage. Treatment with the antibiotic **mupirocin** (2–3 times a day for 5 days) is usually sufficient for decolonization, but rapid recolonization is possible. Administration of mupirocin is only necessary when there is an outbreak of MRSA.

Decolonization of the nose with **PVP-iodine** ointment offers a promising alternative to mupirocin. **Washing the entire body with antiseptic solutions** (like Scinsan scrub foam) could contribute to decontamination of a person colonized with bacteria, but wounds chronically contaminated with MRSA cannot be included in the cleansing. Before this procedure is generally recommended, the results of long-term observations should be evaluated, as a disturbance of the normal skin flora by antiseptic baths can be expected and may result in colonization of the skin with potentially pathogenic organisms.

Measures to be taken for patients with MRSA:
- **Single room**, especially for patients with secreting wounds, tracheostoma, or urinary catheters (with confirmed MRSA at these sites), as well as children or confused individuals with insufficient personal hygiene.
- Oral and written **information** concerning the MSRA-contaminated patients.
- Rational **antibiotic therapy**
- **Good standard hygiene when dealing with any patient:**
  - **Hand hygiene:** hand disinfection during patient care and use of disposable gloves if necessary.
  - **Instruments**, like endoscopes, must be thoroughly disinfected or sterilized between patients. Stethoscopes can be sprayed with an alcohol-based disinfectant. Tourniquets and blood-pressure cuffs should be used on the same patient.
  - Perform **screening** for MRSA weekly on patients at risk on the following body parts: nasal passages, perineum or groin, wounds, skin lesions, sputum (if patient coughs) tracheal secretions (intubation, tracheostoma), and urine (urinary catheter).
  - **Control swabs** can be taken at 24- or 48-hour intervals. The patient can be considered MRSA negative after three negative smears.
- The same **diagnostic and therapeutic options** must be available for patients with confirmed MRSA as for other patients.

- Patients contaminated with MRSA can be **discharged**, as the virulence of MRSA germs differs in no way from normal *S. aureus* bacteria. Relatives of medical personnel are also not exposed to a greater risk due to professional exposure.
- Patients with MRSA can be transferred to **rehabilitation** and **long-term nursing care** facilities and **homes for the aged** as soon as their clinical situation permits. No particular measures are required for transport other than standard hygiene.

- Patients colonized with pathogens should only have single rooms in homes or rehabilitation facilities if they have open wounds and this does not hamper their rehabilitation. Contaminated patients can use all social facilities in the home together with other inhabitants.

Further Reading

Anonymous. Kann die Ausbreitung von multiresistenten Bakterien in Krankenhäusern vermindert werden? Zeitschrift für Chemotherapie 1996;17:9–11

Anonymous. Surveillance nosokomialer Infektionen sowie die Erfassung von Erregern mit speziellen Resistenzen und Multiresistenzen. Bundesgesundheitsblatt Gesundheitsforschung Gesundheitsschutz 2000;43:887–890

Fitzner J, Kappstein I, Dziekan G, Gastmeier P, Daschner F, Rüden H. Hygiene methods for patients with methicillin-resistant Staphylococcus aureus (MRSA). [Article in German] Dtsch Med Wochenschr 2000;125(12):368–371

Gould IM. Antibiotic policies and control of resistance. Curr Opin Infect Dis 2002;15(4):395–400

Holländer R. ORSA, MRSA und ORSE. Humanmedizinische Bedeutung und Biologie der Staphylokokken. Klinikarzt 2002;31:285–289

Kappstein J. Nosokomiale Infektionen. Prävention, Labor-Diagnostik, Antimikrobielle Therapie. 2nd ed. Munich: W. Zuckschwerdt Verlag; 2002

Perl TM, Cullen JJ, Wenzel RP, et al. Mupirocin and the Risk of Staphylococcus aureus Study Team. Intranasal mupirocin to prevent postoperative Staphylococcus aureus infections. N Engl J Med 2002;346(24):1871–1877

5

Surgical Treatment of Osteomyelitis

Acute and Chronic Post-traumatic Osteomyelitis

R. Schnettler

Diagnosis of Acute Osteomyelitis (Early Infection)

NOTE

Early diagnosis of an acute infection depends on clinical signs and regular wound assessment.

NOTE

Clinical suspicion of an early infection after internal fracture fixation or operative joint replacement constitutes an urgent, nondeferable indication for operative revision.

The main clinical symptoms of acute osteomyelitis are the basis of early diagnosis and consist of:

- Redness
- Swelling
- Pain
- Local warmth

Laboratory tests showing continued elevation or renewed rise in inflammatory markers—leukocyte count, erythrocyte sedimentation rate (ESR), and C-reactive protein (CRP)—indicate the presence of an early infection.

Preoperative Preparations

- Radiographs
- Laboratory tests:
  - ESR
  - CRP
  - leukocyte count
  - differential blood count
- Smear
- Blood culture if necessary
- Informed consent:
  - explanation of the entire treatment concept, as well as the risk of
    - recurrence
    - amputation
    - cancer

Emergency treatment in case of:

- Bacteremia
- Septic shock
- Empyema of the joint

Surgical Procedure

Surgical intervention by primary debridement of the bone and soft tissues is the first step in treating osteomyelitis.

This requires not only basic surgical equipment (**Fig. 5.1**), but also special instruments (**Fig. 5.2**). The basic equipment for septic surgery consists of a scalpel and bone forceps (rongeur, Stille-Luer bone rongeur) and, above all, chisels and curettes of different sizes and shapes.

Self-cooling rose-head burrs and bone shavers of different sizes, as well as pulsed jet lavage, complement the basic equipment.

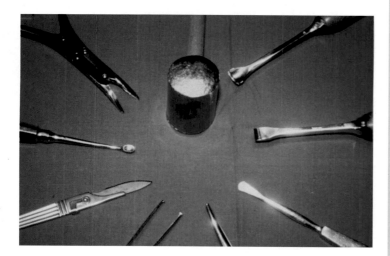

Fig. 5.1 Basic instruments

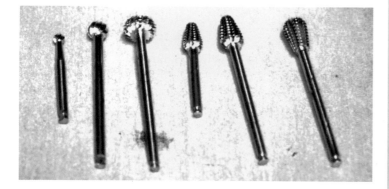

Fig. 5.2 Special instruments

Primary Interventions on Bones and Soft Tissues

Intraoperative filling of a fistulous tract by injecting indigo carmine or methyl blue through a button cannula facilitates dissection (**Figs. 5.3**, **5.4**, **5.5**, **5.6**, **5.7**, **5.8**, **5.9**).

Always take biopsies for histologic examination. Differential diagnoses include: Ewing sarcoma, squamous-

Fig. 5.9 It is essential to take an intraoperative smear for identification of the pathogen(s) and to perform an antibiogram. Additional tissue samples are taken for microbiologic and histologic examination.

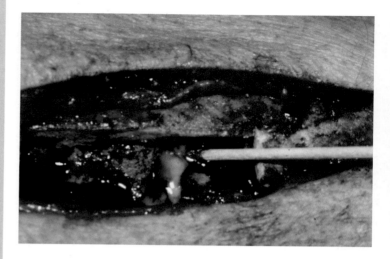

cell carcinoma, and plasma-cell osteomyelitis (**Figs. 5.10, 5.11, 5.12, 5.13, 5.14, 5.15, 5.16**).

Arrest the blood supply with a tourniquet to obtain a clear view for dissection. Before finishing the operation, release the tourniquet to control bone perfusion. Check vital bone for display of punctate bleeding; if this is not seen, further debridement is necessary.

Antibiotic chains should always be placed at the deepest point in the medullary cavity to ensure an adequate antibiotic level.

Use an overflow drain; otherwise the antibiotic will be suctioned off. Fracture stabilization is maintained with external fixation to avoid the risk of reinfection when using plates or nails.

Fig. 5.10 The medullary cavity is radically debrided using special instruments. Necrotic, infected osseous material is completely removed.

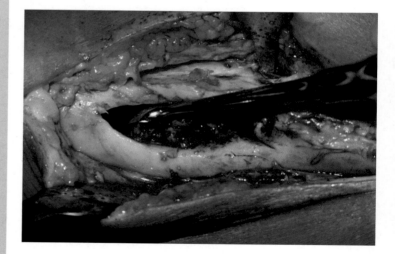

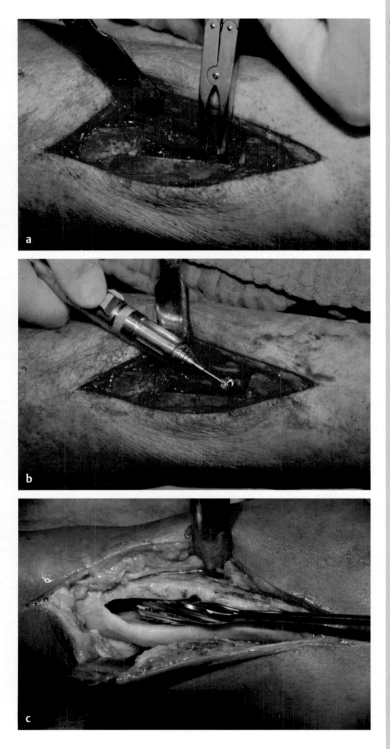

Fig. 5.11a–c Using a rongeur and Stille-Luer bone rongeur (**a**), water-cooled shaver (**b**), and medullary-cavity burr (**c**) facilitates complete debridement of the medullary cavity in both a proximal and distal direction.

Fig. 5.12 For the final removal of tissue debris and reduction of the number of pathogens, the medullary cavity and surrounding soft tissue are irrigated with pulsed jet lavage.

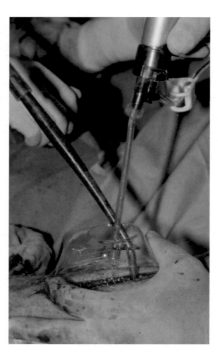

Fig. 5.13 Placement of a local antibiotic chain ensures a highly effective local tissue level of antibiotic.

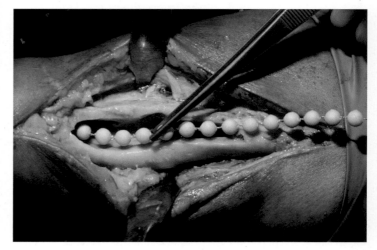

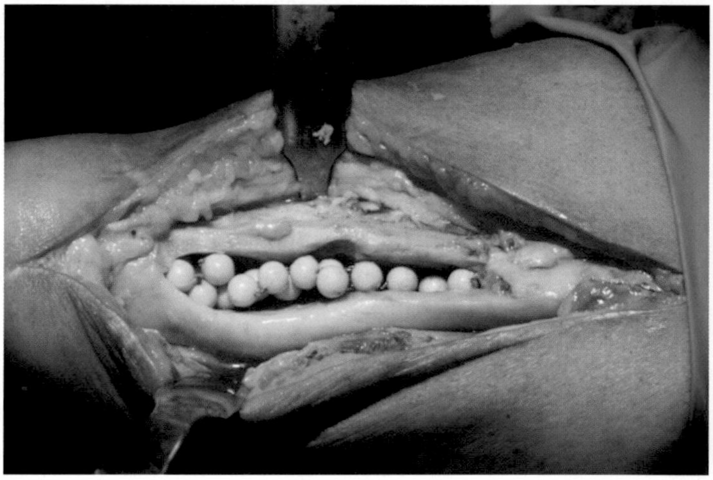

Fig. 5.14 Intraoperative site with gentamicin-PMMA chain in place.

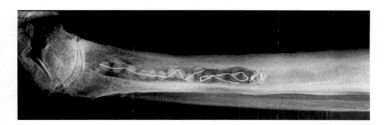

Fig. 5.15 Postoperative radiographic control following implantation of a gentamicin-PMMA chain.

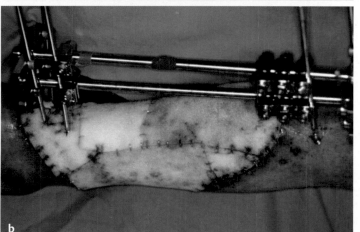

Fig. 5.16a, b Wound closure must always be without tension. This is achieved either with a primary skin suture (**a**) or with the aid of polyurethane foam or a flap (**b**). Wound secretion is removed with an overflow drain.

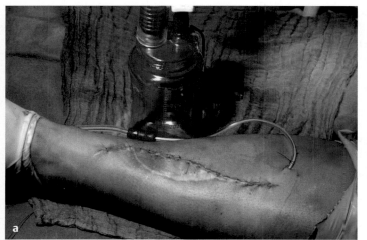

Therapeutic Concept in Acute Osteomyelitis (Early Infection)

The complex problems encountered in acute and chronic osteomyelitis can generally only be treated gradually. Only bone consolidation and reconstruction of the surrounding soft tissues can restore the function of the affected extremity. Early surgical revision is unconditionally indicated at the first appearance of clinical signs of a disturbance in wound healing and beginning infection or

Fig. 5.17a–c Chronic infection of bone and soft tissues.

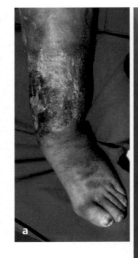
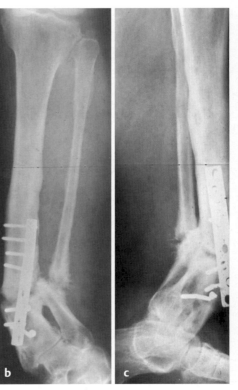

postoperative hematoma formation. Only then will it be possible to maintain the internal fracture fixation and effectively combat the infection. Stability is of great importance for both fracture healing and removal of the focus of infection; stability delays the spread of infection (Burri 1979, Klemm 1979, Klemm & Schnettler 1992, Klemm 1993, Schnettler 1997).

Early Infection of Plate Osteosynthesis

Early surgical intervention combined with local antibiotic treatment has proven useful in the treatment of early infection after internal plate fixation.

Operative revision is a complicated procedure and requires a high level of responsibility and experience. The cause of the infection must be identified and removed. Such operations must always be extensive and not be limited to simply opening an infected hematoma.

Operative revision is always performed in a series of steps, including the sequential removal of biopsies for bacteriologic examination (**Figs. 5.18, 5.19, 5.20, 5.21, 5.22**).

Pathogens can often be identified with the polymerase chain reaction (PCR), even when smears have produced no results. However, PCR is very susceptible to contamination, which can lead to false-positive results.

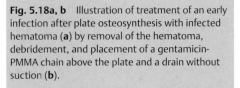

Fig. 5.18a, b Illustration of treatment of an early infection after plate osteosynthesis with infected hematoma (**a**) by removal of the hematoma, debridement, and placement of a gentamicin-PMMA chain above the plate and a drain without suction (**b**).

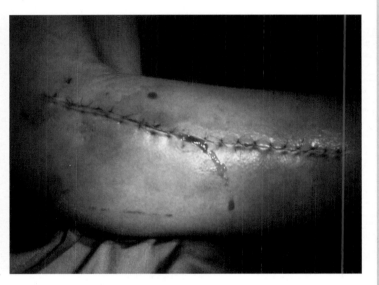

Fig. 5.19 Clinical picture of early infection of a plate osteosynthesis of the humerus with wound drainage 6 days postoperative.

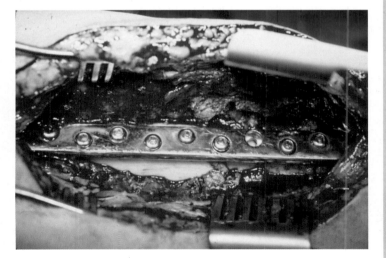

Fig. 5.20 Open the full length of the operative wound, remove all suture material, and take a smear and a biopsy for microbiology and histology.

NOTE

Now is the time to administer antibiotics.

Fig. 5.21 Thorough debridement with complete removal of loose bone fragments and avital tissue.

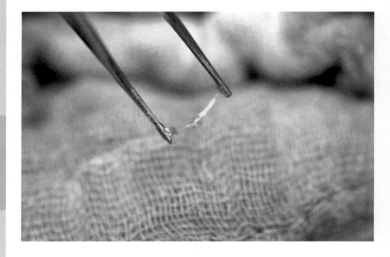

NOTE

If the internal fixation is stable, it can remain in situ. If unstable, an external fixator must be attached before removing the plate to avoid gross dislocations.

Fig. 5.22 Place gentamicin-PMMA chain in a single or double row above the plate (Septopal).

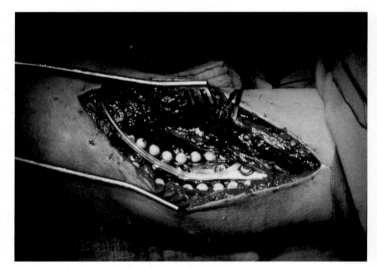

First Step: Clean Out the Infection

Remove the infected hematoma (jet lavage [see also **Fig. 5.12**], brush), test the stability of the implanted material (each individual screw, see also **Fig. 5.20**), and test the viability of all tissues (punctate bleeding from bones and tendons, vital color, and consistency of tissues) (**Figs. 5.23, 5.24**).

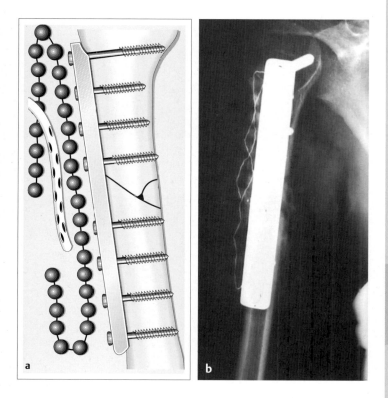

Fig. 5.23a, b An overflow drain (without vacuum) leaves the wound through the skin (**a**). Place a resorbable antibiotic carrier in any of the recesses, if necessary. Take a control radiograph with the gentamicin-PMMA chain in place (**b**).

NOTE

The gentamicin-PMMA (polymethylmethacrylate) chain is left in place until the fracture fixation devices (metal) have been removed.

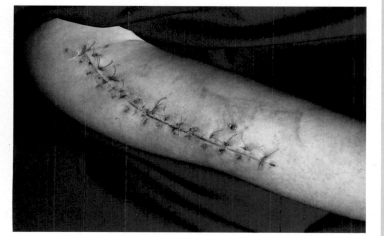

Fig. 5.24 Only the skin should be sutured if an infection exists.

Second Step: Bone Consolidation (Figs. 5.25, 5.26):

Fig. 5.25   Open the operation wound to its full extent. Remove the gentamicin-PMMA chain, the screws, and the plates. Take a smear and biopsies for microbiology and histology. Curette the plate bed and the screw canals. Irrigate the wound cavity (with jet lavage if necessary). Place a resorbable antibiotic fleece in the plate bed if necessary. Drain without vacuum (overflow drain). Suture the skin.

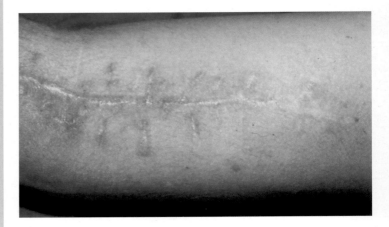

Fig. 5.26a, b   Bone consolidation without infection.

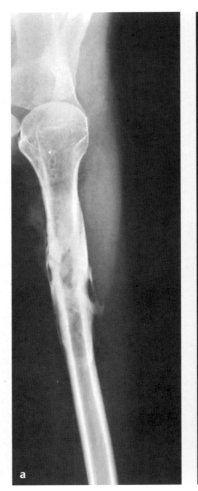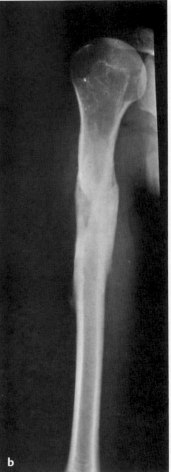

NOTE

Undisturbed healing with complete and lasting eradication of the infection cannot be expected if avital fragments remain under the plate as a result of disturbed periosteal perfusion.

If this is the case, proceed according to the procedure described in Therapeutic Concept in Chronic Osteomyelitis with Defects up to 4 cm, page 115.

Early Infection after Intramedullary Nailing

The treatment strategy for early infection after intramedullary nailing depends on the implant used. Intramedullary nails that have not been reamed should be removed, whereas reamed intramedullary nails should be left in place. Both procedures, as already described for early infection of plate osteosynthesis, involve opening all operative wounds and thorough debridement. This includes opening the proximal and distal incisions for the intramedullary nail.

Nonreamed Intramedullary Nails

Nonreamed intramedullary nails which have become infected early should be removed (**Figs. 5.27, 5.28, 5.29, 5.30, 5.31, 5.32**).

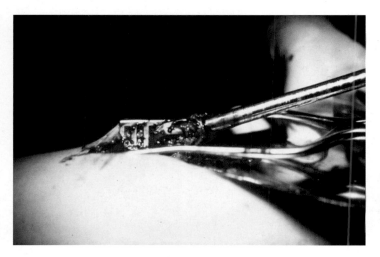

Fig. 5.27 After removal of the nail, debridement of the medullary cavity by drilling with a burr 1–2 mm larger than the diameter of the intramedullary nail. Jet lavage of the medullary cavity.

TIPS AND TRICKS

Remove reaming debris from the drill head for bacteriologic examination.

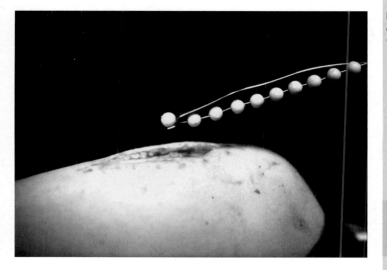

Fig. 5.28 Placement with an applicator of a gentamicin-PMMA chain of appropriate length into the medullary channel.

NOTE

Now is the time to administer an antibiotic.

Fig. 5.29a, b   The end of the gentamicin-PMMA chain should always be placed at the deepest point in the medullary canal to ensure that the antibiotic reaches the entire length of the canal.

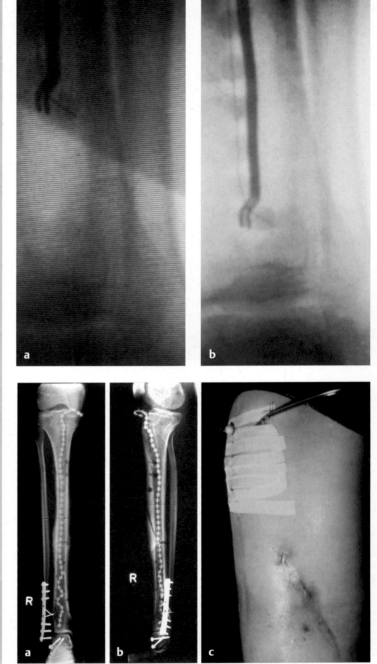

Fig. 5.30a–c   The end of the gentamicin-PMMA chain is left outside of the surgical wound. An overflow drain in placed in the proximal medullary canal. Reosteosynthesis is performed either by means of a reamed intramedullary nail (femur or tibia) or with external fixation (tibia).

NOTE

Reosteosynthesis only after two smears have revealed no pathogens from, for example, irrigation fluid.

Fig. 5.31   Begin gradually removing the chain from the 5th day until complete removal is achieved on the 10th postoperative day, or remove the entire chain on the 10th postoperative day.

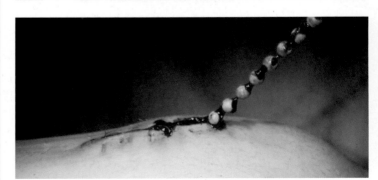

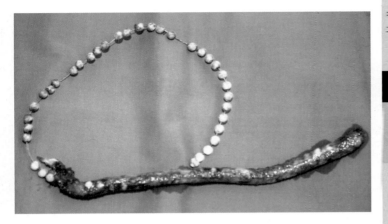

Fig. 5.32 Gentamicin-PMMA chain with granulation tissue (20 days in situ).

ERRORS AND RISKS

The beads can become encased in granulation tissue if the chain is removed too late. In this case the chain cannot be pulled out or it tears.

As an alternative to local antibiotic treatment, suction/irrigation drainage, which has been used for the past four decades, can be applied after removing the intramedullary nail and minimal reaming. This procedure provides mechanical cleaning of the infected region, which is decisive. Not only debris, but also bacteria should be washed away. Prerequisite for the success of the procedure is correct placement of the draining tubes (**Fig. 5.33**).

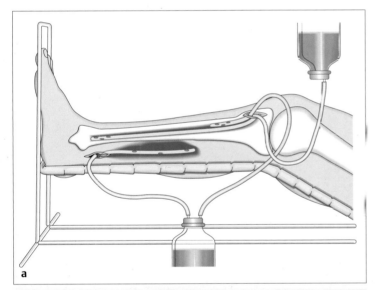

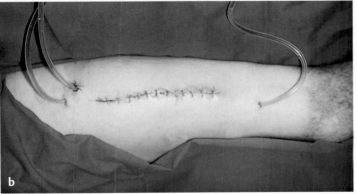

Fig. 5.33a, b
a Place the inflow drainage tube at the deepest point (distal) in the medullary canal and the outflow drain in the proximal medullary canal. Irrigate daily with approximately 3 l.
b Clinical situs

After 3 days, both ends of the drains are attached to Redon bottles.

Smears are taken from the irrigation fluid, but the drains remain in place until the bacteriologic result is available.

If no pathogens have been identified, the drains are removed after 48 hours.

If pathogens have been identified, the suction/irrigation drainage is continued.

Reamed Intramedullary Nails

Reamed intramedullary nails which have become infected early should be left in place. The fundamental operative procedures concerning opening operation wounds and debridement are no different from those of nonreamed intramedullary nails.

First Step: Clean Out the Infection

The status of the infection and the effectiveness of the first operation can be evaluated in the second intervention 24–48 hours later by means of the following procedures:

- Open all wounds
- Remove the gentamicin-PMMA stick
- Irrigate the interior of the intramedullary nail again (with jet lavage if necessary) (**Fig. 5.34**).
- Take a smear of the irrigation fluid (with biopsies if necessary)
- Clean and reimplant the gentamicin stick (**Fig. 5.35**)
- Remove the stick 10 days later without anesthesia (**Fig. 5.36**)

Fig. 5.34 Irrigate the inside of the intramedullary nail with jet lavage if necessary. Take a smear of the irrigation fluid.

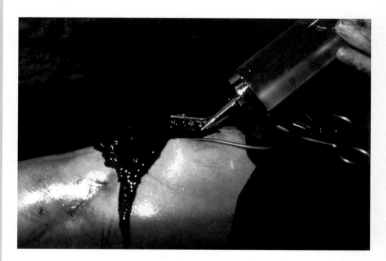

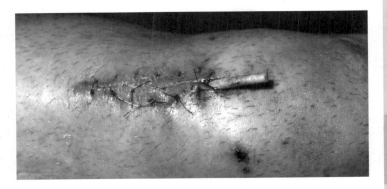

Fig. 5.35 Push a gentamicin-PMMA stick (patient-specific production by Biomet, Berlin, Germany) into the middle of the intramedullary nail. The end of the stick should protrude through the skin. Place an overflow drain in the proximal end of the nail.

NOTE

Planned operative revision is obligatory after 24–48 hours in this procedure.

Next Step: Bone Consolidation

As an alternative to the above procedure, the irrigation-vacuum drainage system can be used as described when the intramedullary nail is left in place.

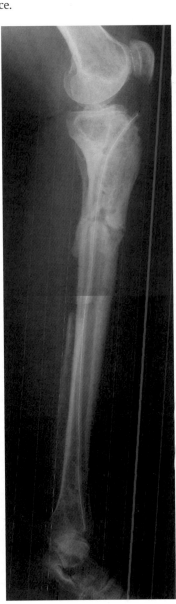

Fig. 5.36 Remove the nail and the locking pins. Carefully ream the medullary cavity. Irrigate again, with jet lavage if necessary. Take a smear from the irrigation fluid and biopsies, if necessary. Insert a gentamicin-PMMA stick into the medullary canal. Remove the stick 10 days later without anesthesia.

NOTE

Open wound treatment or combining local antibiotics with a suction/irrigation drainage system is contraindicated. This leads to loss of an effective antibiotic concentration and the development of resistant pathogens.

Diagnosis of Chronic Osteomyelitis (Late Infection)

Take a thorough medical history including all injuries, operations, hospital stays, and previously identified pathogens.

Physical examination:
- General signs of inflammation:
  - redness
  - swelling
  - pain
  - hyperemia
- Local findings:
  - fistula
  - secretion
  - instability of bone
  - loosening of fracture fixation devices / prostheses
- Laboratory values:
  - ESR
  - CRP
  - blood count
- Preoperative smear of the fistula
- Imaging diagnosis:
  - standard films
  - computed tomography (CT) if necessary
  - magnetic resonance imaging (MRI) if necessary
  - fill fistulous tract with a contrast agent (fistulography) if necessary
- Bone scan (see Chapter 3, Diagnosis of Bone Inflammations with Nuclear Medicine Techniques, p. 54)

Therapeutic Concept in Chronic Osteomyelitis (Late Infection)

Late Infection after Plate Osteosynthesis

The following procedures are recommended for late infection after plate osteosynthesis with bone consolidation:
- Remove the plate and the screws (**Fig. 5.37**)
- Take smears and biopsies (for microbiologic and histologic examination)
- Perform radical debridement of the plate bed and screw holes
- Irrigate (with jet lavage, if necessary)
- Apply local antibiotics (resorbable antibiotic carriers, gentamicin-PMMA chain)
- Insert an overflow drain
- Suture the skin

The further operative procedure depends on the size of the defect (pp. 115–125).

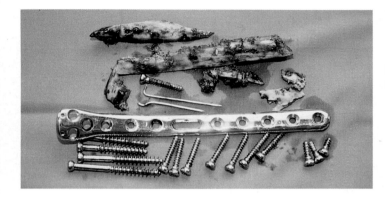

Fig. 5.37 Remove all avital bone particles and all implants.

Late Infection after Intramedullary Nailing

Late infection after intramedullary nailing with bone consolidation is a good indication for short-term local antibiotics (gentamicin-PMMA chain, Septopal).

After removing the intramedullary nail it is very important to carefully ream the medullary canal with a bone-marrow burr 1–2 mm larger than the circumference of the removed nail (gentle debridement). This releases marginal lamellar intramural sequestra, which can then be washed out of the medullary cavity with intensive irrigation (jet lavage, if necessary) (**Figs. 5.38 and 5.39**).

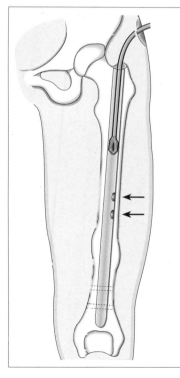

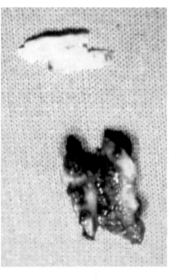

Fig. 5.38 Diagram of lamellar sequester in the medullary cavity.

Fig. 5.39 Lamellar sequester

NOTE

Lamellar, intramural sequestra are avital and therefore constitute the starting point for recurrent bouts of infection.

NOTE

This is a typical late complication following previous infection after intramedullary nailing.

The operative procedure is exactly the same as that described in the section Early Infection after Intramedullary Nailing: Nonreamed Intramedullary Nails, p. 107).

Encapsulated Phlegmons of Medullary Cavities

These are encapsulated foci of infection that are completely surrounded by bone without local signs of inflammation. Pain at rest during the night in the affected extremity and a medical history of intramedullary nailing are indicators of this type of infection. Radiographs often reveal an osteolytic focus. A bone scan is generally positive (**Figs. 5.40, 5.41, 5.42**).
- Localize the encapsulated bone abscess with exploratory drill holes
- Pus often escapes under pressure

Fig. 5.40 Pus from the bore hole.

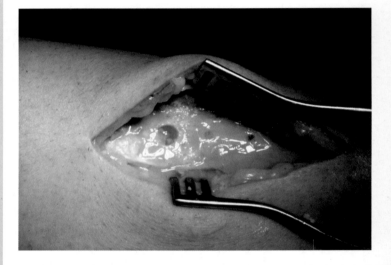

Fig. 5.41 Oval trepanation. Radical debridement.

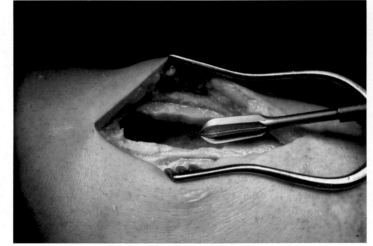

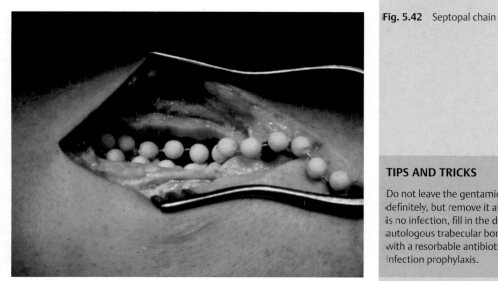

Fig. 5.42 Septopal chain

TIPS AND TRICKS

Do not leave the gentamicin-PMMA chain in indefinitely, but remove it after 4–6 weeks. If there is no infection, fill in the defect, if necessary, with autologous trabecular bone, which can be mixed with a resorbable antibiotic carrier and serves as infection prophylaxis.

- Perform ovular trepanation
- Take smears and biopsies
- Perform radical debridement
- Irrigate (jet lavage if necessary)
- Implant a gentamicin-PMMA chain in the cavity
- Place an overflow drain

Therapeutic Concept in Chronic Osteomyelitis with Defects up to 4 cm

First Step: Clean Out the Infection

1. In the bone:
- Remove metal
- Perform radical debridement and sequestrotomy
- Take smears and biopsies
- Perform stable reosteosynthesis (change of procedure)
- Reduce the number of pathogens with pulsed jet lavage
- Apply local antibiotics (gentamicin-PMMA chain, Septopal) or
- Perform suction/irrigation drainage in exceptional cases

NOTE

Only give an antibiotic after a smear has been taken.

2. In the soft tissues:
- Perform radical debridement
- Close the skin only temporarily (possibly as a vacuum seal)
- Perform serial revisions

TIPS AND TRICKS

Resorbable antibiotic carriers can be broken down into little pieces and mixed with the bone chips.

TIPS AND TRICKS

Perform preoperative angiography to explore possible vascular anastomosis.

Document the vascular status regarding an anastomosis before the operation begins.

The flap must be raised opposite to the vascular pedicle.

Second Step: Reconstruction

1. Of the bone (after 4–6 weeks)

- Perform a revision
- Remove the local antibiotic carrier (Septopal)
- Irrigate intraoperatively (possibly with jet lavage)
- Take smears and biopsies
- Perform autogenous bone grafting
- Perform reconstruction with allografts
- Fill in the defect with iliac-crest bone chips
- Use resorbable bone-replacement materials, possibly mixed with antibiotics
- Use resorbable bone matrix mixed with antibiotics

2. In the soft tissues

Perform the earliest possible definitive skin closure with a

- Split-skin graft
- Local graft, or
- Microvascular free flap (e. g., parascapular flap, latissimus dorsi flap) (see Chapter 6, p. 186 f and 203 f)

There are different ways to cover a bone and soft tissue defect (**Figs. 5.43, 5.44, 5.45, 5.46, 5.47, 5.48, 5.49, 5.50, 5.51, 5.52, 5.53, 5.54, 5.55**).

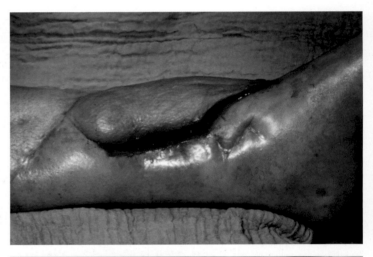

Fig. 5.43 The bone defect is exposed 4 weeks later at the earliest, the local antibiotic is removed, and intraoperative smears are taken. Four weeks earlier radical debridement was performed with administration of a local antibiotic and reconstruction of the soft-tissue defect with a parascapular flap.

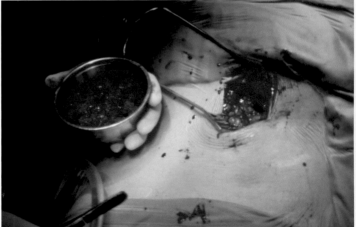

Fig. 5.44 The bone defect can be filled in loosely with autogenic chips of trabecular bone (possibly mixed with antibiotics). Here: harvesting from the posterior iliac crest. The high osteogenetic potency of autogenous trabecular bone generally achieves timely bone consolidation.

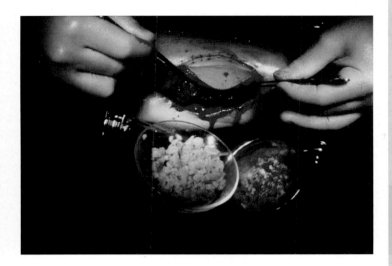

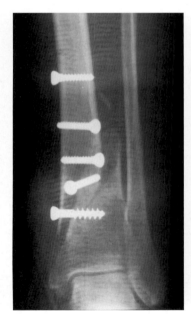

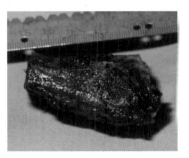

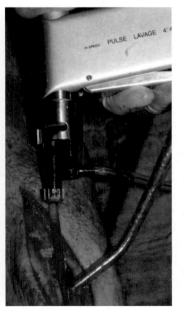

Fig. 5.45 If there are no autogenous trabecular bone chips available, cryoconserved or heat-stabilized trabecular bone can be used.

NOTE

Legally required laboratory tests must be performed.

Fig. 5.46 Bridging the defect with a tricortical bone graft from the iliac crest provides additional stability.

Fig. 5.47 A 54-year-old female with post-traumatic osteomyelitis after insufficient primary osteosynthesis.

Fig. 5.48 Debridement required. Smear taken and irrigation with pulsed jet lavage after metal removal.

Fig. 5.49 Radical debridement of the bone and soft tissues and local implantation of gentamicin-PMMA chain. Temporary wound closure with polyurethane foam and overflow drain. Temporary immobilization in a lower-leg cast and early secondary soft-tissue coverage with microvascular attachment of a parascapular flap.

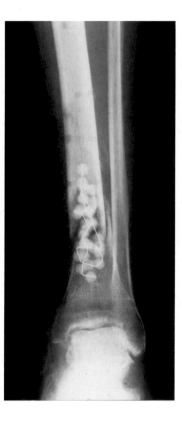

Fig. 5.50 After 4–6 weeks lift the flap across from the vascular anastomosis and remove the gentamicin-PMMA chain.

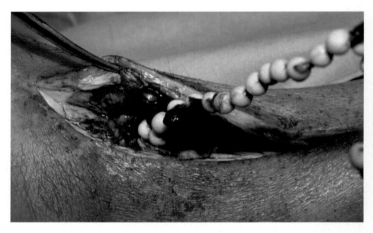

Fig. 5.51 Early secondary coverage of the soft-tissue defect with microvascular attachment of a parascapular flap. Press-fit implantation of a tricortical bone graft from the iliac crest.

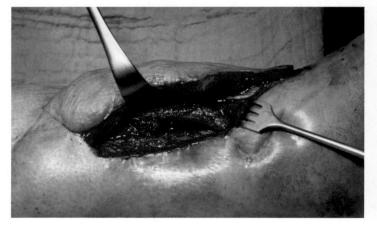

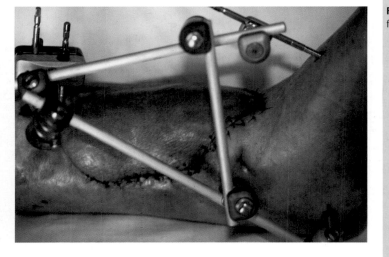

Fig. 5.52 Additional stabilization with external fixation.

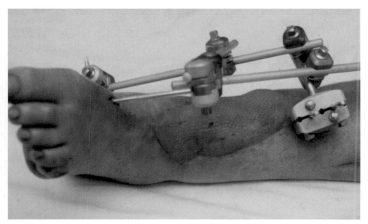

Fig. 5.53 Three months after early secondary flap transplant—soft tissues free of infection.

NOTE

Daily fixateur-pin care necessary.

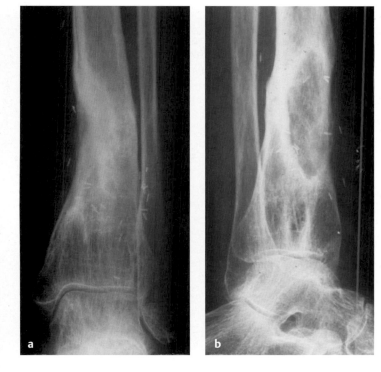

Fig. 5.54a,b One year later there is bone consolidation of the formerly infected nonunion, which is stable on weight bearing. The infection has healed.

Fig. 5.55 Clinical picture of healed area.

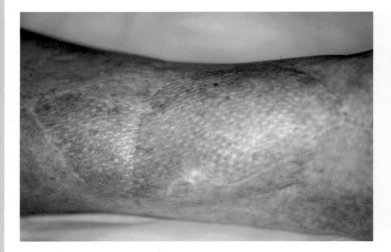

Therapeutic Concept in Chronic Osteomyelitis with a Defect Larger than 4 cm

First Step

Clean the wound as previously instructed.

Second Step

Perform reconstruction.

Of the bone (after 4–6 weeks):
- Perform a revision
- Remove the local antibiotic carrier (Septopal)
- Irrigate intraoperatively—possibly with jet lavage
- Take smears and biopsies
- Use bone chips from the ribs (**Fig. 5.56**)
- Use a free fibular flap (microvascular)
- Perform fibula-pro-tibia transposition (**Fig. 5.57a, b**)
- Perform stable reosteosynthesis with external fixation for callus distraction:
  - monosegmental transport
  - bisegmental transport
  - compression–distraction

Distraction is the method of first choice to bridge large bone defects in comparison to alternatives, like transplantation of rib chips, fibula-pro-tibia transposition, or microvascular bone transplantation. For a detailed discussion, see Callus Distraction, page 133 (**Figs. 5.58, 5.59**).

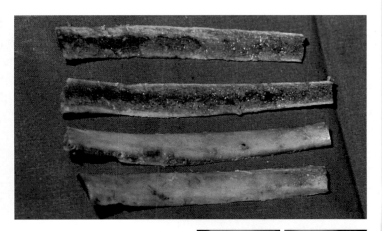

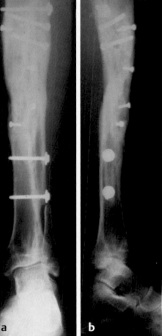

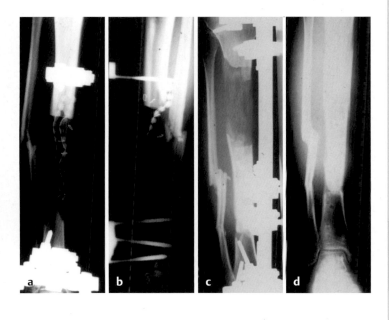

Fig. 5.56 Bone chips from ribs.

Fig. 5.57a, b Fibula-pro-tibia transposition.

Fig. 5.58a–d The monosegmental transport assembly for callus distraction requires proximal or distal corticotomy and stepwise transport of the segment in the defect.

NOTE

The daily transport distance is 1 mm in four individual steps of 0.25 mm each.

Fig. 5.59a–e The bisegmental transport assembly shortens treatment time by transporting both segments toward one another after proximal and distal corticotomy.

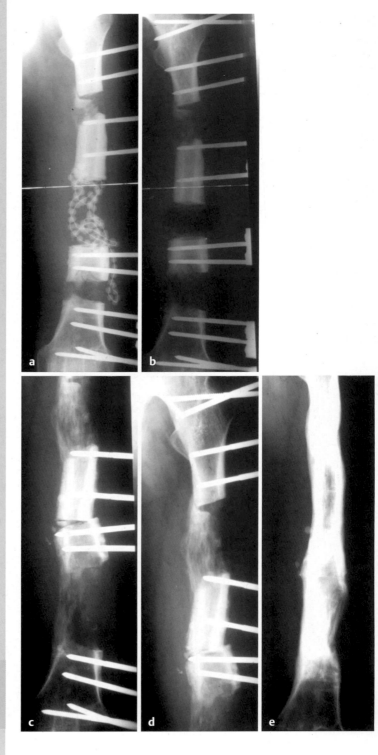

NOTE

Turn the screws 1 mm every day in individual steps of 0.25 mm.

Case Study

By shortening the defect, the compression–distraction assembly releases tension on the soft tissues. The shortened bone is lengthened by means of corticotomy and continuous distraction (**Figs. 5.60, 5.61, 5.62, 5.63**).

After 5 days begin tightening the screws: 4 × 0.25 mm daily

- Train the patient
- Write a plan for daily documentation of screw tightening and give it to the responsible person
- It takes twice as long for callus to mature after it has appeared

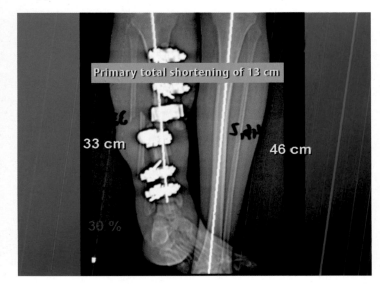

Primary total shortening of 13 cm

33 cm

46 cm

30 %

Fig. 5.60 A 34-year-old male with severe soft-tissue damage and a large bone defect. Chronic post-traumatic osteomyelitis. The compression–distraction assembly was attached after radical debridement of the soft tissue and bone resulted in a shortening of the tibia by 13 cm. Corticotomy.

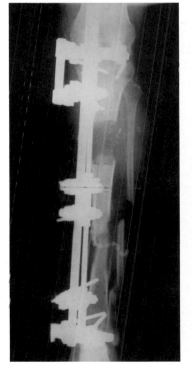

Fig. 5.61 Callus distraction to equalize the leg length by means of a Regazzoni external fixateur took 5 months.

TIPS AND TRICKS

Always choose a medial approach for corticotomy of the proximal tibia due to the good muscle perfusion.

Corticotomy is performed with primary stretching. Protect the periosteum.

Use a chisel. Single diverging drill holes can first be bored with a 2.7-mm drill during continuous rinsing with water for cooling.

Do not use an oscillating saw due to heat damage.

If the leg is shortened by more than one-fifth of the original length, there is risk of a disturbance in the venous drainage and kinking.

Fig. 5.62 Regazzoni fixator. Arrows indicate the Rendel screw, which was turned 0.25 mm 4 × daily.

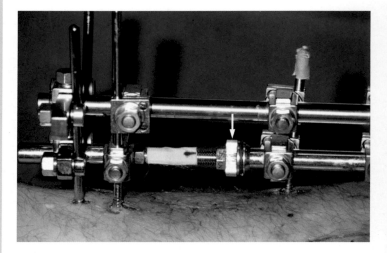

Fig. 5.63a, b No bone consolidation was observed at the docking site. Therefore, plate osteosynthesis was performed with autogenous bone grafting. The antibiotic chains were able to be left in place.

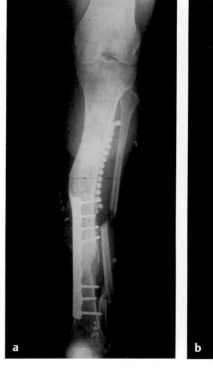
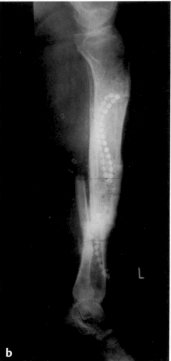

Bibliography

Blaha JD, Nelson CL, Frevert LF, et al. The use of septopal (polymethylmethacrylate beads with gentamicin) in the treatment of chronic osteomyelitis. Instr Course Lect 1990;39:509–514

Blaha JD, Calhoun JH, Nelson CL, et al. Comparison of the clinical efficacy and tolerance of gentamicin PMMA beads on surgical wire versus combined and systemic therapy for osteomyelitis. Clin Orthop Relat Res 1993;295(295):8–12

Bonnaire F, Hohaus T, Cyffka R, Lein T. Bone infections. [Article in German] Unfallchirurg 2002;105(8):716–731, quiz 731, 733

Burri C, Henkemeyer H, Spier W. The treatment of chronic osteomyelitis. Acta Orthop Belg 1975;41(2):235–243

Burri C. Posttraumatische Osteomyelitis. Bern: Huber; 1979

Calhoun JH, Mader JT. Antibiotic beads in the management of surgical infections. Am J Surg 1989;157(4):443–449

Calhoun JH, Henry SL, Anger DM, Cobos JA, Mader JT. The treatment of infected nonunions with gentamicin-polymethylmethacrylate antibiotic beads. Clin Orthop Relat Res 1993;295(295):23–27

Calhoun JH, Anger DM, Ledbetter BR, Cobos JA, Mader JT. The Ilizarov fixator and polymethylmethacrylate-antibiotic beads for the treatment of infected deformities. Clin Orthop Relat Res 1993;295(295):13–22

Cierny G III, Mader JT. Approach to adult osteomyelitis. Orthop Rev 1987;16(4):259–270

Cierny G III. Infected tibial nonunions (1981-1995). The evolution of change. Clin Orthop Relat Res 1999;360(360):97–105

Cottias P, Tomeno B, Anract P, Vinh TS, Forest M. Subacute osteomyelitis presenting as a bone tumour. A review of 21 cases. Int Orthop 1997;21(4):243–248

Dirschl DR, Almekinders LC. Osteomyelitis. Common causes and treatment recommendations. Drugs 1993;45(1):29–43

Gustilo RB, Merkow RL, Templeman D. The management of open fractures. J Bone Joint Surg Am 1990;72(2):299–304

Henry SL, Hood GA, Seligson D. Long-term implantation of gentamicin-polymethylmethacrylate antibiotic beads. Clin Orthop Relat Res 1993;295(295):47–53

Holtom PD, Smith AM. Introduction to adult posttraumatic osteomyelitis of the tibia. Clin Orthop Relat Res 1999;360(360):6–15

Khouri RK, Shaw WW. Reconstruction of the lower extremity with microvascular free flaps: a 10-year experience with 304 consecutive cases. J Trauma 1989;29(8):1086–1094

Klemm K. Gentamicin-PMMA-beads in treating bone and soft tissue infections (author's transl). [Article in German] Zentralbl Chir 1979;104(14):934–942

Klemm K. Indication, technic and results using the external fixator in infected fractures and infected pseudarthrosis. [Article in German] Langenbecks Arch Chir 1982;358:119–124

Klemm K, Schnettler R. The use of gentamicin-PMMA chains in the treatment of infected tibial nonunion. Acta Orthop Belg 1992;58(Suppl 1):222–226

Klemm KW. Antibiotic bead chains. Clin Orthop Relat Res 1993 295(295):63–76

Klemm K. The use of antibiotic-containing bead chains in the treatment of chronic bone infections. Clin Microbiol Infect 2001;7(1):28–31

Lazzarini L, De Lalla F, Mader JT. Long Bone Osteomyelitis. Curr Infec Dis Rep 2002;4(5):439–445

Mader J, Mohan D, Calhoun J. A practical guide to the diagnosis and management of bone and joint infections. Drugs 1997;54(2):253–264

Mader JT, Shirtliff ME, Calhoun JH. Staging and staging application in osteomyelitis. Clin Infect Dis 1997;25(6):1303–1309

Mader JT, Cripps MW, Calhoun JH. Adult posttraumatic osteomyelitis of the tibia. Clin Orthop Relat Res 1999; 360(360):14–21

Mader JT, Shirtliff ME, Bergquist SC, Calhoun J. Antimicrobial treatment of chronic osteomyelitis. Clin Orthop Relat Res 1999;360(360):47–65

Mader JT, Wang J, Calhoun JH. Antibiotic therapy for musculoskeletal infections. Instr Course Lect 2002;51:539–551

Ostermann PA, Henry SL, Seligson D. The role of local antibiotic therapy in the management of compound fractures. Clin Orthop Relat Res 1993;295(295):102–111

Ostermann PA, Seligson D, Henry SL. Local antibiotic therapy for severe open fractures. A review of 1085 consecutive cases. J Bone Joint Surg Br 1995;77(1):93–97

Perry CR, ed. Bone and Joint Infections. London: Martin Duritz; 1996

Schnettler R, Lieser H, Klemm K. Chirurgische Behandlung der posttraumatischen chronischen Osteomyelitis. Akt Chir 1997;32:18–22

Schulte J, Burri C. Treatment results using PMMA-chains in Ulm. [Article in German] Aktuelle Probl Chir Orthop 1979; (12):158–160

Seligson D. Orthopedic infections. Orthopedics 1994;17(5):393–394

Seligson D, Ostermann PA, Henry SL, Wolley T. The management of open fractures associated with arterial injury requiring vascular repair. J Trauma 1994;37(6):938–940

Seligson D, Klemm K. Adult posttraumatic osteomyelitis of the tibial diaphysis of the tibial shaft. Clin Orthop Relat Res 1999;360(360):30–36

Tetsworth K, Cierny G III. Osteomyelitis debridement techniques. Clin Orthop Relat Res 1999;360(360):87–96

Trampuz A, Osmon DR, Hanssen AD, Steckelberg JM, Patel R. Molecular and antibiofilm approaches to prosthetic joint infection. Clin Orthop Relat Res 2003;414(414):69–88

Widmer AF. New developments in diagnosis and treatment of infection in orthopedic implants. Clin Infect Dis 2001;33(Suppl 2):S94–S106

Zumiotti AV, Teng HW, Ferreira MC. Treatment of post-traumatic tibial osteomyelitis using microsurgical flaps. J Reconstr Microsurg 2003;19(3):163–171

Local Surgical Treatment of Osteomyelitis with a Resorbable, Osteoconductive Antibiotic Carrier

R. Kraus, U. Schiefer, R. Schnettler

Introduction

The gold standard in local antibiotic therapy for the treatment of osteomyelitis is presently still the application of PMMA chains containing antibiotics. The main disadvantage of these materials is, among others, the limited choice of commercially added antibiotics (gentamicin and, with limitations, vancomycin). Individual mixing in of several other antibiotics has been described, but the mixture and respective release characteristics of the antibiotics, are uncertain; hence this procedure could involve legal problems. In addition, the chains have to be removed at a later date, and antibiotic chains can only temporarily fill in bone defects as spacers.

Collagen fleece containing an antibiotic has been suggested as an alternative, but the choice of antibiotic for this purpose is limited to gentamicin. The allogenic carrier collagen often causes incompatibility reactions with protracted wound secretion and disturbs wound healing, especially if the fleece is placed near the surface.

For the further development of local antibiotic therapy for osteomyelitis, the following characteristics of carrier materials are desirable:
- applicability of various antibiotics with defined concentrations and reliable elution characteristics
- complete resorbability to avoid the necessity of later surgical removal
- suitability as a bone replacement substance with osteoconductive characteristics to fill in or bridge the defect

PerOssal (aap Implantate AG, Berlin, Germany) offers the required characteristics of a modern local antibiotic carrier and can successfully replace PMMA chains and collagen fleece as an antibiotic carrier in selected indications.

Form of Application, Chemical Composition, and Available Antibiotics

PerOssal is available in the form of pellets. The pellets consist of 51.5% nanocrystalline hydroxyapatite and 48.5% calcium sulfate (POP). In principle, all known antibiotics in a watery solution can be mixed with the carrier substance. A pellet can adsorb approximately 80 μL of fluid, adding up to 4 mL for a standard dose of 50 pellets (10 g).

Reliable in vitro results for antibiotic release and the achievable local and systemic effective drug levels are presently only available for gentamicin, vancomycin, and rifampicin.

Elution Characteristics, Local Effective Levels, Systemic Effective Levels

In vitro comparison of three antibiotic carriers containing gentamicin with PerOssal saturated with gentamicin resulted in a 2.5-fold greater amount of available gentamicin with PerOssal in the first 24 hours. On the second day, the released amount of gentamicin was identical. After 10 days a comparable amount of gentamicin was released from PerOssal as from the collagen carrier Septokoll (Biomet, Berlin, Germany). Whereby antibiotic release from PMMA cement (Septopal [Biomet, Berlin, Germany]) was ten times greater and release from the alternative collagen carrier Sulmycin Implant (Eusa Pharma GmbH, Munich, Germany) was no longer measurable at this point in time (**Fig. 5.64**).

In vivo tests of gentamicin and vancomycin on patients with osteomyelitis of the extremities showed that both antibiotics had extremely high local levels with systemic levels far below the toxicity threshold immediately postoperative and 24 and 48 hours later (**Table 5.1**).

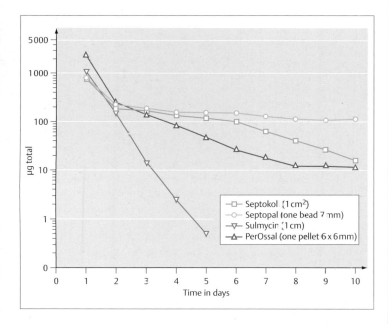

Fig. 5.64 Elution rates of PerOssal for saturation with gentamicin compared with other antibiotic carriers containing gentamicin

Table 5.1 Serum and local antibiotic concentrations in 15 patients with osteomyelitis of the extremities

	Postoperative	Day 1	Day 2
Gentamicin			
Serum concentration	1.1 µg/mL	0.4 µg/mL	0.4 µg/mL
Local concentration	627 µg/mL	305 µg/mL	52 µg/mL
Vancomycin			
Serum concentration	0.34 µg/mL	0.13 µg/mL	
Local concentration	931 µg/mL	130 µg/mL	32 µg/mL

Clinical Application

The implant bed is prepared according to conventional guidelines in septic bone surgery, that is, radical debridement of the infected bone and the affected soft tissues. PerOssal can be applied during two different phases of the surgical treatment. If resistance testing has confirmed that the pathogens are sensitive to vancomycin, clindamycin, and rifampicin, PerOssal can be used during the phase of programmed revisions as the only carrier for these substances with unrestricted availability. At 3- to 5-day intervals PerOssal is then saturated with the appropriate antibiotic and implanted in the bone defect after renewed debridement. As a bone replacement substance with osteogenic characteristics and containing an antibiotic, PerOssal can also be implanted and left in a defect as soon as the clinical findings, laboratory parameters, and microbiologic results indicate that the infection has ceased. After debriding the bone, the pellets are poured into a metal dish on the instrument table. Then the desired antibiotic dose is dissolved in a sterile process. A maximum of 4 mL solvent may be used for 50 pellets to ensure complete adsorption of the antibiotic. In this way, 500 mg of vancomycin, 240 mg of gentamicin, 600 mg of clindamycin, and 600 mg of rifampicin can be applied. After the antibiotic has completely dissolved, the solution is uniformly distributed over the pellets. Within 3–4 minutes the fluid will be completely absorbed by the porous pellets. The substance is then ready for implantation.

Place the pellets intact into the defect, which should be free of blood. Do not suction off residual fluid. Close the implant bed immediately with a sufficient and tensionless soft-tissue cover. If it seems necessary to place a drain, select an overflow, not a vacuum drain.

For large defects it is recommended to mix PerOssal pellets with autogenous trabecular bone chips in a 1:1 to 1:2 ratio. This can reduce wound secretion, which sometimes occurs, especially if PerOssal pellets are placed near the wound surface. Resorption and bony transformation of the substance are also accelerated.

TIPS AND TRICKS

Mixing the pellets with autologous trabecular bone improves resorption and new bone formation.

Case Study 1

At age 42 the patient sustained a fracture of the right tibial plateau. This was treated by open reduction and plate osteosynthesis. The metal was not removed. Three years later the patient presented with clinical signs of acute osteomyelitis. After removing the metal, a large inflamed defect remained in the tibial plateau (**Fig. 5.65a**). Microbiologic testing revealed gentamicin-resistant, coagulase-negative *Staphylococcus aureus*. After repeated surgical debridement and when the clinical examination, laboratory parameters, and microbiologic testing confirmed the absence of infection, 20 g PerOssal with 1000 mg vancomycin was placed in the defect (**Fig. 5.65b**). Radiographs demonstrated increasing resorption of the bone substitute with simultaneous new bone formation (**Fig. 5.65c**). The patient has had no recurrence for the past 5 years.

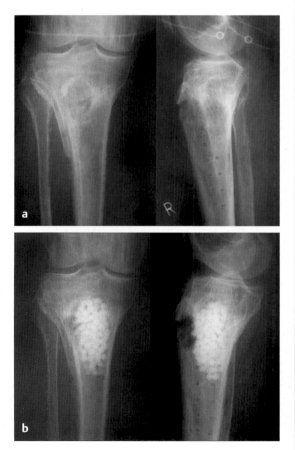

Fig. 5.65a–c
a A 42-year-old patient with fistulous osteomyelitis of the proximal tibia 3 years after plate osteosynthesis of a fracture of the tibial plateau. Microbiologic examination of a smear revealed *S. aureus*.
b After repeated radical surgical debridement of the abscess cavity in the bone, the defect was filled with PerOssal impregnated with vancomycin. The figure shows the postoperative documentation.

Fig. 5.65c ►

Fig. 5.65c Process of resorption: Only approximately 40% of the PerOssal pellets were resorbed after the first 4 weeks (top radiograph), this increased to 90% after 1 year (middle radiograph). After 3 years (bottom radiograph), no more pellets can be seen. The patient remained free of infection during the entire time.

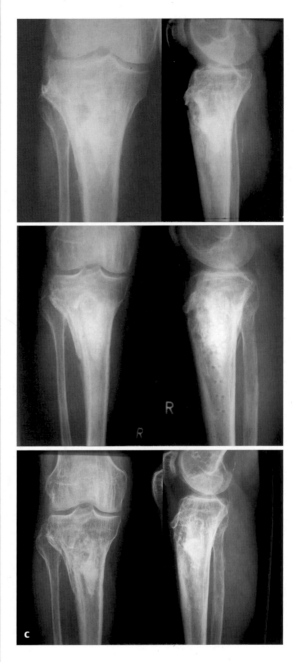

Case Study 2

The patient suffered post-traumatic osteomyelitis with an extensive soft-tissue defect after an open fracture of the first metatarsal of the foot treated by K-wire fixation (**Fig. 5.66a**). Following radical debridement of the bone and temporary placement of a Septopal antibiotic chain (**Fig. 5.66b**), the defect was filled with PerOssal and gentamicin mixed with autogenous trabecular bone in a relationship of 1:2 (**Fig. 5.66c**). Within 1 year the carrier material resorbed completely and new bone formation with subsequent remodeling enabled stable conditions with weight bearing (**Fig. 5.66d**).

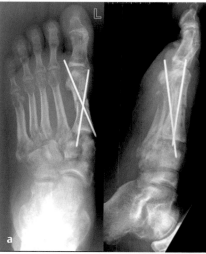
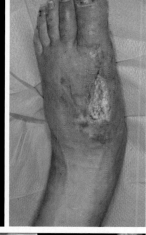

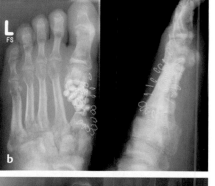

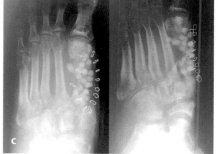

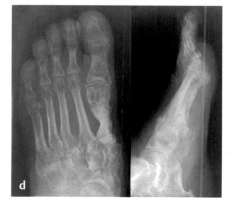

Fig. 5.66a–d
a A grade II open fracture of the first metatarsal was stabilized with Kirschner wires. Post-traumatic osteomyelitis (left) with a soft-tissue defect (right) developed.
b Postoperative radiograph after radical resection of the infected bone and temporary insertion of a Septopal chain.
c After controlling the infection, the antibiotic chain was removed and the defect was filled with a mixture of autogenous trabecular bone and Pe-Ossal pellets impregnated with gentamicin in a 2:1 ratio.
d A year later the bone substitute has been completely resorbed. A new weight-bearing first metatarsal bone has been formed. With kind permission from PD Dr. H. G. K. Schmidt.

Case Study 3

A 9-year-old Afghan boy with an increasing gibbus of the lumbar spine over the previous 2 years was brought to us by a charitable organization. He was suffering from tuberculosis affecting multiple organs, including the lungs, the kidneys, the CNS, and the spine. Radiographs revealed complete destruction of the 4th and extensive destruction of the 3rd lumbar vertebrae (**Fig. 5.67a**). After 3 months of tuberculostatic quadruple therapy, CT-guided drainage of an extensive system of retroperitoneal abscesses, and fitting of a protective support corset, internal fixation was mounted to the posterior spine from L1 and L2 to L5. During the same operation, lumbotomy and debridement of the destroyed vertebral portions were performed. The defect was filled with 10 g of PerOssal saturated with 600 mg of rifampicin (**Fig. 5.67b**). The young patient has now remained free of systemic or local recurrence of tuberculosis for 3 months.

Fig. 5.67a, b
a Lumbar spine of a 9-year-old Afghan boy with tuberculous spondylitis. The 3rd lumbar vertebra is largely destroyed and the 4th lumbar vertebra completely destroyed.
b After posterior stabilization of the lumbar spine with an XIA internal fixator (Stryker, Kalamazoo, MI, US) anterior debridement of the pannus was performed and 10 g of PerOssal with 600 mg of rifampicin was implanted.

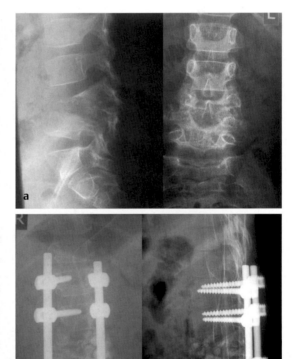

Callus Distraction of the Lower Leg—Ilizarov Method

H. G. K. Schmidt

Below we will discuss only the technical aspects of callus distraction with the Ilizarov method. The clinical application is only mentioned to explain the assembly.

Principle of Segment Transport

Experience gained in lengthening extremities has been very useful for segment transport.

Numerous examiners can confirm that continuous or pulsed stretching stimulation between the two bone ends promotes granulation in which fibroblastlike cells produce collagen fibrils around the central capillaries.

Osteoid-producing osteoblasts arrange themselves uniformly in this matrix and, together with other cells, produce a typical tubular bone (Pesch and Wagner 1974, Monticelli and Spinelli 1981, Paley 1988, Ilizarov 1989, Aronson et al. 1989, Delloye et al. 1990, De Pablos and Canadell 1990, Lascombes et al. 1991, Shearer et al. 1992).

In contrast to lengthening, in segment transport a bone segment is separated from the vital tubular bone and gradually advanced into the defect to be filled in with the help of various traction mechanisms. Finally, the transported segment docks onto the opposite end of the defect in the vital tubular bone and is attached with a so-called fixation ring. For faster and more certain bone consolidation, the transport segment is subjected to compression or autogenic spongiosaplasty is performed (**Fig. 5.68a–d**).

Segment transport can be performed in different ways:
- Simple transport (**Fig. 5.69a**)
- Double transport (**Fig. 5.69b**)
- Tandem transport (**Fig. 5.69c**)

The success of segment transport depends on numerous factors:
- Stability (Aronson et al. 1988, Ilizarov 1989, Pfeil and Niethard 1990, Wolfson et al. 1990, Aronson and Harp 1992, Calhoun et al. 1992, Delprete and Gola 1993, Kenwright and White 1993)
- Number of rings (each fragment must carry two rings)
- Size of rings (as small as possible)
- Number of wires (at least two wires at angles of between 30° and 60° to one another)

NOTE

- Since proximal perfusion is better than distal, this transport direction is preferred
- The tubular bone should be severed (corticotomy) in the metaphysis, if possible
- The essential advantage of double transport is shortening of the distraction time (transport time)
- The removed segment must be pulled at twice the speed in tandem transport
- Double and tandem transport are extremely vulnerable and can only be performed on very select patients

Fig. 5.68a–d Initial situation with defect and stabilization with Ilizarov's external ring fixation (**a**). Installation of the traction mechanism, corticotomy 3–10 cm from the edge of the defect (**b**). Principle of segment transport: distraction in steps (**c**). After docking, removal of the traction mechanism, installation of a fixation ring, and perhaps even cancellous bone grafting (**d**).

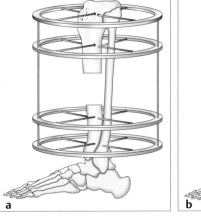

a

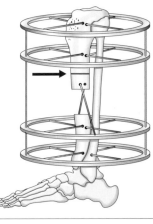

b

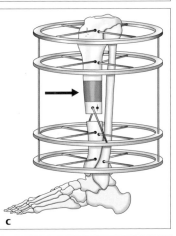

c

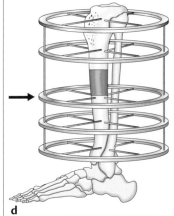

d

Fig. 5.69a–c
a Simple transport: from proximal to distal or distal to proximal
b Double transport. Two segments are transported toward each other:
one segment from proximal to distal and
one segment from distal to proximal
c Tandem transport: both segments are moved from proximal to distal or vice versa

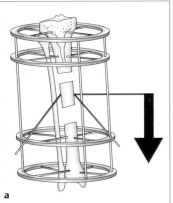

a

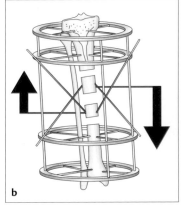

b

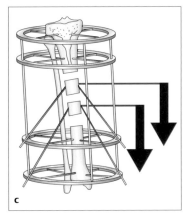

c

- Tension of wires (500–700 N)
- Distance between the rings (as large as possible, with a minimum distance of 4 cm between the rings)
- Corticotomy must preserve both tissue and perfusion (Allan 1948, Anderson 1952, Kawamura et al. 1968, Ilizarov 1989, Brutscher et al. 1992, Kenwright and White, 1993)
- Delay beginning distraction (Bier 1923, Abbott 1927, Barr and Ober 1933, De Bastiani et al. 1987, Ilizarov 1989, White and Kenwright 1991). After corticotomy and moderate separation (maximal 2 mm) of fragment ends, wait 4–12 days (generally 5 days) until granulation tissue has developed which can be stretched
- Extent and timing of distraction (Ilizarov 1989, White and Kenwright 1990)
- Maintenance and/or restitution of function of the extremity (Ilizarov 1989, Schmidt and Wolter 1995)

NOTE

- The more severe the soft-tissue and/or bone damage, the longer you have to wait to begin the distraction.
- The smaller the individual distraction step, the more often it must be performed and the better the new bone formation.
- The most effective daily distraction distance is 1 mm, that is, 4 x ¼ mm/day, and in children, up to 2 mm/day.
- Functional therapy is essential. The treatment goal is not only the radiographic appearance of the tubular bone, but restitution of a functional extremity.

TIPS AND TRICKS

The medial, lateral, and ventral separation of the bone must be performed with a special chisel. Posterior separation is achieved by rotating the fragments in opposite directions. Be sure to preserve the medullary vessels.

Mounting the Ring-Fixator onto the Lower Leg

- With the patient lying supine, disinfect the leg up to the mid-thigh and the foot.
- Place the thigh and foot on pads. The lower leg lies 10 cm above the operating table.
- The "landmarks" are drawn:
  - kneecap
  - medial and lateral joint space of the knee
  - head of fibula
  - tibial tuberosity
  - position of the bone defect
  - lateral and medial malleolus
  - joint space of the upper ankle (talocrural) joint and the proximal joint space of the big toe
- Anterior tibial edge for rotational control

Now choose the required ring size. Hold a ring which has already been screwed together above the proximal tibia asymmetrically (**Fig. 5.70d–f**):
- Ensure that there is a small space (one finger's width) between the inner edge of the ring and the medial and anterior soft tissues.
- Ensure that there is a large space (two fingers' width) lateral and posterior.
- Use a simple assemblage with four rings of equal size for a defect of the middle of the shaft of the lower leg (**Fig. 5.70a, b, d**).
- It is not necessary to construct an assembly for the foot.
- Hold the two groups of rings above the lower leg at right angles to the tibial axis (**Fig. 5.71b, c**).

NOTE

With some practice, intraoperative assemblage can be performed quickly and easily.

NOTE

It is better to choose too large than too small a ring to avoid strangulation of the soft tissues if there is postoperative swelling.

NOTE

Choose a wide distance between the rings in a fragment, as this provides the greatest biomechanical stiffness. The rings are only connected anterior and posterior.

The threaded rods are always placed directly in the first hole next to the ring lock.

Threaded rods should project as little as possible.

- This extends from metatarsal I (olive medial) to metatarsal V, or IV and V (**Fig. 5.74a**).
- This is then connected to the assembly on the lower leg with a half ring by means of diverse small parts so that correction is possible afterward (**Fig. 5.71h–j**; see below).

Fig. 5.70a–h

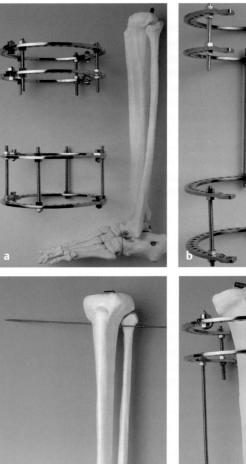

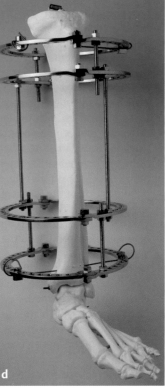

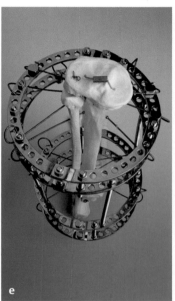

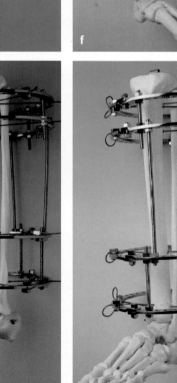

Fig. 5.70e–h

TIPS AND TRICKS

Olive or stopper wires can be attached to the lower leg for bone lengthening, correcting fracture alignment, or segment transport. These wires ensure exact positioning over time, even when there are only short fragments and osteoporotic bones.

ERRORS AND RISKS

- The proximal tibial wire coming from medial is very important.
- It could touch and block tendons of the pes anserinus.
- The wire must be placed behind the tendons toward the popliteal space. There is risk of the wire sliding behind the tibia into the blood vessels.
- After penetrating the soft tissues, the tip of the wire touches the medial edge of the tibia and enters the bone here.
- After the wire has bored through the tibia on the lateral side, never go through the tibial tuberosity to avoid blocking the tendons (**Figs. 5.73a and 5.70e**).

Fig. 5.71a–j

TIPS AND TRICKS

To ensure that the wires near the knee do not obstruct the joint, the knee is fully bent with a rapid movement. If the wire is in the right position, it will not move. If it touches a tendon, it jerks when the knee is suddenly bent, in which case it must be placed in a different position.

The wire may only be fixed and tightened after this test.

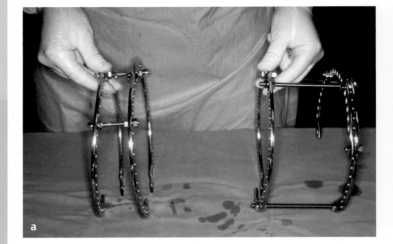

ERRORS AND RISKS

No fibular wire (at approximately 240–260°) may be placed in the second and third fifth of the lower leg to avoid injuring the peroneal nerve.

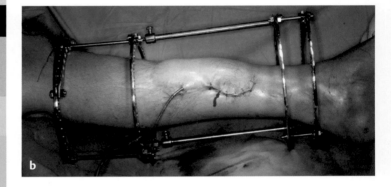

NOTE

When boring through the soft tissues—before entering the bone—all muscles through which wires pass must be stretched against their functional direction by operating assistants. For example, the foot must be held in maximal dorsal flexion if the soleus or the gastrocnemius muscle is crossed from medial. Otherwise the function of the foot could later be blocked.

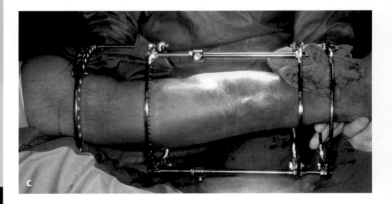

ERRORS AND RISKS

- The posterior tibial artery could be injured if the wire slips in a posterior direction
- The anterior tibial artery or the dorsal artery of the foot next to the tendon of the tibialis anterior muscle could be injured
- The function of the foot could be lost if it is not stretched in the direction opposite its functional direction when the wires cross through the muscles
- If the wire is placed at too steep an angle, it bypasses the tibia or enters the tendon of the tibialis anterior muscle

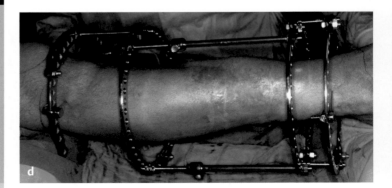

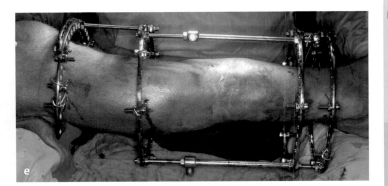

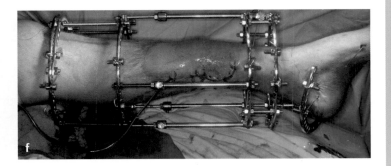

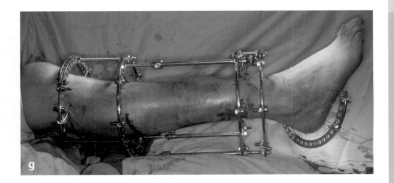

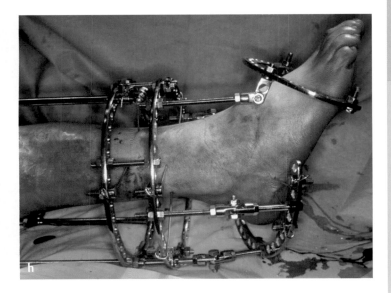

Fig. 5.71e–h

NOTE

- When placing a wire, existing wires can be struck. It the wire is displaced by more than 1 cm, it should be removed and replaced.
- A deviation of up to 1 cm can be compensated by means of a long slotted screw and one or two thick washers without a slot.
- Distances of greater than 1 cm from the ring must never be compensated by pressing the wire against the ring.
- If the wire cannot be attached directly to the ring because other wires are in the way, choose an entry point 1 cm from the ring. The wire is then attached to the ring with washers.
- If the distal fragment/segment is not aligned, this can be corrected by means of the attached wires.

TIPS AND TRICKS

- Simple fixation between the nut on the threaded rod and the ring always results in a right angle.
- The cone-shaped plates ensure a fixation of 15° at all levels (**Fig. 5.72d, e**).
- Even slightly slanting positions are automatically brought into right angles without conical plates. Corrections are not possible without bolts.
- The threaded rods between ring 2 (proximal segment) and ring 3 (distal segment) are removed.
- Corrections are performed with image-intensifier control.
- The conical plates make fixation in slanted positions between the threaded rods and the ring possible (**Fig. 5.72d, e**).

Fig. 5.71i–j ▶

Fig. 5.71i–j

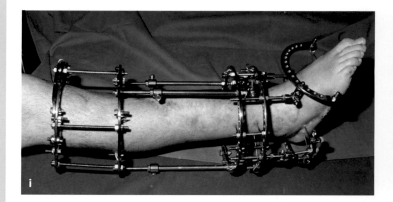

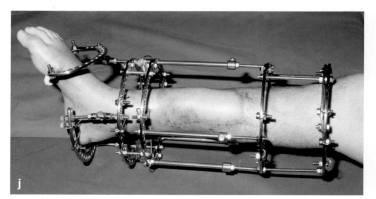

NOTE

- If the distal fragment is shorter than 4 cm, 2-ring assembly is impossible because the inner distance would be far less than 4 cm.
- From a biomechanical standpoint, 4 cm is the smallest distance which still ensures sufficient stability.
- If the distal fragment or the malalignment of the foot (often contractures causing pes equines in supination) is < 4 cm, the back of the foot is included in the assembly.

Fig. 5.72a–e

NOTE

If the assembly is not sufficiently tightened, the wire will slide, and the assembly will be unstable and lead to pain and the risk of a pin infection.

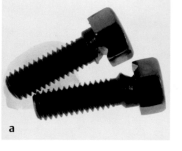

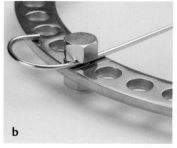

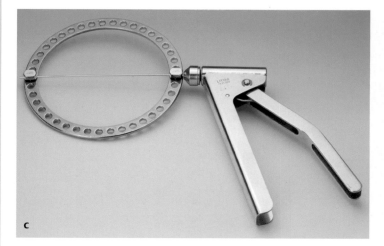

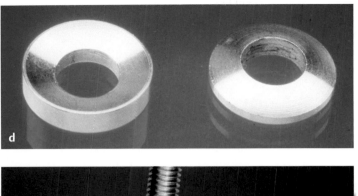

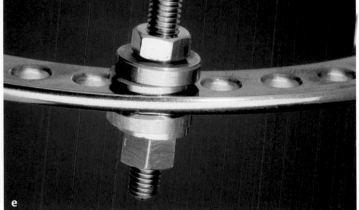

Fig. 5.72d–e

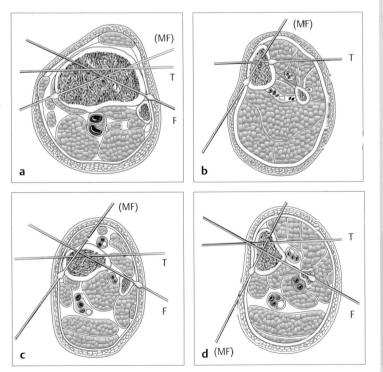

Fig. 5.73a–d T = transversal, F = fibular, MF = medial tibial facet

NOTE

- This assembly provides a stable construction, which ideally replaces the second ring in the tibial pilon when the fragment is short.
- Stretching the ankle joints in advance results in a slight dehiscence of the joint surfaces in the upper and lower ankle and subtalar joints and prevents ankylosis.

Fig. 5.74a, b The forefoot wire is attached to the not too small half ring (risk of swelling, leave room for dressing). (**b**) Connection to lower leg (**Fig. 5.71h–j**) and to the correction of the malalignment. Very complex malalignments can be corrected stepwise with these three wires (**Fig. 5.67g, h**).

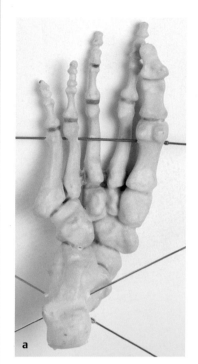

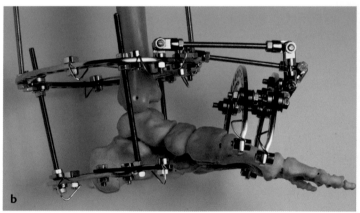

Corticotomy

The so-called transport segment is created by means of corticotomy.

- Install the traction mechanism, for example with crossed olive wires.
- Perform corticotomy 3–10 cm from the edge of the defect, in the metaphysis.
- Drill holes in a fan-shaped pattern. The bone is then severed from anterior, medial, and lateral with a corticotomy chisel. The remaining posterior bony bridge is fractured.

Performing Segment Transport

The following can be used as traction mechanisms (**Fig. 5.75a**):

- The outer ring
- Crossed olive wires
- Cerclage wires on screws
- Cable traction
- Place the transport ring between the second and third fixation rings. It is transported in a distal or proximal direction on exactly parallel threaded rods.
- Crossed olive wires are bored at an oblique angle through the tip of the transport segment, advanced through the soft tissues, and, depending on whether traction is to be distal or proximal, attached to the threaded rods with a slot (**Fig. 5.75b**).
- Cerclage wires attached to the transport segment with screws (**Fig. 5.75a**) are advanced through the soft tissues, either from distal or from proximal, and attached to the above-mentioned traction mechanism (**Fig. 5.75b**).
- Cable traction according to Weber (2003)
- Traction cables are used instead of cerclage wires because they are more flexible (**Fig. 5.76a**).
- Distal traction cables can be diverted to proximal with a diversion reel.

An example of an open transport segment is shown in **Fig. 5.77**.

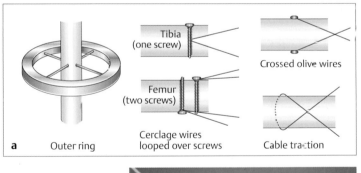

a   Outer ring

Tibia (one screw)

Femur (two screws)

Cerclage wires looped over screws

Crossed olive wires

Cable traction

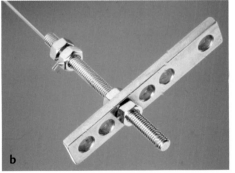

Fig. 5.75a, b
a Traction mechanisms in segment transport. Possible transport mechanisms include wires, cerclage, or traction cable.
b Concept of the wire transport with a slotted threaded rod.

Fig. 5.76a, b   System of traction cables in use: initial transport of the radius with the cable (**a**) and later (**b**).

Note: in **Fig. 5.76a, b** the traction cable is not threaded through the bone in a figure-of-eight. The later image shows that it can dislocate.

TIPS AND TRICKS

Two oblique holes of 2 or 2.7 mm are bored through the distal end of the transport segment. The traction cable is threaded through the holes from one side in a figure-of-eight.

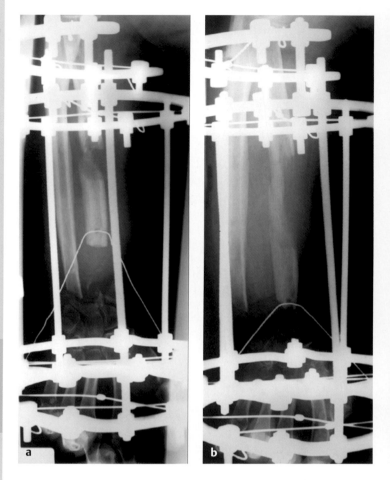

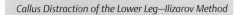
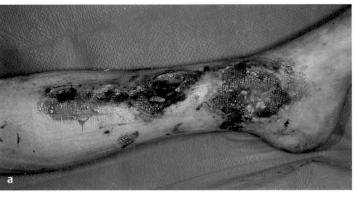

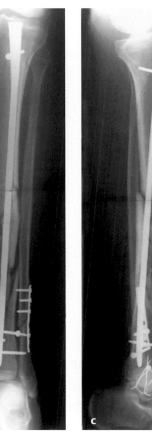

Fig. 5.77a–q

a–c Chronic osteomyelitis with a soft-tissue defect after placement of an intramedullary nail for a complete fracture of the lower leg.

Fig. 5.77d–q ▶

Fig. 5.77d–j

d–f Radical debridement, segment resection, local antibiotics (Septopal), temporary coverage of the soft tissues with artificial skin, and stabilization in a ring fixator.

g–j Transport with a cerclage wire looped over a screw in the lateral tibia. 4 × 1/4 mm/day transport speed (**g, h**). Follow-up (**i, j**).

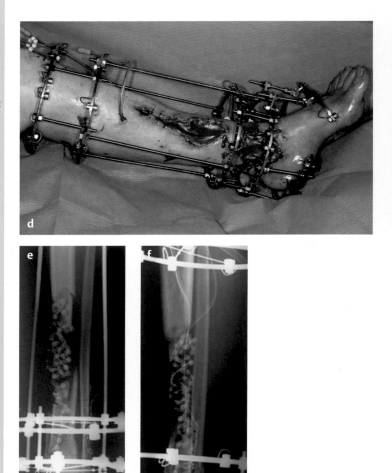

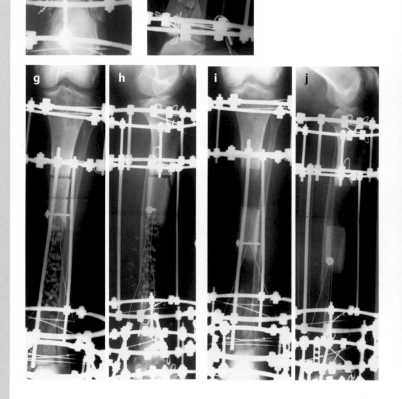

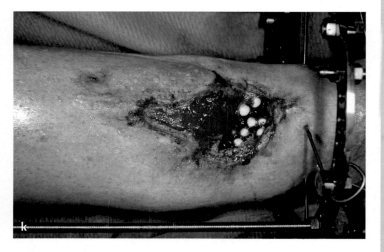

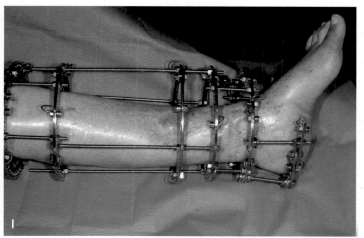

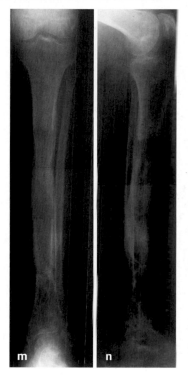

Fig. 5.77k–n
k The soft-tissue defect is beginning to close spontaneously.
l, n Closure of a large soft-tissue defect is achieved with open transport.

Fig. 5.77o–q ▶

Fig. 5.7 o–q Healed wound. The remaining defect was covered with a split-skin graft.

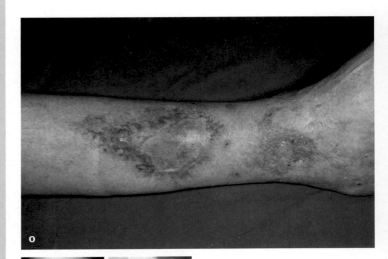

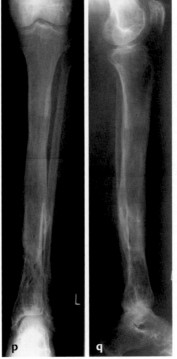

Bibliography

Abbott LC. The operative lengthening of the tibia and fibula. J Bone Joint Surg Am 1927;9:128–152

Allan FG. Bone lengthening. J Bone Joint Surg Am 1948;30:490–505

Anderson MV. Leg lengthening. J Bone Joint Surg Br 1952;34:150

Aronson J, Harrison B, Boyd CM, Cannon DJ, Lubansky HJ. Mechanical induction of osteogenesis: the importance of pin rigidity. J Pediatr Orthop 1988;8(4):396–401

Aronson J, Harrison BH, Stewart CL, Harp JH Jr. The histology of distraction osteogenesis using different external fixators. Clin Orthop Relat Res 1989;241(241):106–116

Aronson J, Harp JH Jr. Mechanical considerations in using tensioned wires in a transosseous external fixation system. Clin Orthop Relat Res 1992;280(280):23–29

Bagnoli G, Paley D. The Ilizarov Method. Philadelphia: B.C. Decker; 1990

Barr JS, Ober FR. Leg lengthening in adults. J Bone Joint Surg Am 1933;15:674–678

Bier A. Über Knochenregeneration, über Pseudarthrosen und über Knochentransplantate. Archiv klin Chir 1923;127:1–135

Brutscher R. Die Behandlung ausgedehnter Defekte an langen Röhrenknochen durch Segmentverschiebung. University of Munich: Habilitationsschrift; 1989

Brutscher R, Rüter A, Rahn B, Perren SM. The significance of cortocotomy or osteotomy in callus distraction. [Article in German] Chirurg 1992;63(2):124–130

Calhoun JH, Li F, Ledbetter BR, Gill CA. Biomechanics of the Ilizarov fixator for fracture fixation. Clin Orthop Relat Res 1992;280(280):15–22

Calhoun JH, Li F, Bauford WL, Lehman T, Ledbetter BR, Lowery R. Rigidity of half-pins for the Ilizarov external fixator. Bull Hosp Jt Dis 1992;52(1):21–26

De Bastiani G, Aldegheri R, Renzi-Brivio L, Trivella G. Limb lengthening by callus distraction (callotasis). J Pediatr Orthop 1987;7(2):129–134

Delloye C, Delefortrie G, Coutelier L, Vincent A. Bone regenerate formation in cortical bone during distraction lengthening. An experimental study. Clin Orthop Relat Res 1990;250(250):34–42

Delprete C, Gola MM. Mechanical performance of external fixators with wires for the treatment of bone fractures—Part I: Load-displacement behavior. J Biomech Eng 1993a;115(1):29–36

Delprete C, Gola MM. Mechanical performance of external fixators with wires for the treatment of bone fractures—Part II: Wire tension and slippage. J Biomech Eng 1993b;115(1):37–42

de Pablos J Jr, Canadell J. Experimental physeal distraction in immature sheep. Clin Orthop Relat Res 1990;250(250):73–80

Giebel G. Kallusdistraktion, klinische Anwendung. In: Hierholzer G, Weller S, eds. Traumatologie aktuell. 2nd ed. Stuttgart: Thieme; 1993

Green SA. The Ilizarov method: Rancho technique. Orthop Clin North Am 1991;22(4):677–688

Ilizarov GA. The tension-stress effect on the genesis and growth of tissues. Part I. The influence of stability of fixation and soft-tissue preservation. Clin Orthop Relat Res 1989a;238(238):249–281

Ilizarov GA. The tension-stress effect on the genesis and growth of tissues: Part II. The influence of the rate and frequency of distraction. Clin Orthop Relat Res 1989b;239(239):263–285

Ilizarov GA. Transosseous Osteosynthesis. Berlin: Springer; 1992

Kawamura B, Hosono S, Takahashi T, et al. Limb lengthening by means of subcutaneous osteotomy. Experimental and clinical studies. J Bone Joint Surg Am 1968;50(5):851–878

Kenwright J, White SH. A historical review of limb lengthening and bone transport. Injury 1993;24(Suppl 2):S9–S19

Lascombes P, Membre H, Prévot J, Barrat E. Histomorphometry of bone regenerate in limb lengthening by Ilizarov's technique. [Article in French] Rev Chir Orthop Repar Appar Mot 1991;77(3):141–150

Monticelli G, Spinelli R. Distraction epiphysiolysis as a method of limb lengthening. I. Experimental study. Clin Orthop Relat Res 1981;154(154):254–261

Paley D. Current techniques of limb lengthening. J Pediatr Orthop 1988;8(1):73–92

Pesch H-J, Wagner H. Histomorphological findings of bone regeneration under distraction in diaphysial "extension osteotomy" (author's transl). [Article in German] Verh Dtsch Ges Pathol 1974;58:305–308

Pfeil J, Niethard FU. Lower leg lengthening using the Ilizarov system. Presentation of the various surgical techniques and analysis of lower leg lengthening procedures performed 1986-1989. [Article in German] Orthopade 1990;19(5):263–272

Pfeil J, Grill F, Graf R. Extremitätenverlängerung, Deformitätenkorrektur, Pseudarthrosenbehandlung. Berlin: Springer; 1996

Reichel H. Der diaphysäre Knochen nach Kallusdistraktion. Munich: Zuckschwerdt; 1998

Rüter A, Kohn D, Correll J, Brutscher R. Kallusdistraktion. Munich: Urban & Schwarzenberg; 1998

Hecker WC, Ring-Mrozik E, Limmer S, Mantel K. Risk score and postoperative complications in pediatric surgery. [Article in German] Langenbecks Arch Chir 1995;380(4,4)239–246

Shearer JR, Roach HI, Parsons SW. Histology of a lengthened human tibia. J Bone Joint Surg Br 1992;74(1):39–44

Weber M. Segmenttransport mittels Kabelrollentechnik. Trauma u. Berufskr 2003;5:264

White SH, Kenwright J. The timing of distraction of an osteotomy. J Bone Joint Surg Br 1990;72(3):356–361

White SH, Kenwright J. The importance of delay in distraction of osteotomies. Orthop Clin North Am 1991;22(4):569–579

Wolfson N, Hearn TC, Thomason JJ, Armstrong PF. Force and stiffness changes during Ilizarov leg lengthening. Clin Orthop Relat Res 1990;250(250):58–60

Hematogenous Infection of Bones and Joints

K. Parsch

Terms

Pathogenic bacteria that enter the body through portals in the skin or mucous membranes can spread to bone by various routes that include hematogenous seeding. The organisms tend to colonize well-perfused metaphyses and occasionally the diaphyses of the tubular bones as well as the carpus, tarsus, clavicle, scapula, and vertebral bodies. Acute and subacute osteomyelitis and septic arthritis may have a variety of clinical manifestations, depending on patient age, anatomy, and especially on local and systemic host resistance.

The authors have chosen to place surgical treatment at the forefront of this book. Nevertheless, or perhaps for this very reason, it is important to emphasize the urgency of surgical treatment on the one hand while also setting limits in cases where surgery is unlikely to benefit the patient.

Acute osteomyelitis is distinguished from subacute and chronic forms of the disease. We treat hematogenous septic arthritis as a third pathologic entity. This condition requires differentiation from rheumatoid arthritis and also from transient arthritis, both of which warrant an entirely different therapeutic approach.

Acute hematogenous osteomyelitis develops when local and systemic host defenses are compromised. This entity is becoming increasingly rare in Central Europe. Up to ten cases per year were being treated at our hospital in the 1980s and 1990s. While our facility still serves a total population of approximately 3 million people, the number of cases has decreased to just three to five annually during the past 5 years.

The most severe form of acute, multifocal osteomyelitis with accompanying arthritis has always been rare, at least in central Europe. Multiorgan involvement leads to a life-threatening situation. A weakened immune status may be a predisposing factor.

Subacute or primary chronic osteomyelitis (bone abscess) develops in children who are in good general health but have local compromise of host resistance. Bacteria that reach the metaphyses via the bloodstream multiply slowly and form a localized abscess over a period of weeks or months. Besides the metaphysis, which is a site of predilection, subacute bone infections may also develop in the diaphysis and sometimes within the epiphysis. A smear from the affected site is usually found to contain staphylococci and may occasionally yield Gram-positive or Gram-negative organisms.

Plasma cell osteomyelitis is the mildest form of bone infection. The body is able to mount an effective immune response marked by an intense infiltration of plasma cells. Causative pathogens are not identified from blood samples or wound smears in plasma-cell osteomyelitis.

A special form of subacute osteomyelitis is **Garrè sclerosing osteomyelitis**, which is characterized by recurrent, painful inflammatory flare-ups in the bone. Localized hypertrophic bone growth leads to angular limb deformities and elongation.

Another important entity is **chronic recurrent multifocal osteomyelitis** (CRMO), a self-limiting disease that may involve various skeletal sites. Today the diagnosis is based primarily on radiographic and MRI findings and a mild elevation of inflammatory markers. Bone scintigraphy was the former imaging modality of choice. A causative organism is not identified in biopsy samples. The disease is treated with anti-inflammatory drugs. The only primary indication for surgery would be a biopsy to exclude skeletal lymphoma.

Septic arthritis: The hematogenous spread of bacteria into bone—osteomyelitis—is closely linked to a similar process that affects joints—arthritis. Thus, osteomyelitis of the head or neck of the femur in infants is usually the result of primary colonization of the joint by infectious organisms (coxitis), with progression to osteomyelitis occurring over a period of several days.

Hematogenous arthritis affects the hip joint (coxitis) and knee joint (gonitis) with approximately equal frequency. Staphylococci and streptococci are chiefly responsible, but other Gram-positive and Gram-negative organisms are sometimes identified. Although the incidence of hematogenous septic arthritis has been declining during the past few years, an average of five children still present with primary septic arthritis at our hospital each year.

Septic arthritis may also develop from the spread of osteomyelitis in the metaphysis or epiphysis. It usually results from the delayed or inadequate treatment of an acute periarticular osteomyelitis.

The sections below deal with the **surgical treatment** of different types of hematogenous bone and joint infection.

Acute Hematogenous Osteomyelitis

Indications

- Acute phlegmon of the medullary cavity
- Acute subperiosteal abscess
- Accompanying arthritis

Contraindications

- Incipient osteomyelitis that has not yet formed an abscess or spread beneath the periosteum
- Osteomyelitis that is detectable by early signs in MRI only
- Uncertain differential diagnosis (e. g., Ewing sarcoma)

Operative Procedure

The periosteum is incised, the medullary cavity is opened, and smears and tissue samples are obtained from both sites. This is immediately followed by the institution of parenteral antibiotic therapy with a second-generation cephalosporin, preferably cefuroxime (100 mg/kg).

The optimum treatment of acute hematogenous osteomyelitis should include meticulous curettage and irrigation of the subperiosteal infected area and of the medullary cavity. Antibiotic-impregnated PMMA beads are implanted, and the wound is closed over a drain (**Fig. 5.78a–f**).

Principal Signs and Symptoms

- Localized pain, usually in the metaphysis but occasionally in the diaphysis of a tubular bone
- Inability to bear weight on the affected limb
- Local warmth
- Soft-tissue swelling around the painful site

Laboratory Findings

- Quantitative elevation of CRP (usually > 10 mg/L)
- ESR elevated above 50 mm in the first hour (Westergren)
- Leukocytosis: white blood cells > 10 000/mL (value uncertain)
- Venous blood culture
- Antistaphylolysin titer in venous blood
- Antistreptolysin titer in venous blood
- PCR may reveal positive findings in cases of culture negative samples (Chometon et al. 2007).

Preoperative Preparations

- Confirm agreement between clinical presentation, laboratory values, and MRI findings.
- Explain the need for acute intervention.

- Explain anticipated pain control measures.
- Explain the proposed PMMA bead implantation and later removal.
- Explain the risk of recurrence.
- Institute antibiotic therapy only after the infection site has been opened and smears taken.
- Prepare a plaster cast or prefabricated splint to facilitate postoperative care (**Fig. 5.78c**).

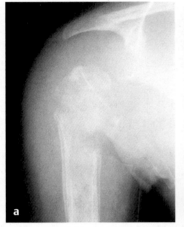

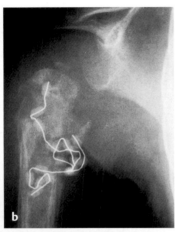

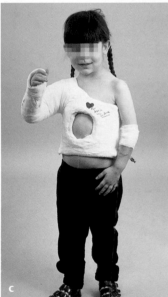

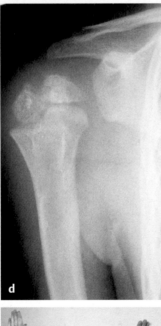

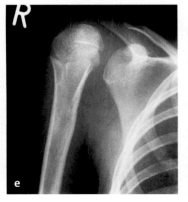

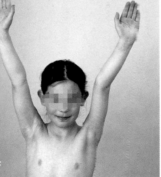

Fig. 5.78a–f
a Acute osteomyelitis of the right proximal humerus. A previously healthy 4-year-old girl was admitted with a 1-week history of severe pain and high fever. Radiograph shows a moth-eaten pattern of destruction in the humeral metaphysis and epiphysis. MRI was withheld as clinical and radiographic findings were clear. Treatment consisted of surgical debridement and PMMA bead implantation. Cefuroxime was initially administered parenterally.
b Radiograph of the right proximal humerus after a second surgical revision with the PMMA beads in place. *S. aureus* was identified, this was followed by parenteral antibiotic therapy with cefuroxime.
c A thoracic abduction cast was used to protect the proximal humerus after successful surgical and antibiotic treatment (CRP < 5 U/mg). Residual elevation of the ESR.
d Radiograph of the right humerus 8 months after acute osteomyelitis. Inflammatory parameters have returned to normal. The metaphysis has healed. The bipartite condition of the proximal humeral epiphysis is a result of the infection.
e Radiograph of the right proximal humerus 4 years after resolution of osteomyelitis. No significant residual changes are detected.
f Normal shoulder function 4 years after osteomyelitis of the right proximal humerus.

The end of the PMMA chain should protrude very slightly from the periosteum so that it can be easily located for removal.

Parenteral antibiotic therapy is initiated after the second smear is taken.

Bone should be removed sparingly to avoid postoperative structural weakening with fractures.

The advantage of removing the PMMA beads in a second intervention provides better skin conditions.

Removing the beads in small steps leads to retracted scars which is difficult for pediatric patients to tolerate.

Removing the beads in a second sitting allows for a second curettage of the infected area.

Early mobilization on a continuous passive motion (CPM) splint will hasten recovery.

Acute osteomyelitis with abscess formation is characterized by severe pain, increased infection markers, and MRI evidence of an abscess.

Early surgical exposure, irrigation, curettage, PMMA bead implantation, and postoperative parenteral antibiotic therapy will lead to rapid pain relief and normalization of inflammatory signs.

Reintervention is mandatory in case of a recurrence. The antibiotic may need to be changed based on sensitivity results.

The patient should be mobilized early, but full weight bearing is not allowed until laboratory values have returned to normal.

Surgical Treatment Principles for Bone and Soft-Tissue Infections

- Do not use a tourniquet or exsanguinating wrap on the affected limb.
- Place the incision at the site of maximum pain and swelling, also paying attention to radiographic and MRI findings.
- Incise the periosteum and take a smear and biopsy.
- Drain and irrigate the abscess cavity.
- Tap the cortex to locate the abscess perforation site.
- Open the cortical bone at the most suspicious site.
- Take a smear and histologic sample from the medullary cavity.
- Debride and irrigate the medullary cavity.
- Implant PMMA mini-beads or ordinary PMMA beads, depending on the cavity size.
- Close the wound in layers over a drain.
- Place the limb in a prefabricated plaster cast or plastic splint for immediate postoperative immobilization.
- Remove the PMMA beads in a second surgical procedure. This is done an average of 2 weeks after the first procedure after clinical symptoms (pain) have subsided and elevated CRP and ESR levels have returned to normal.
- Immobilize the limb in a plaster or plastic cast for peripheral inflammations and in a Keeler splint for proximal infections.
- Nonweight-bearing limb exercises are begun early and are supported by physical therapy.
- Weight bearing is gradually increased according to laboratory findings. Normal activities can generally be resumed by 6 weeks.

Complications

- Recurrence
- Multifocal involvement especially in small infants
- Subperiosteal abscess, cellulitis
- Bone necrosis, sequestrum, involucrum
- Fistula formation
- Longitudinal growth disturbance (osteomyelitis in infants)
- Pathologic fractures

Subacute or Chronic Osteomyelitis (Bone Abscess)

Indications

- Clinical manifestations of an abscess (pain and swelling)
- Radiographic detection of an abscess
- MRI detection of an abscess

Contraindications

- Minimal pain
- MRI features of subacute to chronic osteomyelitis with no radiographic abnormalities

Differential Diagnoses

- Trauma or presumed trauma with a fracture, fissure, or ligamentous lesion (**Fig. 5.79**)
- Soft-tissue masses such as a cavernous hemangioma of the distal thigh near the joint
- Eosinophilic granuloma
- Unicameral bone cyst with or without pathologic fracture
- Aneurysmal bone cyst with or without fracture
- Osteosarcoma
- Ewing sarcoma
- Acute lymphatic leukemia with lymphoma formation

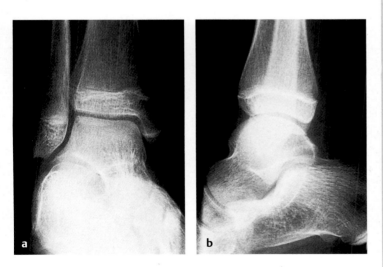

Fig. 5.79a–g
a, b Radiographs of the distal tibia and ankle joint are normal in this 13-year-old girl, who complained of severe right ankle pain. She has a history of a sports-related injury.

Fig. 5.79c–g ▶

Fig. 5.79c–g
c MRI shows increased fluid in the medullary cavity of the distal tibia signifying osteomyelitis with an associated periosteal reaction.
d Radiographic findings after debridement, culture specimen, PMMA bead implantation, and parenteral antibiotic therapy with cefuroxime. The inflammatory reaction is subsiding while the PMMA beads are still in place.
e, f Radiographs 8 months after the inflammation has subsided. There is still some demineralization of the distal tibia.
g Clinical appearance of feet and ankles. Mild swelling over the medial malleolus with a scar.

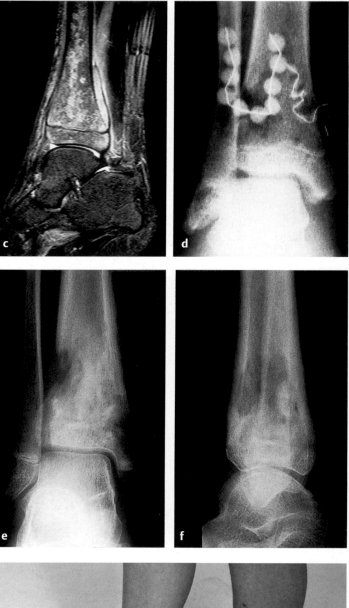

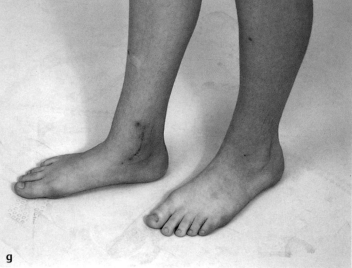

Operative Procedure (Fig. 5.80a–f)

First determine whether the subacute or chronic inflammation really requires surgical debridement or can be managed by specific antibiotic therapy.

The decision for conservative or operative treatment is based on clinical signs and symptoms, laboratory values, and radiographic and MRI findings. Surgical treatment is not indicated if clinical, laboratory, and MRI findings indicate only a mild illness. Surgical debridement is indicated for a painful bone abscess, regardless of whether it has perforated into the subperiosteal space.

Principal Signs and Symptoms

- Periarticular pain
- Pain on weight bearing
- Pain at rest and night pain
- Periarticular swelling
- Local warmth

Laboratory Findings

- ESR elevated to average values of 20–40 mm in the first hour
- Mild CRP elevation (>10 to 50 mg/L)
- Differential blood count (distinguish from malignancies)

Preoperative Preparations

- Radiographs
- MRI
- Laboratory tests
- Informed consent. The patient should be informed about the risk of recurrence and the implantation of a local antibiotic delivery system, especially if the differential diagnosis is uncertain.

Chronic Recurrent Multifocal Osteomyelitis (Fig. 5.81)

Fig. 5.81a–j

a, b Technetium bone scans show inflammatory foci in the 2nd metacarpal, the lateral portion of the distal femoral metaphysis, and the metaphysis of the medial malleolus. This 9-year-old girl complained of nocturnal pain at all three sites. ESR was moderately elevated and CRP was slightly elevated at 2 mg/L.

c Expansion and periosteal thickening of the second metacarpal.

d, e Radiographs of the distal tibia show metaphyseal rarefaction in the medial malleolus.

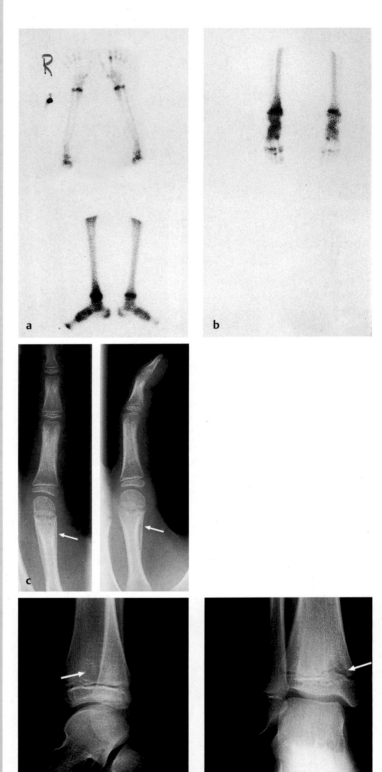

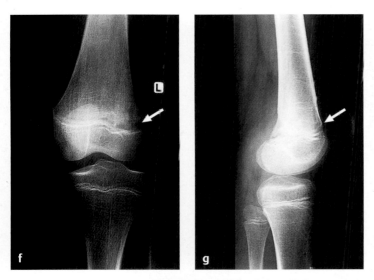

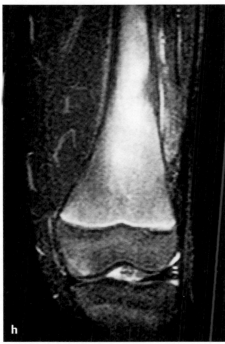

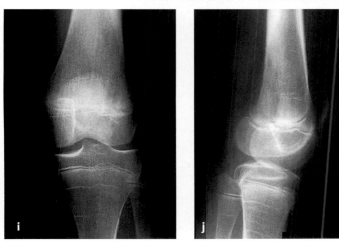

Fig. 5.81f–j
f, g Radiographs of the distal femur show rarefaction of the metaphysis and adjacent epiphysis.
h MRI of the distal femur in a 13-year-old girl, 4 years after resolution of trifocal CRMO symptoms. Clinical involvement was now limited to the distal femoral region. There was no need for reintervention as the patient responded well to oral antibiotics and anti-inflammatory drugs.
i, j Radiographs 1 year after MRI show a normal appearance of the metaphysis and epiphysis. The girl, now 14 years of age, is free of clinical complaints.

Septic Arthritis

Indications

- Clinical, laboratory, and sonographic or MRI findings that confirm septic arthritis
- Aspiration of pus or puslike material from a joint
- Spread of infectious organisms from adjacent osteomyelitis

Contraindications

None

Differential Diagnosis

- Post-traumatic effusion—excluded by laboratory findings. (Hemarthrosis or post-traumatic effusion does not cause abnormal inflammatory values.)
- Rheumatoid arthritis—excluded by the severity of complaints. (Despite effusion, the pain of rheumatoid arthritis is mild compared with septic arthritis.)
- Transient synovitis of the hip or knee joint—excluded by negative laboratory values and relatively mild pain in the presence of effusion.

Operative Procedure

Bacterial septic arthritis poses a serious threat to the affected joint. The infection may spread rapidly to the adjacent epiphysis and metaphysis, especially in neonates and small infants, resulting in destructive changes and growth disturbance .

Early detection is essential for providing appropriate surgical and antibiotic therapy.

Principal Signs and Symptoms

- Severe to very severe malaise
- Temperature elevation ranging to septic febrile episodes
- Initially severe or excruciating pain on motion and weight bearing

- Pain or pseudoparalysis in infants caused by the slightest touch—of the arm in shoulder arthritis, of the leg in arthritis of the hip or knee joint
- Local swelling, which is most conspicuous in the peripheral joints and less obvious in the hip or shoulder joint

Laboratory Findings

- Elevated CRP. If findings are ambiguous, repeat the test a short time later (e. g., 8 hours) to check for rising values.
- Maximal elevation of the ESR
- Leukocytosis (less significant parameter)
- Detectable antistaphylolysin or antistreptolysin titers, for example
- PCR may reveal positive findings in case of culture-negative samples.

Imaging Studies

- Plain radiographs are always required, if negative in the early phase, they can be repeated with soft-tissue contrast slightly increased.
- Ultrasound is used mainly on deeper joints like the hip and shoulder. It can easily detect joint effusion as well as secondary capsular changes.
- MRI can detect effusion and any infectious foci in the adjacent metaphyses or epiphyses.
- CT is equivalent to ultrasound in the detection of effusion.
- Technetium scintigraphy shows a cold spot in the acute phase. Scans in chronic arthritis show increased uptake in subchondral or metaphyseal areas.

Preoperative Preparations

- Clinical findings (considerable pain and limited motion)
- Laboratory findings: elevated CRP and ESR
- Imaging: ultrasound and MRI
- If ultrasound or MRI cannot be performed, aspirate the joint.
- The urgency of the intervention is explained to the patient and family members.

Fig. 5.83c–g
c, d Surgical exploration revealed copious inflammatory material. *S. aureus* was identified as the cause. Antibiotic-impregnated PMMA mini-beads were implanted. Parenteral administration of cefuroxime 100 mg/kg.
e, f Radiographs 1 month later show partial necrosis of the distal femoral epiphysis and metaphysis.
g Radiograph of the distal femur at 18 months demonstrates complete loss of the lateral distal femur.

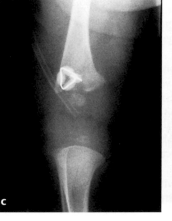

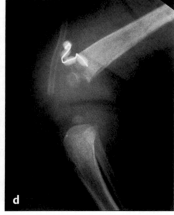

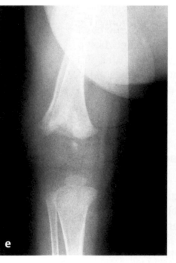

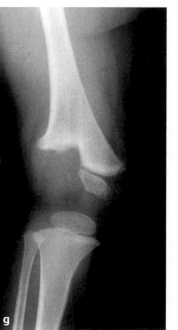

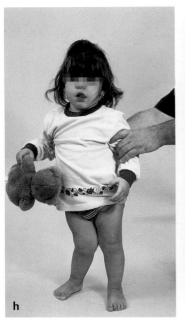

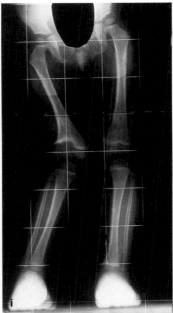

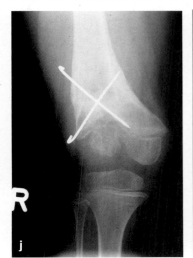

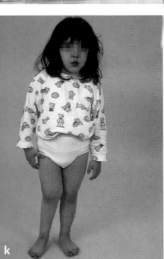

Fig. 5.83h–k
h Clinical appearance of postinfectious valgus deformity of the right leg.
i Standing radiograph documents massive valgus deformity on the right side.
j Radiograph of the right knee after corrective supracondylar osteotomy demonstrates a straight limb axis. The lateral distal femoral epiphysis has partially reformed and appears mineralized.
k Clinical appearance at 4 years of age. The right leg axis is still acceptable but will probably require future corrections since valgus deformity tends to recur.

Bibliography

Bergdahl S, Ekengren K, Eriksson M. Neonatal hematogenous osteomyelitis: risk factors for long-term sequelae. J Pediatr Orthop 1985;5(5):564–568

Blyth MJG, Kincaid R, Craigen MA, Bennet GC. The changing epidemiology of acute and subacute haematogenous osteomyelitis in children. J Bone Joint Surg Br 2001;83(1):99–102

Choi IH, Pizzutillo PD, Bowen JR, Dragann R, Malhis T. Sequelae and reconstruction after septic arthritis of the hip in infants. J Bone Joint Surg Am 1990;72(8):1150–1165

Chometon S, Benito Y, Chaker M, et al. Specific real-time polymerase chain reaction places Kingella kingae as the most common cause of osteoarticular infections in young children. Pediatr Infect Dis J 2007;26(5):377–381

Deely DM, Schweitzer ME. MR imaging of bone marrow disorders. Radiol Clin North Am 1997;35(1):193–212

Diedrich O, Kraft CN, Sasse J, Zhou H, Lüring C. Primary subcutaneous hematogenous osteomyelitis in childhood. [Article in German] Unfallchirurg 2002;105(7):651–655

Dormans JP, Drummond DS. Pediatric Hematogenous Osteomyelitis: New Trends in Presentation, Diagnosis, and Treatment. J Am Acad Orthop Surg 1994;2(6):333–341

El-Sayed AM. Treatment of early septic arthritis of the hip in children: comparison of results of open arthrotomy versus arthroscopic drainage. J Child Orthop 2008;2(3):229–237

Ezra E, Cohen N, Segev E, et al. Primary subacute epiphyseal osteomyelitis: role of conservative treatment. J Pediatr Orthop 2002;22(3):333–337

Gordon JE, Huang M, Dobbs M, Luhmann SJ, Szymanski DA, Schoenecker PL. Causes of false-negative ultrasound scans in the diagnosis of septic arthritis of the hip in children. J Pediatr Orthop 2002;22(3):312–316

Hamdy RC, Lawton L, Carey T, Wiley J, Marton D. Subacute hematogenous osteomyelitis: are biopsy and surgery always indicated? J Pediatr Orthop 1996;16(2):220–223

Kallio P, Ryöppy S, Jäppinen S, Siponmaa AK, Jääskeläinen J, Kunnamo I. Ultrasonography in hip disease in children. Acta Orthop Scand 1985;56(5):367–371

Kocher MS, Zurakowski D, Kasser JR. Differentiating between septic arthritis and transient synovitis of the hip in children: an evidence-based clinical prediction algorithm. J Bone Joint Surg Am 1999;81(12):1662–1670

Kocher MS, Zurakowski D, Barnewolt C, Kasser JR. Validation of a clinical prediction rule for the differentiation between septic arthritis and transient synovitis of the hip in children. J Bone Joint Surg Am 2004;86(8):1629–1635

Levine MJ, McGuire KJ, McGowan KL, Flynn JM. Assessment of the test characteristics of C-reactive protein for septic arthritis in children. J Pediatr Orthop 2003;23(3):373–377

Mandell GA. Imaging in the diagnosis of musculoskeletal infections in children. Curr Probl Pediatr 1996;26(7):218–237

Manzotti A, Rovetta L, Pullen C, Catagni MA. Treatment of the late sequelae of septic arthritis of the hip. Clin Orthop Relat Res 2003;410(410):203–212

Mazur JM, Ross G, Cummings J, Hahn GA Jr, McCluskey WP. Usefulness of magnetic resonance imaging for the diagnosis of acute musculoskeletal infections in children. J Pediatr Orthop 1995;15(2):144–147

Nade S. Acute haematogenous osteomyelitis in infancy and childhood. J Bone Joint Surg Br 1983;65(2):109–119

Parsch K, Savvidis E. Coxitis in the newborn infant and infant. Diagnosis and therapy. [Article in German] Orthopäde 1997;26(10):838–847

Parsch K, Nade S. Infections of bones and joints. In: Benson MKD, Fixson JA, MacNicol MF, Parsch K, eds. Children's Orthopaedics and Fractures. London: Churchill Livingstone; 2002:119–145

Parsch K. Die septische Arthritis des Hüftgelenkes (Coxitis septica). In: Wirth CJ, Zichner L, eds. Orthopädie und orthopädische Chirurgie: Becken und Hüfte. Stuttgart: Thieme; 2003:229–235

Peltola H, Vahvanen V, Aalto K. Fever, C-reactive protein, and erythrocyte sedimentation rate in monitoring recovery from septic arthritis: a preliminary study. J Pediatr Orthop 1984;4(2):170–174

Rasool MN. Primary subacute haematogenous osteomyelitis in children. J Bone Joint Surg Br 2001;83(1):93–98

Salter RB, Bell RS, Keeley FW. The protective effect of continuous passive motion in living articular cartilage in acute septic arthritis: an experimental investigation in the rabbit. Clin Orthop Relat Res 1981;159(159):223–247

Stanitski CL, Harvell JC, Fu FH. Arthroscopy in acute septic knees. Management in pediatric patients. Clin Orthop Relat Res 1989;241(241):209–212

Vienne P, Exner GU. Garré sclerosing osteomyelitis. [Article in German] Orthopäde 1997;26(10):902–907

6 Plastic and Reconstructive Surgery

M. Lehnhardt, H.-H. Homann, H.-U. Steinau

General Comments

Primary Treatment and Prevention of Post-traumatic Osteomyelitis

Insufficient primary debridement of fractures with soft-tissue damage, delayed revascularization, and extensive exposure of the bone for fracture stabilization result in a vicious cycle, which is promoted and sustained by ischemia of the wound edges, postprimary infections, and compartment syndromes. If the clinical signs of a beginning infection are recognized at a later stage or not at all, this leads to a loss of soft tissue caused by infection, which spreads to the exposed bones. This results in an increase in surgical interventions, treatment days, inability to work, and psychological problems.

Therefore, systematic treatment strategies are required to help identify and remove potential sources of error.

The extent of soft-tissue trauma is often underestimated in open injuries due to the visible destruction of soft tissues in defined areas. The actual soft-tissue damage is far more extensive.

There is only a gradual difference between closed and open soft-tissue damage. Initially in closed soft-tissue trauma, only indirect signs indicate the severe tissue damage. Dislocations, diastasis of fragments, severe lateral displacements, and comminuted fractures, as well as foreign bodies and air inclusions identified in radiographs indicate massive disintegration of the tissue structures. Underestimation of the damage, failure to treat sufficiently, traumatic surgical techniques, and increasing disturbance in perfusion caused by forced wound closure are classic triggers that magnify the primary injuries. These complex injuries require an all-encompassing concept in which soft-tissue reconstruction takes precedence.

Cleaning out the Infection and Covering the Soft-Tissue Defect

Basic surgical training teaches that only wounds with smooth edges and without contusion zones, recesses, and foreign-body contamination can be expected to heal primarily after adaption without tension. Friedrich's (1898) and von Reyher's (Lehnhardt et al. 2002) recommendations based on empirical and clinical observations have since been scientifically confirmed. The essential parameters of wound healing, like angiogenesis in soft tissues and bones, cell proliferation, collagen synthesis, protein production, reepithelization, and cellular hormone activity, depend on a constant supply of oxygen and nutrients. Moreover, sufficient elimination of bacteria by means of increased macrophage activity can only be expected with physiologic oxygen concentrations in the tissues.

The surgeon supports these natural functions by performing primary radical excision of devitalized or insufficiently perfused bones and soft tissues.

If the extent of the resulting defect does not permit primary wound closure (**Figs. 6.1 and 6.2**), local and microvascularly attached flaps are used to provide complete biologic coverage with restitution of the natural skin barriers.

If large open wounds with exposed bones remain, granulation tissue usually loses the battle against bacterial contamination and infection. In particular, bradytrophic tissues, edematous soft tissues, and bone fragments separated from their origins cannot recover their normal perfusion. The well-known surgical concept of restraint (wait until demarcation appears) in chronic peripheral circulatory disturbances (peripheral arteriovenous disease, diabetes mellitus) is not acceptable under these circumstances.

NOTE

Neither antibiotics nor local enzymatic treatment can replace radical surgical debridement.

NOTE

If it is not possible to interrupt the beginning vicious cycle consisting of primary tissue damage, local hypoxia, infection, and secondary tissue damage early by excising tissue and providing final skin closure, this can result in far more extensive damage and even loss of the affected part of the extremity.

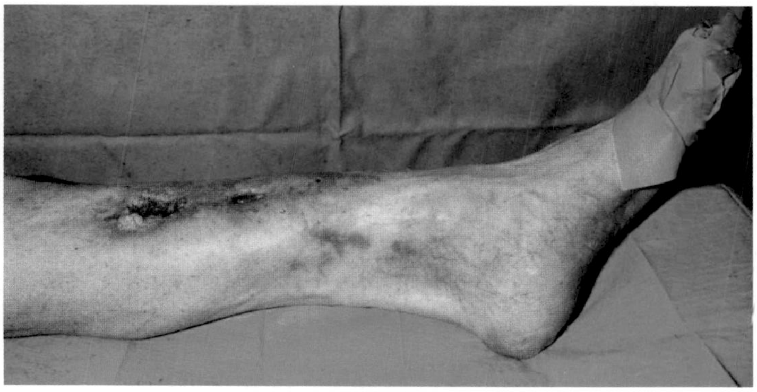

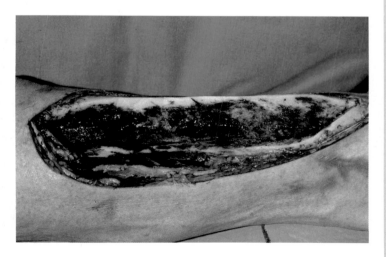

Fig. 6.1 Typical finding in fistulous osteomyelitis of the tibia with chronic secretion.

Fig. 6.2 Operation site after radical debridement of the tibia and the soft tissues.

Depending on the damage, one must often exchange preservation of the limb for loss of function. If amputation is unavoidable, transfer of distal portions of the amputated extremity onto the stump for improvement of functional rehabilitation with a prosthesis should be discussed.

Problems accompanying microvascular tissue transplantation:
- Exaggerated indication
- Vascular anastamosis in the infected region, position of the vessels (kinking)
- Wound closure under tension
- Strangulating dressings (swelling, compression due to incorrect positioning)
- Delayed revision
- Unnecessary lengthening of the operation by individual surgeons (the standard is two teams)

Owing to tactical and technical improvements, the success rate of microvascular transplants is approximately 95%. Analysis of failures has identified the causative problems listed here. Aside from the choice of appropriate procedure for the patient's specific local problem, tactical errors and delayed revisions constitute the main causes. Timely secondary interventions can usually preserve transplanted flaps.

Since microvascular techniques make up only one, albeit a very essential, factor in the treatment of chronic osteomyelitis, interdisciplinary cooperation is necessary to reduce the error rate in general management.

The most effective prophylactic and therapeutic measures for chronic osteomyelitis depend on early plastic surgery of the soft tissues following radical debridement for success. Moreover, these are ideal prerequisites for secondary osteoplastic interventions and measures to improve function.

Problems in the treatment of soft-tissue damage on the extremities:
- Evaluation of the wound: underestimation of the extent of damage
- Evaluation of the peripheral perfusion: delayed revascularization, failure to slit the compartment in time, unfavorable incisions
- Instead of programmed serial debridement: waiting for demarcation, leaving wound recesses and bone cavities
- Insufficient interdisciplinary cooperation

Radical, extended wound debridement is a fundamental prerequisite for long-term eradication of infection. In a clinically manifest infection, any devitalized bone fragment is to be considered contaminated with bacteria and removed. Fistulous tracts can be filled with blue dye. Compromises cause recurrences.

Unstable fracture fixation disturbs bone healing, and stable fixation accelerates bone consolidation. The treatment principle is to remove nonstabilizing material and to leave osteosynthetic material which is stably anchored. External fixation normally fulfills all requirements for renewed fracture fixation.

Flaps

In the presence of an acute infection, the first step is to clean out the focus of infection by means of debridement. After the acute signs of infection and concomitant edema have abated, a second debridement increases the certainty of a successful outcome. The defect should only be covered after several sequential cleansing operations have been performed (lavage in stages).

Several different principles are available for surgical coverage of the defect (**Fig. 6.3**).

Direct wound closure is only seldom possible—in small defects and areas with stretchable surrounding soft tissues—and should be completely tension-free.

Skin Grafting

Since revascularization is of central importance in surgical toilet, skin grafting alone has declined in importance. Only fascia or muscle flaps ensure a distinct improvement in perfusion. Skin grafting alone should only be

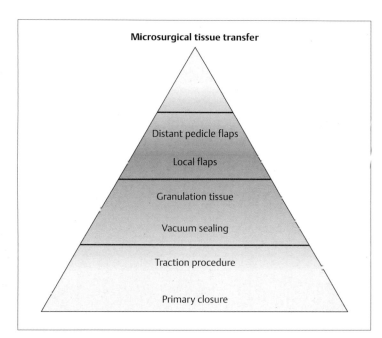

Fig. 6.3 Reconstruction ladder for defect coverage.

Microsurgical tissue transfer

Distant pedicle flaps

Local flaps

Granulation tissue

Vacuum sealing

Traction procedure

Primary closure

NOTE

Reverdin's (pinch) grafts with small, mixed islands of skin have been completely abandoned due to their vulnerability and unaesthetic appearance, especially at the donor sites.

NOTE

The average thickness of a split-skin graft should be approximately 0.3 mm.

performed in exceptional cases in aged patients with impaired vascular systems after granulation tissue has sufficiently covered the bare site. The introduction of modern continuous drainage methods (e. g., Vacuseal, K.C.I., Wiesbaden, Germany) improves the outcome of procedures combining culturing granulation tissue and secondary split-skin grafting for parts of extremities which are not subjected to mechanical stress. A well-vascularized and noninfected recipient site is the prerequisite for a successful split-skin graft. In special cases coverage can also be achieved with the aid of Integra artificial skin (Integra Lifescience, Mainsborough, NJ, US).

Free skin grafts, especially as mesh grafts, are considered simple and sure procedures, and the rate of healing is high even if the receiver site is slightly infected. Aside from lacking a revascularization effect and unsatisfactory cosmetic results, decreased ability to withstand stress, especially on mechanically vulnerable areas, are large disadvantages. Following slight traumas, these areas tend to develop pressure sores and cracks (**Fig. 6.4**).

Free, full-thickness skin grafts require good perfusion and lack of infection in the recipient region and are used in particular for the correction of large scars. The groin offers a good harvest site, where donor sites of up to 28 × 8 cm corresponding to an abdominal flap can be closed with a primary suture.

Split-skin grafts can be harvested in various thicknesses.

Sufficient germinal material remains, especially in the hair follicles, for spontaneous healing of the donor site. Harvesting is ideally done on the buttock or thigh. A mesh (accordion) graft is usually used to increase the size and ensure drainage of secretions. The donor site can be dressed with simple fatty gauze; however, use of an occlusive foil is preferable, which leads to faster healing in a liquid milieu and causes less pain.

A split-skin graft receives nutrients by means of diffusion and perfusion (plasmatic imbibition) within the first 3 days if the recipient area has sufficient blood supply. This is followed by capillocapillary docking (inosculation) and

Fig. 6.4 Insufficient soft-tissue coverage in a split-thickness graft transplanted directly over the bone.

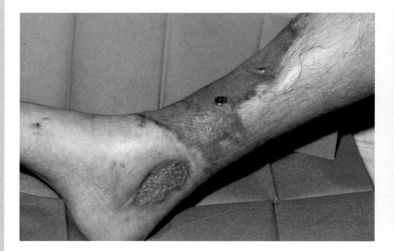

capillary proliferation, developing rapidly in muscle and fascia and slowly in the periosteum and tendon sheath. There is no angiogenesis in bones without periostea and exposed tendons.

The graft is secured with single sutures or staples. To prevent shearing forces, apply a foam tie-over pressure bandage.

The first dressing change takes place after approximately 5 days because the graft is then adherent. If the recipient site is infected, the dressing should be changed earlier if odor indicates a complication.

Skin Flaps

If the recipient site is not suitable for a split-skin graft or if this kind of coverage would produce a poor functional result, a flap is indicated.

McGregor and Morgan's classification is used for practical reasons (Krupp 2002). The determining factor is the form of perfusion in the flap. Accordingly, skin–fat flaps with vascular circulation from the subdermal and dermal plexes (**random pattern flaps**) are differentiated from flaps with axial perfusion (**axial pattern flaps**).

The first group is raised without particular attention to the vascular anatomy. They usually contain 1–2 or more angiosomes. An angiosome is an area of skin perfused by an anatomically defined blood vessel. For this reason the relationship between the length and the width of the pedicle should not exceed 2:1, otherwise the perfusion of the periphery of the flap may be disturbed.

In axially perfused skin flaps the incision is based on the course of the anatomically identified vascular system. The relationship between the length and the width of the pedicle can be up to 5:1, depending on the cross-section of the supplying vessel. A gain in length can also be achieved by a properly prepared incision around the vessel. **Fasciocutaneous or perforator flaps** represent the further development of the principle of axially defined blood supply of soft-tissue flaps. The principle is the dissemination of perforating vessels above and immediately below the deep facia and the muscle septa (e. g., radial flaps).

The form of flap perfusion plays a key role. A major pedicle has blood vessels that can nourish the flap alone. Additional smaller vessels, which cannot nourish the flap alone, are referred to as minor pedicles. There are, of course, flaps with several major pedicles, that is, each of these pedicles could nourish the flap alone. Some minor pedicles that are able to nourish the flap together if the major pedicle fails are called secondary, segmental pedicles. The localization and distribution of major and minor pedicles of individual muscles in the human body is very consistent.

NOTE

Performing careful hemostasis prior to placement of the skin graft prevents the development of a hematoma, which could cause the graft to fail due to lack of direct contact with the recipient site.

NOTE

The decisive factor is the perfusion of the flap. Accordingly, skin–fat flaps with blood supply from the subdermal and dermal plexes (**random pattern flaps**) are differentiated from flaps with axial perfusion (**axial pattern flaps**).

TIPS AND TRICKS

Random pattern flaps can be conditioned by a preparatory incision around the flap and partial or complete mobilization followed by replacement of the mobilized portion. Peripheral necroses 12–14 days later when the final wound closure is performed are far rarer.

NOTE

Random pattern flap: length to width = < 2:1.
Axial pattern flap: length to width = < 5:1.

NOTE

Always attempt to leave the flap on its major pedicle.

Fig. 6.5b, c
b To prevent osteomyelitis of the top of the skull, the wound edges are debrided and the tabula externa removed tangentially with a Lexer chisel until petechial bleeding appears. A contralateral pedicled temporoparietal scalp rotation flap is raised and covers the defect without any tension.
c Defect coverage 1 week after the operation.

TIPS AND TRICKS

If the skull is exposed, the external layer of bone should be tangentially removed with a chisel until punctuate bleeding appears before the defect is covered.

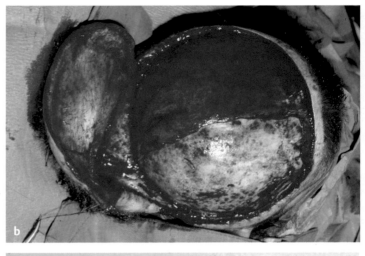

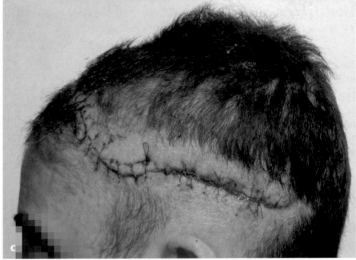

Fig. 6.6 Burns on the head and other regions. Seven months after the trauma a 22 × 8 cm defect remains with a yellowish tabula externa. The entire occipital and skullcap region has only been thinly covered with a split-skin graft.

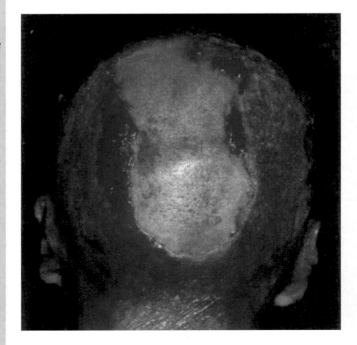

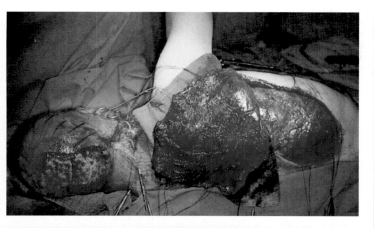

Fig. 6.7 Radical debridement with abrasion of the superficial bone and multiple trepanations in the skull until petechial bleeding appears. A latissimus dorsi flap has been raised.

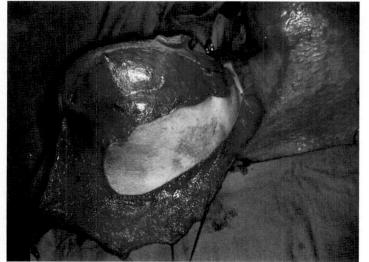

Fig. 6.8 Coverage of the skullcap and the occiput with a partial myocutaneous latissimus dorsi flap measuring 32 × 36 cm. Revascularization is achieved with an end-to-end anastamosis of the right superior thyroid artery and the external jugular vein (for the technique see Latissimus Dorsi Flap, p. 203).

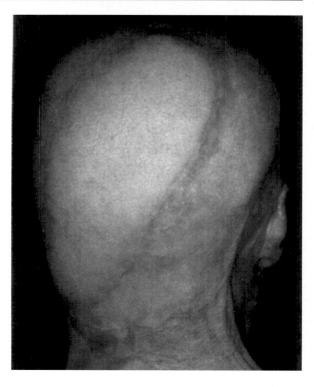

Fig. 6.9 Final result 4 years later. The skin over the occiput is normal with good soft-tissue coverage, over which a wig can be comfortably worn.

Shoulder Girdle and Upper Arm

In septic bone surgery, the pectoralis major and the latissimus dorsi muscles, as well as scapular and parascapular flaps, are primarily used to cover defects in this area.

Pectoralis Major Flap

In principle, the whole muscle with adjacent skin and soft tissues can be raised as a flap due to the intramuscular branches. Numerous anatomical norm variants exist. In 30% there is no pars abdominalis, and a smooth transition to the deltoid muscle (no deltoideopectoral sulcus) often exists.

Indications:
- Defects in the lateral head/neck
- Defects in the mouth
- Defects in the thoracic wall/shoulder

Vascular and nervous supply:
Thoraco-acromial artery and vein:
- The blood vessels cross the clavipectoral fascia with one to two large branches and the accompanying nerves and proceed on the lower surface of the muscle in a mediocaudal direction. The trunks divide into several lateral branches.
- The muscle and the skin above it is reached from medial by terminal branches of the anterior intercostal arteries II–V from the region fed by the internal thoracic artery.
- Venous drainage occurs through several veins running parallel to the arteries.
- The motor innervation of the myocutaneous pectoral flap derives from the medial (C5–C7) and lateral (C8–T1) pectoral nerves.

The length of the neurovascular pedicle depends on the distribution of vessels and nerves on the lower surface of the muscle. In 40% of cases there is only one neurovascular pedicle. In the remaining 60% there is a further pedicle to the pars clavicularis or abdominalis.

The main neurovascular pedicle proceeds in a cranial direction and is prevented from kinking by the clavicle. The vascular course should prevent twisting of the pedicle in flaps rotated in a ventrocranial direction. This portion of the muscle receives very little additional blood supply from segmental skin vessels (**Figs. 6.10, 6.11, 6.12, 6.13**).

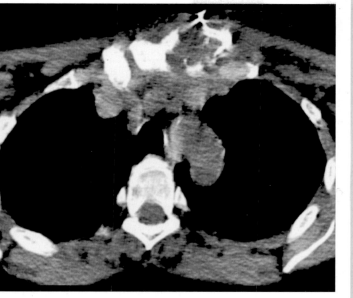

Fig. 6.10 Empyema of the left sternoclavicular joint with osteomyelitis after a cortisone injection.

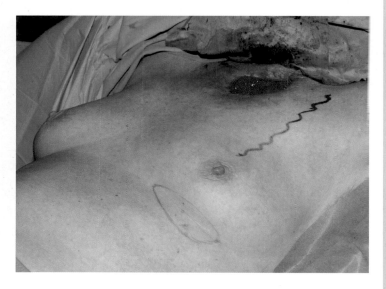

Fig. 6.11 Radical debridement with partial resection of the sternum, clavicle, and the first rib resulting in a defect measuring 8 × 10 cm. The pleura and mediastinum are exposed at the donor site. The course of the thoracoacromial artery and vein has been drawn.

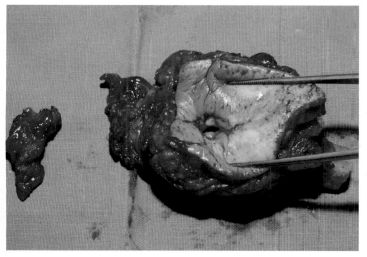

Fig. 6.12 The joint and the first rib have been resected en bloc. The fistulous sinus is shown.

Fig. 6.13 Coverage of the defect with an ipsilateral pectoralis major island flap. The skin island is raised from the fold under the breast. After removal of mammary-gland tissue the muscle is removed from the pectoralis minor muscle beneath it and dissected from caudad to craniad. Following subcutaneous tunneling the pedicled myocutaneous graft is placed in the defect.

TIPS AND TRICKS

In this case it is not necessary to remove the attachment of the major pectoral muscle from the humerus because the pedicle only needs to cover a short distance.

NOTE

Complications at the donor site are few; scar tissue in the fold under the breast is generally not visible.

If a large defect requires covering, it may be necessary to cover the donor region with a split-skin graft.

If it is necessary to mobilize the flap, the muscle attachment on both the humerus and the clavicle can be severed. After dissection of the afferent vessels to their origins, a flap can be harvested to cover defects in the lower face and inside the mouth.

NOTE

Combined flaps can be obtained from the scapular region; a combination of parascapular, scapular, and latissimus flaps enable coverage of very large defects.

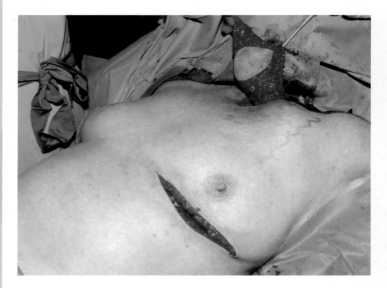

Parascapular Flap

Although flaps from the scapular region have no sensory nerves, this is an ideal donor region because the blood supply is reliable and the skin is thick and resistant to trauma.

A parascapular flap and a variation thereof (scapular flap) can be used either as a free flap or a pedicle flap (**Fig. 6.14**).

Indications:
- A pedicle flap is used to cover defects in the armpit.
- A free flap is especially suited to cover areas requiring a hearty skin graft (foot, distal portion of the lower leg).

Vascular Supply:
These flaps contain a main branch of the circumflex scapular artery (see also **Fig. 6.39**). This originates from the subscapular artery and proceeds between the teres major and teres minor muscles. The subscapular artery divides into two branches. Besides the branch described above, there is the thoracodorsal artery, which supplies the latissimus dorsi muscle (see Latissimus Dorsi Flap, p. 203) on the lateral margin of the scapula. The thoracodorsal artery branches here into the parascapular artery, which runs in a caudad direction, and the scapular artery, which runs in a medial direction.

A small branch also runs in a caudad direction.

The arteries are accompanied by veins. The flaps can have a separate pedicle for each artery, or both arteries can be in one pedicle.

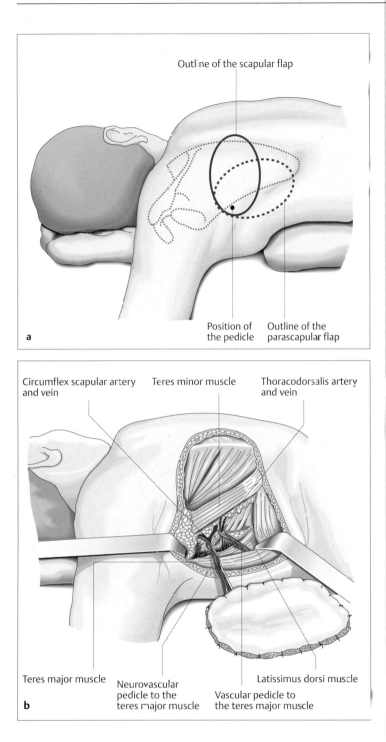

Outline of the scapular flap

Position of the pedicle

Outline of the parascapular flap

a

Circumflex scapular artery and vein

Teres minor muscle

Thoracodorsalis artery and vein

Teres major muscle

Neurovascular pedicle to the teres major muscle

Vascular pedicle to the teres major muscle

Latissimus dorsi muscle

b

Fig. 6.14a, b Planning a flap

a The skin island is elliptical. The possibility of primary closure of the donor site after harvesting the graft can be tested preoperatively by pinching the folds of skin together in an axial direction. Dissection should always begin from medial with visualization of the vascular pedicle, because this is the safer method. Alternatively, the flap can be completely incised and dissected from the periphery to the center until the vascular pedicle is visible. Only choose this method if it is possible to precisely evaluate the relationship between the medial armpit and the top of the scapula.

b The flap is principally raised in the epifascial layer. Some fascia should also be raised around the vascular pedicle, because the first branching off of the vessels could lie just below the fascia. Tie off lateral branches of the circumflex scapular artery. Further anterior dissection of the pedicle is easy.

NOTE

The parascapular artery is larger and anatomically more consistent than the scapular artery.

187

Elbow and Forearm

Large, infected defects with exposed bones in the elbow region are best covered with a radial flap with a proximal pedicle. Defects in the forearm can be closed with a flap from the groin. Defects in the distal forearm, wrist, and hand can be covered well with a radial flap with a distal pedicle.

Radialis Flap

A radial (forearm) flap is a fasciocutaneous flap that is harvested from the anterior aspect of the forearm. It can be transplanted as a free or a pedicled flap. Its versatility is due to the fact that it can have either a proximal or a distal pedicle (retrograde arterial flow).

Indications:
- Proximal pedicle: defects in the elbow region
- Distal pedicle: defects in the wrist, hand, and finger
- Free flap: bridging vascular defects, defects on the heel and distal tibia

Rare indications:
A free flap incorporating bones from the radius is rarely indicated.

Vascular and nervous supply:
- Branches of the radial artery penetrate the antebrachial fascia.
- Sensory innervation is provided by the lateral antebrachial cutaneous nerve. Discriminatory sensation is, however, limited so that a free forearm flap cannot be considered a true neurovascular flap.

The flap limits are the edge of the ulna on the medial aspect and the middle line of the posterior forearm, including the palmar skin.

Radial Flap with a Distal Pedicle
See **Figs. 6.15, 6.16, 6.17, 6.18, 6.19.**

NOTE

There is retrograde venous flow through the comitans veins and the superficial venous network of the forearm. If an island flap with a distal pedicle is used, it is not necessary (but advantageous) to include a superficial vein.

NOTE

Before removing this flap, an Allen test must confirm sufficient perfusion of the hand through the ulnar artery. This test should be confirmed intraoperatively by clamping off the radial artery.

ERRORS AND RISKS

Disturbances in the perfusion of the thumb have been reported in rare cases. These require reconstruction of the radial artery with a venous imposition graft.

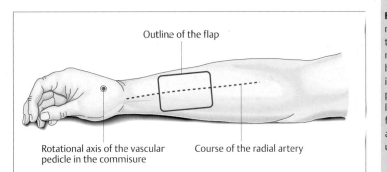

Outline of the flap

Rotational axis of the vascular
pedicle in the commisure

Course of the radial artery

Fig. 6.15 Drawing the planned flap over the middle third of the anterior forearm. Planning the length of the pedicle and determining the rotational axis. For a defect on the back of the hand, the rotational axis is at the base of the dorsal interosseus muscle (immediately proximal of the point where the radial artery branches off). For a long pedicle, the rotational axis is at the tip of the first commissure. The deep branch of the radial artery is included in the pedicle, which is tunneled under the tendons of the thumb.

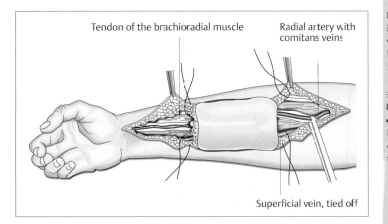

Tendon of the brachioradial muscle

Radial artery with comitans veins

Superficial vein, tied off

Fig. 6.16 Dissection of the pedicle with a distal incision along the radial artery. Superficial veins which enter the pedicle are ligated. Dissection begins on the ulnar side and continues to the lateral edge of the flexor carpi radialis muscle and includes the fascia. The muscle is held on the ulnar side and dissection proceeds in the deep layers of tissue. The flap is now separated from the superficial branch of the radial nerve on the radial aspect. Deep dissection is performed on the medial edge of the brachioradial muscle until reaching beneath the radial artery.

Fig. 6.17 After ligating the proximal blood vessels, the flap can be separated from the flexor muscles below it and mobilized.

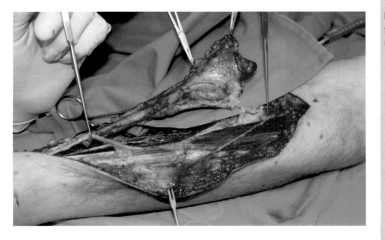

Fig.6.18 The flap is fitted into the defect. The example shows the possible rotational arch, which reaches up to the fingertips.

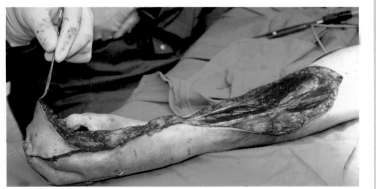

Fig. 6.19 The final steps involve covering the donor site with a split-skin graft and tunneling the pedicle subcutaneously.

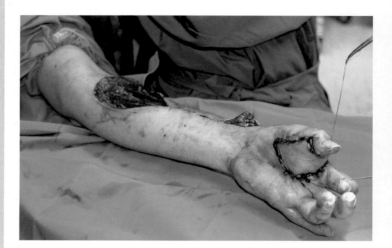

Radial Flap with a Proximal Pedicle

The surgical technique corresponds to that of flaps with distal pedicles. The flap is marked out over the distal third of the forearm. A short distal incision is made to check the position of the radial artery. From proximal the pedicle can be dissected up to its origin from the brachial artery. See **Figs. 6.20, 6.21, 6.22**.

Fig. 6.20 Cutting out the radial flap in the anterior forearm with proximal dissection of the vessels. The fasciocutaneous flap is raised on the vascular pedicle.

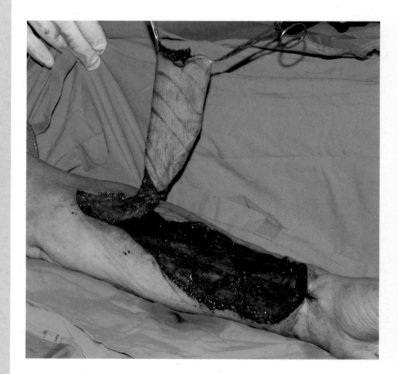

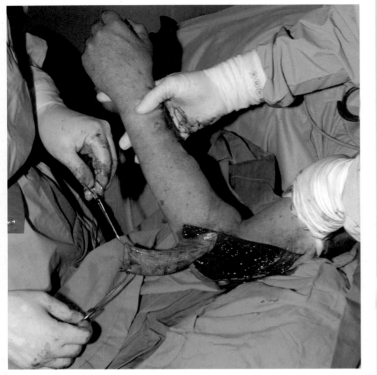

Fig. 6.21 Tunneling the skin and pulling through into the defect.

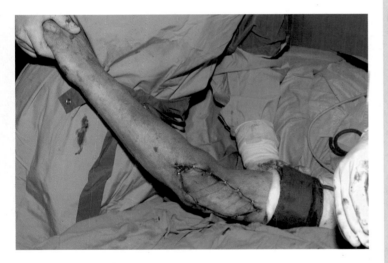

Fig. 6.22 Fitting the flap into the defect. Covering the donor site with a split-skin graft.

Groin Flap

Groin flaps are among the most frequently used grafts for reconstructive surgery. Large defects, especially on the upper extremities, can be covered well with groin grafts with vascular pedicles. Because of the high variability in the diameter of its blood vessels, a groin flap is rarely used as a free flap.

NOTE

Identifying the course of the artery is facilitated by orientation aids. Doppler ultrasound can help localize the site where the artery penetrates the medial edge of the sartorius muscle.

TIPS AND TRICKS

If the skin pedicle is not too thick, it is recommended to form a tube. (Be careful not to damage the vessel!)

NOTE

The flap is one-third above and two-thirds below the inguinal ligament.

Fig. 6.23   U-shaped flap

Indications:
- A distant pedicle flap is appropriate for soft-tissue defects in the upper extremities, especially the elbow, forearm, and hand.
- A free flap offers the advantage of few complications at the donor site.

Vascular Supply:
The superficial circumflex iliac artery and the comitans veins supply groin flaps.

This artery is a long cutaneous vessel. It originates from the femoral artery approximately 2 cm distal to the inguinal ligament, penetrates the fascia at the medial edge of the sartorius muscle, continues at an oblique angle in the subcutaneous tissue, and curves around the iliac crest approximately 2.5 cm below the anterior superior iliac spine.

The flap can usually be raised far above its vascular territory because there is generally a rich vascular network in the distal portion. This means the distal portion can be considered a random pattern flap. Flaps with a length of up to 30 cm and a width of 15 cm can be harvested.

Hand surgery often requires very long flaps to have sufficient play for early physiotherapeutic exercises. This necessitates dissection of the base. In this area the fascia of the sartorius muscle should be included in the flap to avoid damage to the vascular pedicle.

Flap design / orientation aids:
See **Figs. 6.23, 6.24, 6.25.**

The flap is U-shaped, and the longitudinal axis follows the superficial circumflex artery.

The flap design is determined so that one-third of the flap is above and two-thirds below the inguinal ligament.

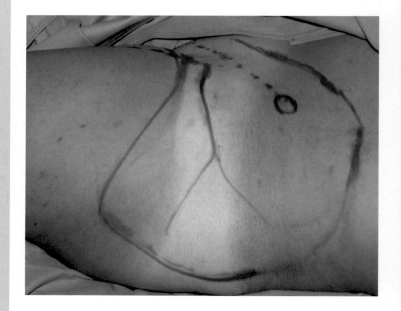

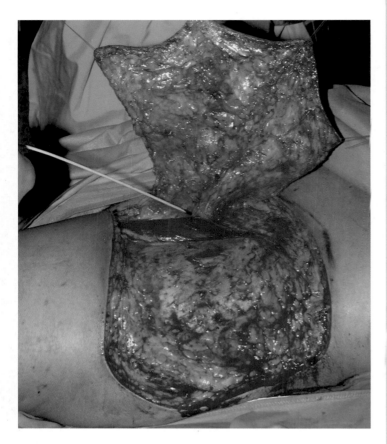

Fig. 6.24 Dissection begins on the distal portion and is not difficult. It proceeds on the lower edge of the subcutaneous fatty tissue; the muscle fibers remain intact. Carefully identify the lateral edge of the sartorius muscle. Incise the fascia of the sartorius muscle and include in the flap to avoid injury to the vascular pedicle. Continue dissection to the origin of the artery. The wooden stick shows the vascular pedicle.

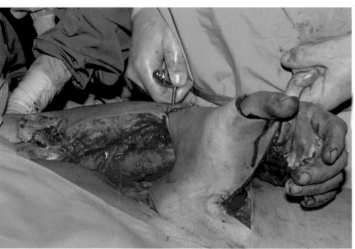

Fig. 6.25 Fitting the flap into the defect. The edges of the donor site are mobilized and sutured.

A palpable pulse over the femoral artery, inguinal ligament, anterior superior iliac spine, and sartorius muscle serve as orientation points.

The pedicle is severed after 2–3 weeks. Conditioning is recommended from the beginning of the second week. The pedicle is initially clamped off with a soft intestinal clamp for an hour at a time. The clamping time can then be increased.

NOTE

If the edges of the skin are mobilized, the donor site can always be primarily sutured.

TIPS AND TRICKS

After severing the pedicle and suturing the base, the pedicle should not be immediately sutured into the defect, but left as a long trunk to wait for demarcation. Two to three days later the portions with sufficient perfusion can be sutured into the defect.

Pelvis/Thigh/Knee

Because of the mechanism of injury and the extensive soft-tissue cover, osteomyelitis is relatively rare in the thigh. It occurs after the extremity has been run over, after infected osteosyntheses, and after changing prostheses.

There are several flaps that can be used to cover defects in the pelvic region and the thigh.

Pelvis:
- **Gracilis muscle:** The flap is raised on its proximal pedicle approximately 7 cm below the pubic branch. It is suitable for defects of the sacrum and perineum.
- **Biceps femoris muscle:** This can be combined with the semitendinosus muscle and be used as an extended musculocutaneous flap to cover a defect in the sacral region and in the groin and abdomen.
- **Tensor fascia latae muscle:** This is used for small defects above the trochanter and in the groin.

Vastus Lateralis Flap

The vastus lateralis muscle provides an excellent flap for cover of defects over the greater trochanter. Its proximal pedicle permits a large rotational arch and filling in of large holes (e.g., exchanging a total hip replacement [THR]).

Functional loss in the muscle, which is only one of four muscles constituting the quadriceps femoris muscle, is negligible.

Vascular and nervous supply:
This muscle coincides with Type II blood supply in the Mathes–Nahai classification. It is perfused by numerous arterial branches which originate mainly from the deep artery of the thigh.

Proximal portion:
Here the muscle is perfused by two large arteries:
- By the lateral circumflex femoral artery, which lies beside the femoral origin of the muscle
- By the lateral circumflex femoral artery or from a common trunk which arises from the deep artery of the thigh.

Middle portion:
Blood is supplied here by the perforating arteries from the deep artery of the thigh.

Distal portion:
Blood is supplied by a branch of the popliteal artery.

NOTE

The vastus lateralis muscle contains a substantial vascular connection between the deep artery of the thigh and the popliteal artery as a collateral circulation to the superficial artery of the thigh. A preoperative angiography must clarify the necessity of this collateral circulation in patients with arteriovenous disease.

NOTE

The two proximal branches are sufficient to supply the entire muscle.

The nerves come from the motor branches which accompany the lateral circumflex femoral artery and enter the middle third of the muscle.

Indications:
This flap is used to cover defects in the proximal thigh, above the trochanter, over the pubis, and in the lower ipsilateral abdominal wall (**Figs. 6.26, 6.27, 6.28**).

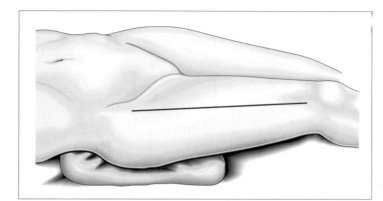

Fig. 6.26 The incision is shown along a line beginning 10 cm distal of the anterior superior iliac spine to the lateral edge of the patella. After subcutaneous dissection sever the fascia lata parallel to the skin incision.

ERRORS AND RISKS

The vascular pedicle of the tensor fasciae latae muscle can be injured.

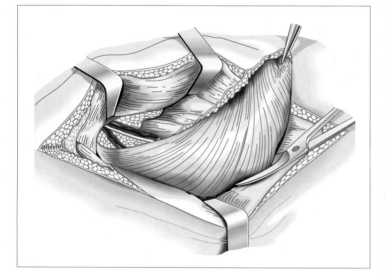

Fig. 6.27 Now the layer between the rectus femoris and the vastus lateralis muscles is severed. The tendon is incised distally and separated from the rectus femoris muscle. The lateral superior arteries and veins of the knee may need to be ligated and severed. Now push the index finger between the vastus lateralis muscle and the periosteum of the femur and carefully raise the muscle. Further dissect the muscle in a proximal direction with a raspatory and scissors. Perforated vessels are ligated and severed. The muscle can now be released from the linea aspera from both distal and proximal directions.

ERRORS AND RISKS

The vascular pedicle of the vastus lateralis muscle can be injured. It runs under the rectus femoralis muscle and crosses the proximal third of the operation site.

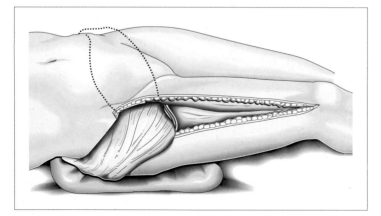

Fig. 6.28 Possible rotational arch of the vastus lateralis flap.

Chronic Osteomyelitis Following Infection of Fracture Fixation with a Femoral Intramedullary Nail

See **Figs. 6.29, 6.30, 6.31.**

Fig. 6.29 Groove-shaped opening of the femoral medullary cavity on the lateral side. Radical debridement and jet lavage. Three muscle flaps are dissected: the lateral head of the gastrocnemius muscle, the vastus lateralis muscle, and the biceps femoris muscle.

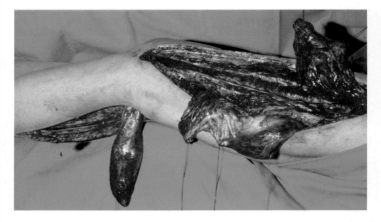

Fig. 6.30 The muscle is rotated into the groove-shaped defect, thereby creating a so-called muscular seal.

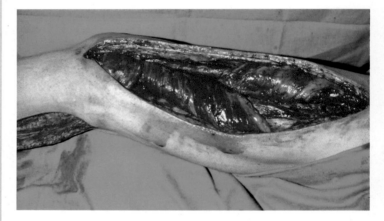

Fig. 6.31 Covering the donor site with a split-skin graft. The figure shows the healed leg with function of the knee joint.

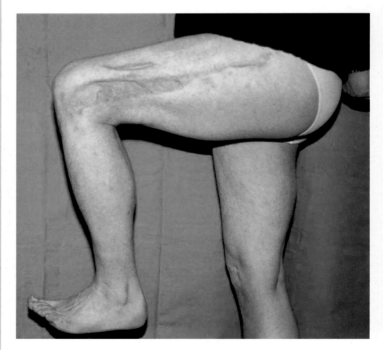

Gastrocnemius Flap

The gastrocnemius muscle with its two heads is the muscle flap most often used for reconstructions of the knee and lower leg. Harvesting is not difficult, and the blood supply is reliable. Even if there is peripheral arterial occlusive disease, each head can be removed with a separate incision without great risk of causing skin necroses.

The gastrocnemius muscle has a medial and a lateral head and is supplied by the sural arteries, which originate from the popliteal artery and are accompanied by motor nerve branches.

This muscle has Type I vascular supply (Mathes–Nahai classification) (**Fig. 6.32**).

NOTE

Each head can be mobilized individually on its neurovascular pedicle.

Fig. 6.32 Anatomy and vascular supply of the heads of the gastrocnemius muscle.

ERRORS AND RISKS

If there is patchy undermining of the wound or there has been a contusion, the vascular supply through the perforans arteries or the axial and segmental vascular system must be tested for patency.

NOTE

Segmental occlusions of the popliteal artery, which can lead to necroses of the tips of the flap, can appear following implantation of a knee prosthesis. Therefore, it is recommended to always perform a preoperative angiography on these patients.

NOTE

Performing an angiography of the femoropopliteal transitional segment is essential prior to transplanting a gastrocnemius flap.

The supplying arteries branch off above the joint space of the knee.

If the gastrocnemius muscle is mobilized from distal, it loses its additional perfusion through the perforans arteries at calf level and the saphenus artery, which has an axial course.

If the femoropopliteal segment is replaced during vascular reconstruction, the arterial and venous supply should be tested by angiography before raising the flap.

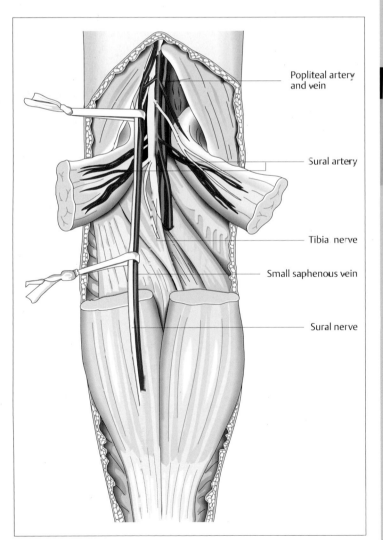

Popliteal artery and vein

Sural artery

Tibia nerve

Small saphenous vein

Sural nerve

Medial Head

The medial head is longer than the lateral head and is therefore used more often.

Indications:
- Defects of the proximal part of the middle third of the tibia, the anterior and medial sides of the knee, and the femoral condyle
- Defects above the anterior and medial side of the knee joint
- Defects near the medial femoral condyle
- Defects (holes) in the distal portions of the femur

Chronic Osteomyelitis after Infection of Internal Plate Fixation of the Proximal Tibia (Fig. 6.33)

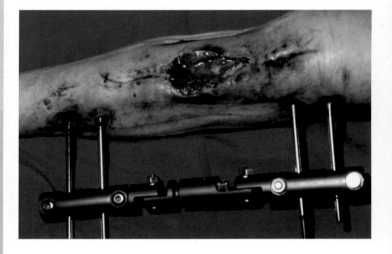

Fig. 6.33 Repeated radical debridement after removal of plates. Temporary skin closure with artificial skin (Vacuseal, K.C.I., Wiesbaden, Germany) and local antibiotic administration (Septocoll, Biomet, Berlin, Germany). Stabilization with external fixation.

TIPS AND TRICKS

Since the medial gastrocnemius head is longer than the lateral one, it is used more often. The connection with a cutaneous flap in the distal portion of the muscle and on the distal portion of the aponeurosis can further lengthen the flap so that even defects in the distal thigh can be covered.

Rotation beyond the knee joint can be improved by tunneling the muscle beneath the tendons of the biceps, semitendinosus, and gracilis muscles (for holes in the distal portions of the femur).

Surgical Steps for Mobilizing the Medial Gastrocnemius Head

See **Figs. 6.34, 6.35, 6.36, 6.37**

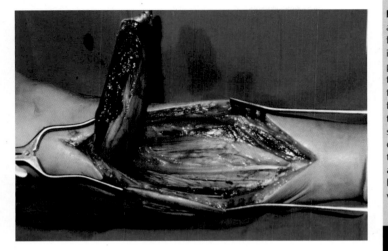

Fig. 6.34 With the patient in a supine position and the knee slightly bent, the incision is performed 4 cm posterior to the posterior tibial edge in the middle of the calf and proceeds up to the popliteal fossa. The intermuscular layer between the soleus muscle and the medial head of the gastrocnemius muscle is manually widened with the fingers after incision of the thin aponeurosis. The tendon of the plantar muscle becomes visible. The surreal nerve is then exposed on the posterior side of the medial head. Dissect the layer between the two heads. Now sever the tendon at the distal end and dissect stepwise from distal to proximal. Mobilize the common fibular nerve, identify the neurovascular pedicle, then sever the motor branch.

ERRORS AND RISKS

Injury to the great saphenous vein with its accompanying nerves and lymph nodes must be avoided during subcutaneous dissection.

NOTE

The motor branch is carefully exposed and severed. It accompanies blood vessels and is usually found lateral to the proximal portions of the muscle.

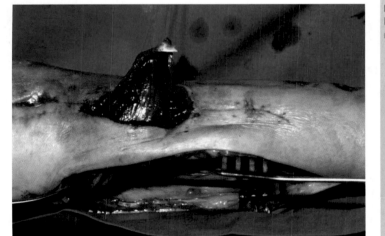

Fig. 6.35 Rotation of the medial gastrocnemius head into the defect. Releasing the origin of the muscle widens the rotational arch.

TIPS AND TRICKS

The isolated muscle attached to its vascular pedicle must be tunneled under the tendons of the semitendinosus and gracilis muscles to enable it to reach the medial and lateral condyles or the anterior aspect of the knee.

Fig. 6.36 Covering the rotated flap with a split-skin graft. Stabilization of the site with external fixation.

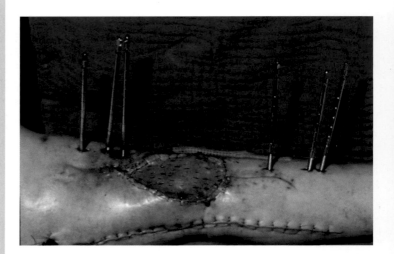

Fig. 6.37 Several transverse incisions in the aponeurosis on the lower side of the muscle (be very careful not to injure the axial vessels) enlarge the rotational arch. Sever the proximal tendon attachment, and release the popliteal segment from the posterior tibia.

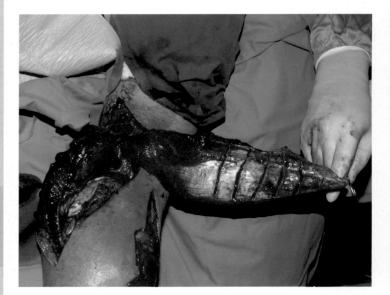

TIPS AND TRICKS

Several transverse incisions in the aponeurosis on the posterior side of the muscle increase the rotational arch.

TIPS AND TRICKS

Small defects in the lateral patella can be closed. By rotating the graft 180° and tunneling it under the peroneal nerve, the muscle can reach the distal fourth of the femur.

Lateral Head

Indications:
- Defects over the lateral side of the knee
- Defects near the lateral femoral condyle

Surgical steps for mobilization of the lateral head of the gastrocnemius muscle:
- The patient lies supine with slight medial rotation of the leg
- Incise the skin over the posterior fibula from the middle of the calf to the popliteal fossa.
- Perform a longitudinal incision in the deep fascia of the leg and expose the sural nerve.
- Perform a longitudinal incision in the aponeurosis between the two gastrocnemius heads.
- Perform lateral dissection between the tendons of the soleus and gastrocnemius muscles.

- After severing the tendon, dissect the lateral head in a proximal direction.
- Mobilize the common fibular nerve and identify the neurovascular pedicle prior to severing the motor branch.

Lower Leg

Choice of Soft-Tissue Graft

The differential therapeutic options in choosing a suitable soft-tissue graft depend on the size of the defect and extent of damage. The following text lists the different possible reconstructive methods.

Differential therapeutic options for soft-tissue closure on the lower leg:
1. Direct closure, relaxation incision, fasciocutaneous bridging flaps
2. Dermotraction procedure (be careful not to disturb the perfusion)
3. Vacuum seal and split-skin graft
4. Local flap, fascia flap, turn-over flap
5. Pedicled muscle flap, vascular-pedicled island flap
6. Microsurgical tissue transfer
7. Microvascular attachment of amputated parts
8. Cross-leg transplantation

Wound closure should always be without tension, possibly achieved with relaxation incisions or fasciocutaneous bridge flaps. Dermotraction procedures can also be useful. If the tibia, blood vessels, and nerves are exposed, early coverage with fasciocutaneous flaps or muscle flaps is indicated.

Primary shortening of the lower leg in the fixator after segment resection considerably broadens the indication for a gastrocnemius flap by diverting the action radius toward distal. If the tibia is shorted by approximately 6 cm, the medial gastrocnemius flap reaches the distal third of the lower leg if a proximal disinsertion is performed on the femur condyle. Careful dissection of the dominant vascular pedicle and severing of the branches of the motor nerve enable an increase in length of approximately 2–4 cm (**Table 6.1**).

Among the at least 25 anatomically suitable donor sites in the human body, the latissimus dorsi muscle has achieved central importance in microsurgical soft-tissue reconstruction of the lower leg, especially for large defects. Its consistent vascular system, its size, the esthetically favorable primary closure of the donor site, and the negligible functional deficit make it an ideal graft. The microsurgical latissimus transplantation has ushered in

NOTE

The oblique fibers of the soleus muscle, which stretch between the tibia and the fibula, compress the fourth compartment and comprise the most important muscle pump system in the lower leg.

Therefore, this muscle may only be used to cover soft-tissue defects in special cases among older patients.

This undoubtedly provides a clearly defined indication for microsurgical tissue transfer instead of a soleus flap with a distal or proximal pedicle in younger patients.

Raising local muscle flaps from the lower leg can cause deficits in pronation and supination strength with decreased gait stability.

Table 6.1 Local flap in the knee and lower leg

Knee	Gastrocnemius flap
	Saphenous artery flap
	Medial fasciocutaneous saphenous flap
Proximal third	Gastrocnemius flap
	Sartorius flap
	Gracilis flap
	Semimembranosus flap
Middle third	Gastrocnemius flap
	Tibialis anterior flap
Distal third	Soleus flap
	Sural flap
	Flexor hallucis longus flap
	Extensor hallucis longus flap
	Dorsalis pedis flap
	Flexor digitorum communis flap

a decisive change in therapy with a reduction in amputation rates and fistula quotas to fewer than 10%. Primary shortening of the lower leg enables microvascular attachment in the proximal segment of the lower leg, usually without requiring a venous interponate.

Chronic Osteomyelitis of the Distal Tibia (Fig. 6.38)

Fig. 6.38 The bone and soft tissues have been repeatedly debrided. The entire distal portion of the lower leg and the upper ankle joint are covered with a microvascularly attached myocutaneous latissimus dorsi flap. Bone shifting begins 5 days after flap transplantation and corticotomy.

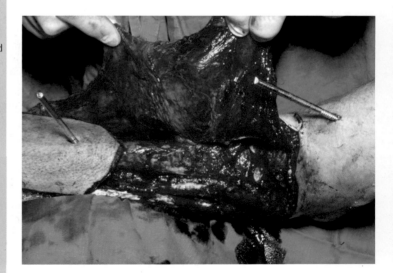

NOTE

Soft-tissue flaps, bone shortening, and bone regeneration are closely connected.

Convalescence up to full weight bearing is considerably shortened following soft-tissue grafting.

Soft-Tissue Flaps and the Venous System

Serial examinations after second- and third-degree open fractures of the lower leg confirm that a posttraumatic reduction in the venous drainage of up to 50% can be expected in most patients in their 20s and 30s. If the changes with age which occur without accidents (valve insufficiency, perforans insufficiency) are added, a much higher incidence of chronic venous drainage disturbances, that is, post-thrombotic syndrome, must be expected. Taking these factors into consideration, it is necessary to protect the superficial and deep venous systems and lymph nodes during all surgical interventions.

Latissimus Dorsi Flap

There are numerous indications for a latissimus dorsi flap, both as a free myocutaneous and as a pedicled flap, to cover defects and for functional restitution. The functional deficits at the donor site are unimportant in comparison to the amount of tissue gained. Defects of up to 20 × 40 cm can be covered (**Figs. 6.39, 6.40, 6.41, 6.42, 6.43, 6.44**). A vascularized rib segment (ninth or tenth rib) can be removed with the muscle.

Indications:
- A vascular pedicled flap is used to cover defects on the shoulder, upper arm, posterior side of the elbow, and chest wall up to the clavicle. A distal pedicle can also be used.
- A free flap is used to cover extensive soft-tissue defects, especially in the distal lower leg.

Vascular and nervous supply:
- Thoracodorsal artery and vein
- Thoracodorsal nerve

TIPS AND TRICKS

Transport corticotomy alone is not adequate to solve soft-tissue problems. The result of a tibia segment reconstruction must be not only a stable bone, but also functional, sufficient soft-tissue coverage of the anterior edge of the tibia, which is subjected to considerable mechanical stress.

ERRORS AND RISKS

A split-thickness graft over the ankle leads to a potentially unstable and vulnerable scar. Therefore, this reconstructive procedure is not used.

Fig. 6.39 Anatomy of the latissimus dorsi muscle: the neurovascular bundle passes through the axilla and lies on the posterior side of the muscle, covered by the fascia. The length of the vascular pedicle after leaving the circumflex scapular artery averages 4 cm (2–5 cm, maximally 12 cm) before the first branches enter the muscle. The main artery is the thoracodorsal artery, which is accompanied by the thoracodorsal vein and nerve. Normally five to seven branches of segmental arteries T6–L5 feed the aponeurosis of origin. They play only a minor role in the blood supply of the muscle.

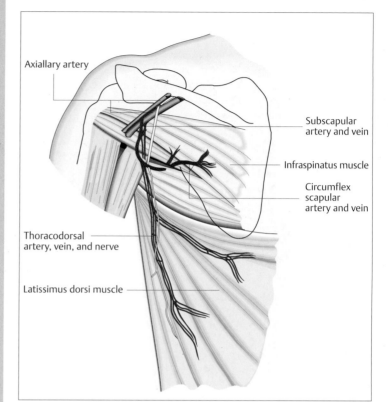

Fig. 6.40 Placing the patient in an oblique or lateral position for removal of the flap. The arm is elevated.

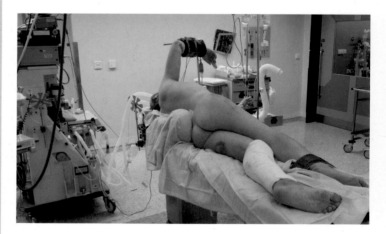

Fig. 6.41 The dimensions of the incision depend on the size of the required skin island. The dotted line marks the anterior edge of the muscle.

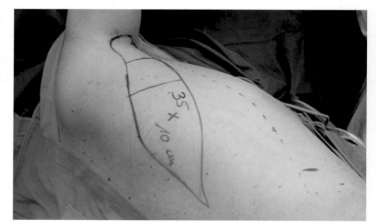

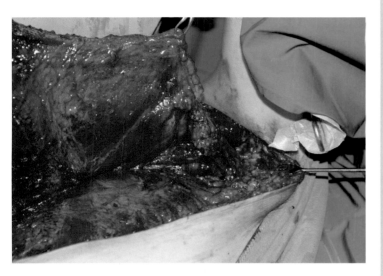

Fig. 6.42 First dissect the anterior edge of the muscle with the vascular pedicle at the axilla. On the distal aspect the origin of the muscle is dissected and severed from its insertion on the iliac crest and spine. The flap is now raised from distal to proximal and the insertions on the scapula are severed.

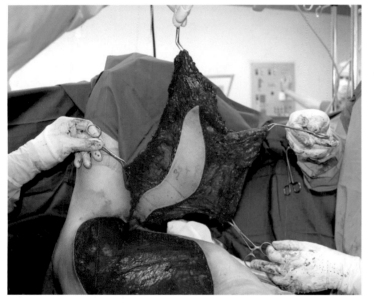

Fig. 6.43 After releasing the muscle completely, remove the insertion in the armpit and, after identifying the axillary artery and vein, ligate and sever the neurovascular pedicle.

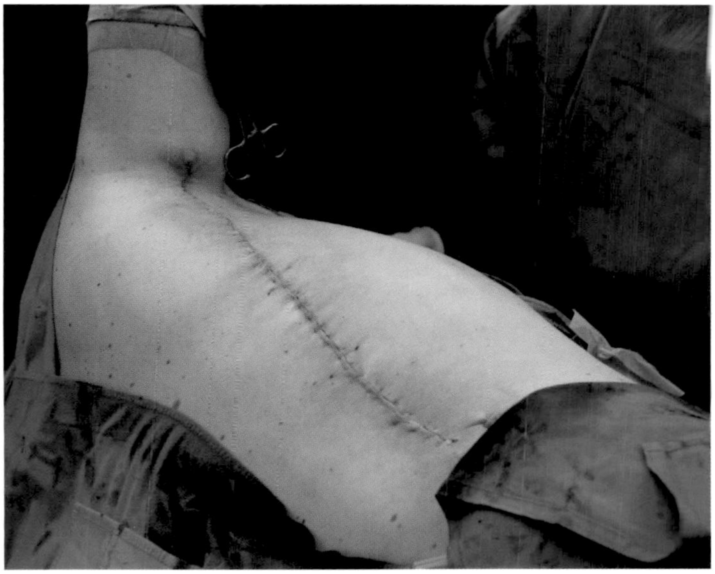

Fig. 6.44 Mobilization of the edges of the skin enables a tension-free closure. Insertion of two drains, one anterior and one posterior.

TIPS AND TRICKS

The wound edges can be attached to the thoracic wall to reduce postoperative seromas, which otherwise frequently occur.

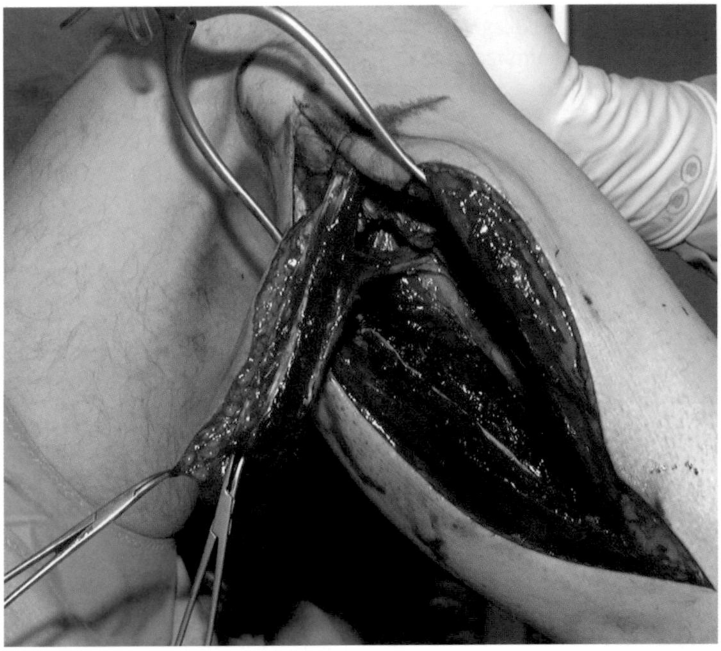

Fig. 6.55 The flexor hallucis longus muscle is retracted, and the fibular artery and vein are further exposed.

TIPS AND TRICKS

A small amount of the posterior tibial muscle should also be left on the anterior side to avoid injuring the vascular bundle.

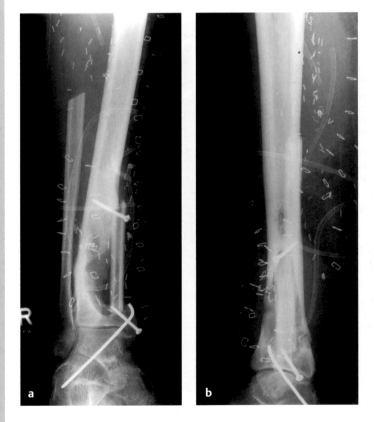

Osteotomy of the fibula can be performed after severing and retracting the periosteum.

The posterior tibial artery and an accompanying vein are anastomosed end-to-side.

The transplant is attached with screws and a Kirschner wire (**Figs. 6.56, 6.57, 6.58**).

Fig. 6.56a, b Postoperative radiographs.

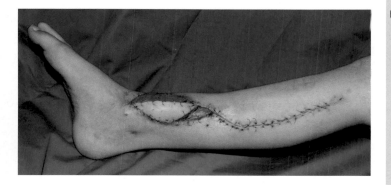

Fig. 6.57 Postoperative clinical result.

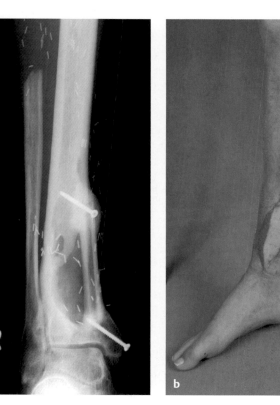

Fig. 6.58a, b Radiographic and clinical results 6 months later.

Ankle and Foot

Defects on the ankle and foot can be covered by a large number of regional perforator flaps, which will not be described in detail here.

- The **lateral supramalleolar flap** can be used to cover defects on the back of the foot and the posterior part of the heel.
- The **medial plantar artery flap** (a neurovascular graft) is suitable for covering small defects on the heel.
- The **extensor brevis muscle** covers the lateral side of the tibial epiphysis if it remains attached to the lat-

Fig. 6.59 Drawing of the flap with pedicle in the middle of the calf. The patient is supine. For a sural flap with a distal pedicle, the slightly curved course of the sural nerve to the rotational axis is drawn from the lower end of the flap.

eral tarsal artery pedicle and there is no lesion of the dorsalis pedis artery.

- The **peroneus brevis muscle** is suitable for covering the middle of the Achilles tendon. Fasciocutaneous flaps can be used either from lateral or medial to cover distal soft-tissue losses above the attachment of the Achilles tendon to the calcaneus.
- The **flexor hallucis longus muscle** with a proximal pedicle can cover the lower Achilles tendon.

Sural Flap

Indications:
A sural flap is taken from the posterior aspect of the calf. It is used to cover the heel, the area around the medial malleolus, and the medial distal lower leg.

Vascular and nervous supply: Sural artery and nerve.

Arterial blood is supplied by the sural artery and innervation by the sural nerve.

The descending neurovascular bundle penetrates the deep fascia of the leg approximately in the middle of the calf and continues subcutaneously. The artery becomes a vascular network at the level of the retromalleolar region.

There are numerous anastamoses between this vascular axis and the fibular artery.

The pedicle consists of subcutaneous tissue, the fascia, the sural nerve with its vascular axis, and the accompanying small saphenous vein. The flap cannot be stretched much further proximal than the musculotendinous border of the gastrocnemius muscle because the vascular pedicle lies subfascial and further proximal (**Figs. 6.59, 6.60, 6.61, 6.62, 6.63, 6.64, 6.65**).

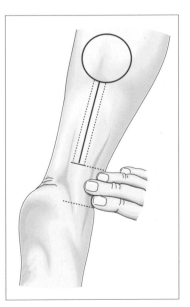

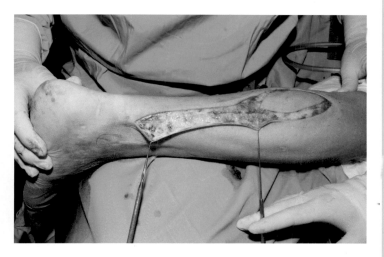

Fig. 6.60 Dissection of the flap begins at the section distant from the pedicle. Sharp, short, transverse skin incisions are made in the skin and fascia. Now the nerve with its accompanying arteries can easily be identified and severed. Sever the small saphenous nerve between ligatures. It is included in the flap. Cut out the skin island. Next it is essential to fixate the fascia and subcutis with resorbable sutures to prevent dissection. Further incision only severs the skin on the pedicle (sural nerve).

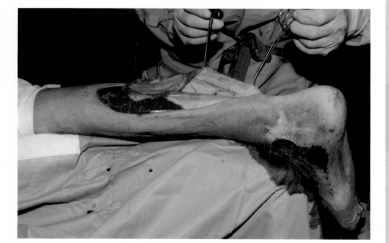

Fig. 6.61 Further dissection of the sural nerve and small saphenous vein must be performed with the subcutaneous fat en bloc and include the fascia up to the rotational axis.

TIPS AND TRICKS

The fascia can be pushed up (blunt dissection) from the belly of the gastrocnemius muscle.

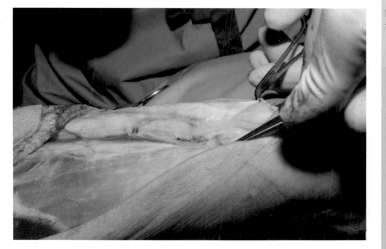

Fig. 6.62 Perforans vessels that enter the flap on the lateral side of the Achilles tendon.

TIPS AND TRICKS

To avoid compression of the flap, the patient must lie on his/her side after the operation. Alternatively, prepare a special splint to protect the sural flap and its pedicle from compression.

After rotating the sural flap into the defect, cover the vascular pedicle with a split-skin graft to prevent compression and the risk of flap failure.

If a defect on the lateral malleolus is covered with a sural flap, this can be placed upside down without twisting the pedicle. In this case, the entire flap, including the pedicle, must be covered with a split-skin graft.

Fig. 6.63 Dissection to the distal perforans vessel. This is the exact rotational axis of the flap.

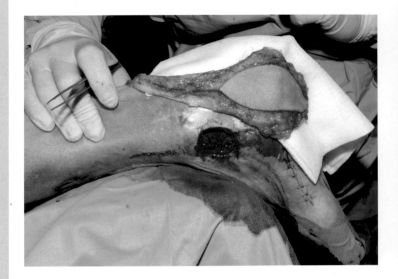

Fig. 6.64 Longitudinal skin incision above the future pedicle to the proximal edge of the defect.

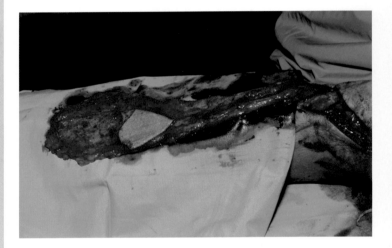

Fig. 6.65 The raised island flap can be rotated into the debrided soft-tissue defect without tension and attached with single sutures. A soft silicone drain is recommended. The pedicle is now covered with a split-skin graft. Primary wound closure is usually possible if the edges of the donor site are mobilized. Otherwise it can be covered with a split-skin graft.

NOTE

To prevent venous congestion and flap failure, be very careful not to twist the pedicle or bend it when rotating the flap into the defect .

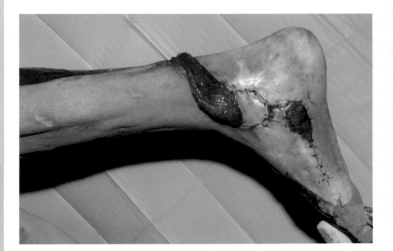

Dorsalis Pedis Flap

The dorsalis pedis flap (graft from the back of the foot) is one of the earliest known neurovascular flaps, which can be transplanted either as a free or a pedicled flap. Today the indication for this flap is rare due to the considerable morbidity at the donor site and the availability of alternative flaps.

Indications:
- Defects on the edges of the foot, the distal third of the lower leg, and the heel (as a pull-through procedure)
- As a free sensory flap

Vascular and nervous supply:
Blood is supplied by the dorsalis pedis artery, and branches of the superficial fibular nerve provide sensory perception.

The dorsalis pedis artery, which is a continuation of the anterior tibial artery, crosses the anterior section of the joint capsule of the upper ankle joint, the talus, the navicular bone, and the intermediate cuneiform bone from proximal to distal (**Fig. 6.66**).

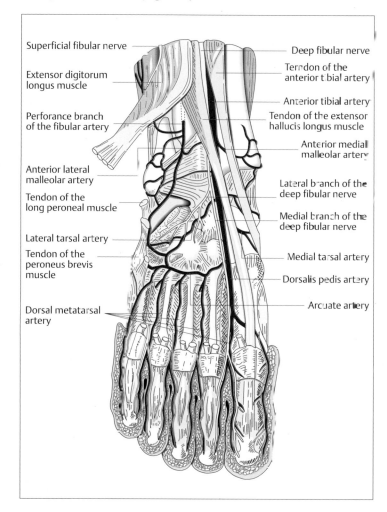

Superficial fibular nerve

Extensor digitorum longus muscle

Perforance branch of the fibular artery

Anterior lateral malleolar artery

Tendon of the long peroneal muscle

Lateral tarsal artery

Tendon of the peroneus brevis muscle

Dorsal metatarsal artery

Deep fibular nerve

Tendon of the anterior tibial artery

Anterior tibial artery

Tendon of the extensor hallucis longus muscle

Anterior medial malleolar artery

Lateral branch of the deep fibular nerve

Medial branch of the deep fibular nerve

Medial tarsal artery

Dorsalis pedis artery

Arcuate artery

Fig. 6.66 Anatomy of the anterior aspect of the foot.

NOTE

The artery lies directly on the bone, especially at the level of the first intermetatarsal space. This makes dissection of this flap difficult.

When dissecting the artery in the distal (digital) portion, the tendon of the extensor digitorum brevis muscle must be severed where it inserts into the tendon of the extensor hallucis longus muscle.

Including the first head of the extensor digitorum brevis muscle in the flap increases its viability. The corresponding segment of the lateral tarsal artery is thus included in the flap.

Branches of the superficial fibular nerve which lie within the flap provide sensory perception.

The tendon of the extensor hallucis longus muscle lies on the medial side of the dorsalis pedis artery. The extensor digitorum longus muscle and the deep fibular nerve lie on the lateral side of the artery. The artery has several branches which proceed between the metatarsal bones to the plantar arch.

The dermal branch, which supplies the flap, originates from a short segment of the artery lying between the extensor hallucis longus muscle and the first head of the extensor digitorum brevis muscle.

Chronic Osteomyelitis of the Distal Tibia

See **Figs. 6.67, 6.68, 6.69, 6.70, 6.71, 6.72.**

Fig. 6.67 Repeated radical debridement of the bone and soft tissues is required for necrotic bones. Local antibiotics are administered and defect coverage with a dorsalis pedis flap is planned.

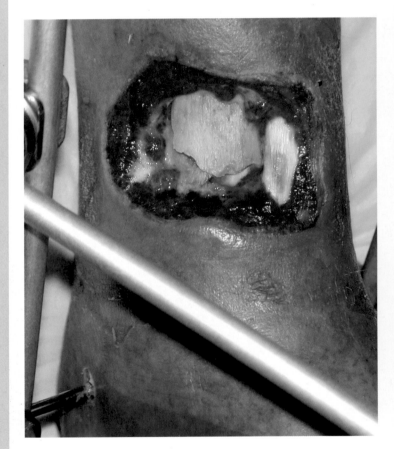

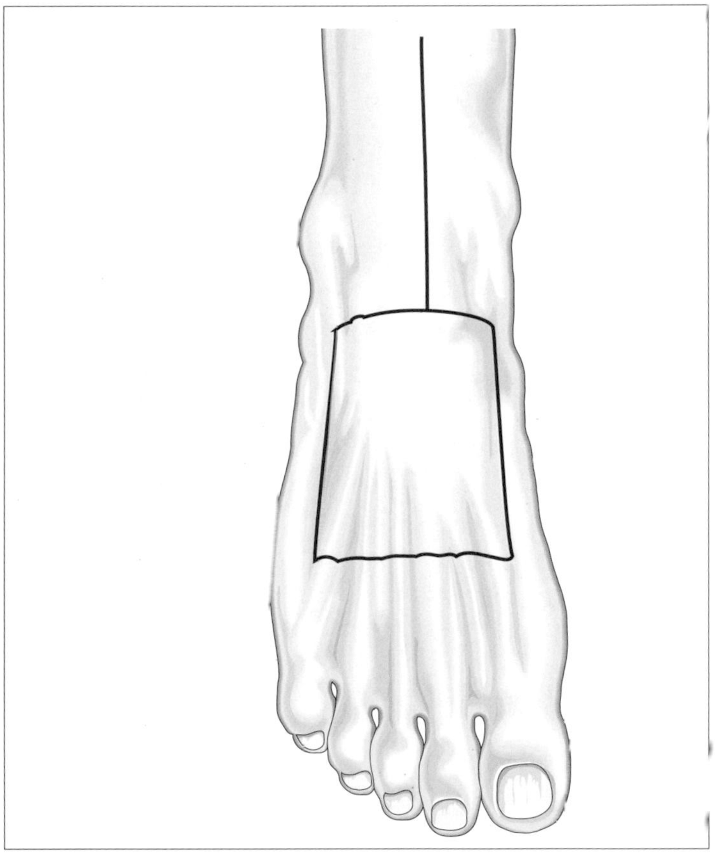

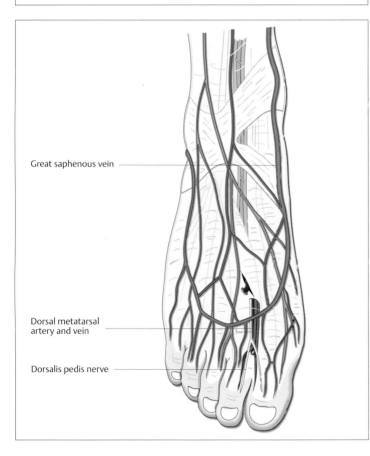

Fig. 6.68 Drawing the flap. Landmarks: on the proximal side, above the distal leg of the inferior extensor retinaculum and medial, above the tendon of the extensor hallucis longus muscle. The veins which flow into the great saphenous vein are included. On the lateral side, the flap extends down to the tendon of the extensor digitorum longus muscle. The flap should end in the middle of the metatarsal bones.

Fig. 6.69 Dissect the artery above the upper ankle joint on the medial side of the tendon of the extensor hallucis longus muscle. Tie off the veins on the medial side, and dissect the medial edge of the flap. Lateral of the tendon of the extensor hallucis longus muscle is the tendon of the extensor digitorum brevis muscle, which is severed and attached to the lower surface of the flap. The distal branches of the superficial fibular nerve are also severed.

Great saphenous vein

Dorsal metatarsal
artery and vein

Dorsalis pedis nerve

ERRORS AND RISKS

There is risk of injury to the branches of the superficial fibular nerve.

Fig. 6.70 Dissect the first intermetatarsal space and expose the intermetatarsalis dorsalis superficialis artery (if there is one). This is then ligated and severed, and the proximal stump integrated in the flap. Now identify the deep branch of the dorsalis pedis artery.

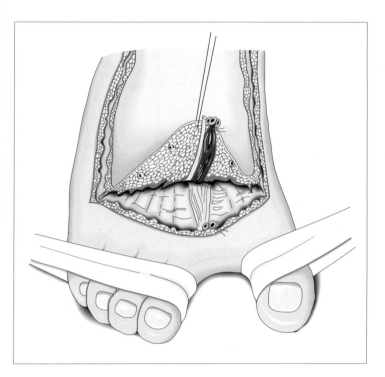

Fig. 6.71 Retraction of the extensor digitorum longus muscle and exposure of the extensor digitorum brevis muscle. The first head of this muscle can be left in place together with the tissue above it and is separated from the rest of the musculature. Tie off the lateral tarsal artery below the muscle. If the medial portion of the muscle is not to be included in the flap, the motor branch can be preserved. Now ligate the distal end of the artery. Also ligate the first tarsalis dorsalis artery and, if it is located superficially, integrate it in the flap. If the artery lies beneath the interosseus muscle, tie off and sever the dorsalis pedis artery at the point where it enters the plantar branch. Finally, suture together the tendons of the extensor digitorum longus and the extensor hallucis longus muscles.

NOTE

When dissecting the flap, the paratendinous tissue must be left in place because the donor site has to be covered with a split-skin graft.

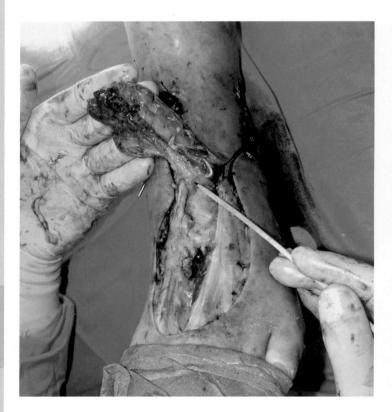

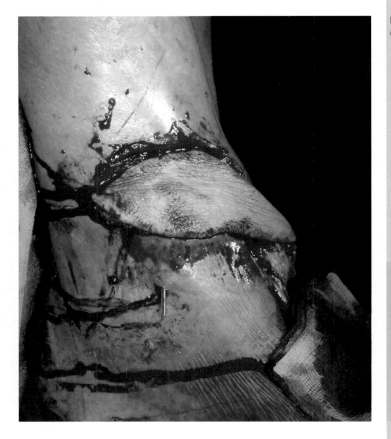

TIPS AND TRICKS

If perfusion is uncertain, as shown in the example, a bridge of skin can be left on the pedicle. This considerably decreases the flap rotation, but improves its venous drainage.

Because of the consistent anatomy of the artery and its caliber, blood supply is rarely a problem. Venous congestion is a more common problem which can, however, be solved by leaving a skin bridge or several superficial veins.

Adductor Digiti Minimi (VY) Flap

This is indicated to cover distal defects on the lateral edge of the foot. This flap can still be used even after unsuccessful attempts to cover the defect with flaps with a medial pedicle, as in the following example.

Indications:
Defects on the distal, lateral edge of the foot can be covered by this flap.

Vascular supply:
The lateral branch of the plantar artery provides blood.

The blood supply of the flap comes from the lateral branch of the plantar artery. This can be either a muscle flap or a musculocutaneous flap. The blood vessel runs parallel to the adductor digiti minimi muscle, but somewhat medial in a distal direction.

NOTE

When planning this flap, take into consideration the later scar formation in the weight-bearing area of the sole of the foot.

Chronic Fistulous Osteomyelitis with a Skin Defect in Congenital Clump Foot

See **Figs. 6.73, 6.74, 6.75, 6.76.**

Fig. 6.73 Clinical picture after amputation of metatarsal V and failed coverage of the defect with a sliding flap. In this patient with congenital varus malposition of the foot, the incision is more lateral. The entire heel remains intact.

Fig. 6.74 After incising the flap, V-shaped dissection is performed in the deeper layers of tissue. The plantar aponeurosis and the plantar muscle are included in the flap. The vessels are preserved. The abductor digiti minimi has already been dissected and its blood vessel identified.

Fig. 6.75 Removal of the muscle at its insertion on the calcaneus and the intermuscular septa in the back of the foot. The flap is advanced into the defect without tension.

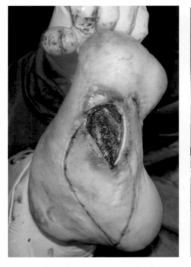
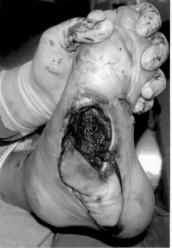
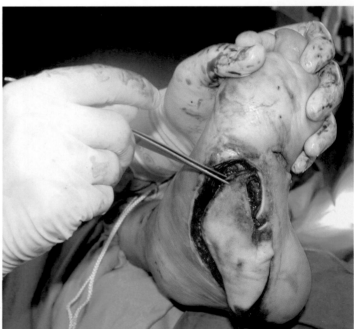

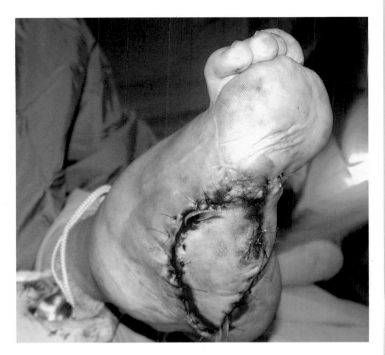

Fig. 6.76 Before suturing the flap into the defect, the tourniquet is opened and the flap perfusion checked. After careful hemostasis, the flap is sutured and a drain inserted.

NOTE

Further treatment includes 4 weeks without weight bearing on forearm crutches. Sutures should not be removed earlier than 3 weeks when soft tissues are endangered, as in the case study.

Lateral Upper-Arm Flap

The fasciocutaneous flap can be either a free or a pedicled flap. It is harvested from the lateral aspect of the upper arm and has a septal pattern.

Indications:
- A flap with a proximal pedicle can be used to cover defects over the shoulder (up to the coracoid and axilla).
- A flap with a distal pedicle can be used to cover defects on the elbow (anterior and posterior regions).
- The free lateral upper-arm flap is mostly used to cover defects on the hand. It can be harvested from the same arm.

The lateral upper-arm flap with a proximal pedicle is an alternative to a parascapular flap.

Vascular and nervous supply:
- The septal arteries from the posterior descending branch of the deep artery of the arm provide blood.
- The posterior antebrachial cutaneous nerve and a branch that originates from the radial nerve provide sensory perception.

The posterior antebrachial cutaneous nerve perforates the deep fascia somewhat proximal of the lateral epicondyle (perfuses the skin of the posterior forearm). A small nerve originates directly from the radial nerve and provides sensory perception of the skin on the flap.

NOTE

Donor sites of up to approximately 6 cm can be closed primarily. Hairy upper arms can be cosmetically disadvantageous.

NOTE

Blood is supplied to the flap by septal arteries which anastamose with the posterior recurrent interosseous artery in the subcutaneous tissue on the lateral side of the elbow.

The pedicle should always be dissected to the origin of the profunda brachii artery from the brachial artery. This provides a pedicle with a length of up to 8 cm.

The technique for a free and a pedicled graft is identical.

Technique for a Proximal Pedicled Upper-Arm Flap

See **Figs. 6.77, 6.78, 6.79.**

Fig. 6.77 The planned flap is drawn in the distal lateral third of the upper arm, as well as the incision for dissection of the pedicle. The dotted line runs between the acromion and the lateral epicondyle. Dissection begins from posterior, including the fascia of the triceps muscle. The posterior descending branch of the deep brachial artery runs in the exposed intermuscular septum. This is now freed from anterior. The layer between the deltoid and the triceps brachii muscles is exposed and the muscles are held apart.

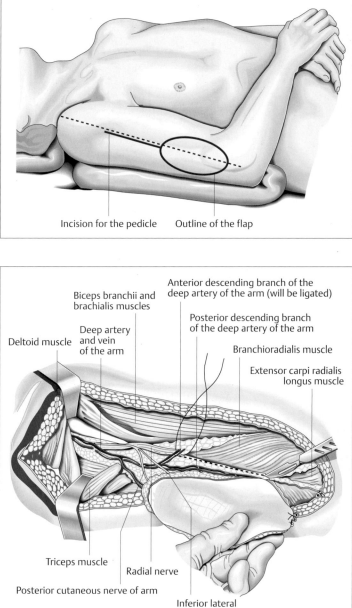

Incision for the pedicle   Outline of the flap

Fig. 6.78 The radial nerve and vascular pedicle are now visible. The anterior descending branch is ligated. The septum is severed just above the bone and the flap is raised. The blood vessels are tied off at the distal edge of the flap.

Biceps branchii and brachialis muscles

Anterior descending branch of the deep artery of the arm (will be ligated)

Deep artery and vein of the arm

Posterior descending branch of the deep artery of the arm

Deltoid muscle

Branchioradialis muscle

Extensor carpi radialis longus muscle

Triceps muscle

Radial nerve

Posterior cutaneous nerve of arm

Inferior lateral cutaneous nerve of arm

ERRORS AND RISKS

There is risk of injury to the radial nerve.

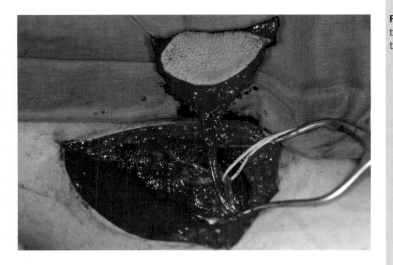

Fig. 6.79 The proximal pedicle is exposed when the deltoid and triceps brachii muscles are retracted.

Osteomyelitis of the Heel with Bilateral Fistulas and an Ulcer after Frostbite

See **Figs. 6.80, 6.81, 6.82, 6.83**.

Upper-arm flap with a distal pedicle:

- The island of skin is raised somewhat further distal on the lateral aspect of the upper arm compared with a flap with a proximal pedicle.
- A short distal incision permits mobilization of the distal pedicle.
- Dissection is the same as for a flap with a proximal pedicle.
- The descending branch of the profunda brachii artery is severed and tied off at its origin.
- The septum is separated from the humerus, and a short fasciocutaneous pedicle is dissected and mobilized distal to the flap

NOTE

A flap with a distal pedicle can be rotated either in an anterior or posterior direction.

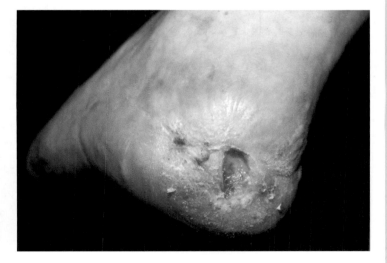

Fig. 6.80 Serial radical surgical debridement has been performed on this heel. Both bone and tissue were biopsied for microbiologic examination. After an antibiogram, systemic antibiotics were administered and a local resorbable antibiotic carrier (e.g., Septocoll) was inserted.

Fig. 6.81 Dissection of a 4 × 5-cm fasciocutaneous flap from the lateral upper arm. The posterior tibial artery and vein are dissected and tunneled subcutaneously and attached by end-to-side anastamoses.

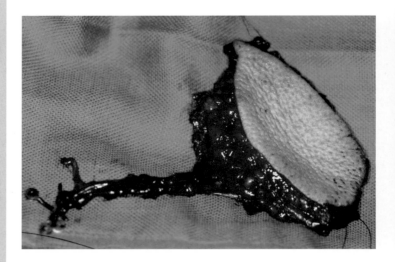

Fig. 6.82 Clinical result 1.5 years later with well-contoured padding of the heel.

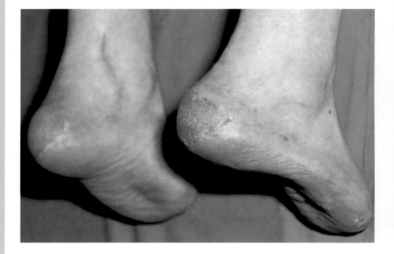

Fig. 6.83 Clinical result after primary closure of the donor site.

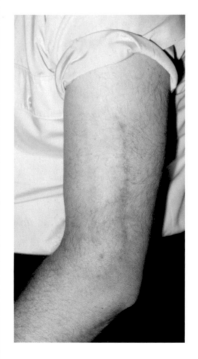

Maintaining and Lengthening an Amputation Stump in Chronic Osteomyelitis

Even with modern reconstruction procedures amputation remains an essential procedure in the surgical spectrum.

If clinical conditions require a proximal amputation and there is insufficient soft tissue, there is a probability of lifelong functional deficits.

Chronic pain, intolerance of cold, skin irritations and ulcers, tendency to swell, recurrent erysipelas, spinal complaints, uncertain gait, reduced functional capacity, and increased energy requirements are typical problems. With increasing age and cardiorespiratory deficits, energy requirements cannot be met when the patient has to walk with a prosthesis. He or she then has to use a wheelchair.

If the clinical condition requires amputation of the knee joint, carry out a test to determine whether it would be possible to perform a transgenicular or transcondylar amputation, thus preserving the original muscle strength.

Always consider using the foot. The tibial nerve could be rolled up like a modified Borggreve graft. The weight-bearing parts of the arch in particular, above all the unit consisting of the calcaneus and the soft tissues of the heel, can be used as a stump end and can provide a gain in length of approximately 10 cm.

If there are long segmental defects in the thigh or knee, the described methods can be applied. Aside from hinged flaps with a lengthening of the tibia with a vascular pedicle as a femur replacement, a Borggreve rotation flap in particular offers obvious functional advantages. If the length of the lower leg is precisely adjusted to that of the thigh stump, the ankle can serve as a knee replacement. A modification of this technique is to use parts of the foot or lower leg to form a Chopart stump and achieve at least a length corresponding to exarticulation of the knee joint.

Circular traction sutures can provide a considerable gain in length with a tensionless wound closure. The foundation for every preoperative plan is an interdisciplinary analysis of the weight-bearing zones on the prosthesis-bearing stump, which should be covered with well-padded, thin flaps with sensory innervation if possible. It this is not possible due to unfavorable local conditions, employing microvascular techniques before shortening the stump is justified.

NOTE

If the extent of osteomyelitis permits the formation of a long, well-padded stump on the lower leg, functional rehabilitation and social reintegration can generally be successfully achieved.

NOTE

A fundamental principle is to attempt to preserve a lower-leg stump with adequate length (> 10 cm) if the knee joint is mobile.

TIPS AND TRICKS

When forming a thigh stump, the entire spectrum of surgical reconstruction procedures must be employed to preserve as much length as possible. The form of the stump must not always conform to conventional expectations. Even after loss of the function of the quadriceps muscle or the long knee flexor or with a high lesion of the ischiadic nerve, if there is sufficient soft-tissue coverage, a long, atypical thigh stump is preferable. The area innervated by the saphenous nerve guarantees a stump with sensory sensation at the level of the knee.

NOTE

The use of amputated body parts is an important principle among the available technical techniques.

NOTE

Besides the use of amputated parts, conventional skin grafts make up the majority of reconstructive procedures.

Infected Nonunion of the Defect with Circular Constriction due to Scar Tissue (Case Study)

See **Figs. 6.84, 6.85, 6.86, 6.87**.

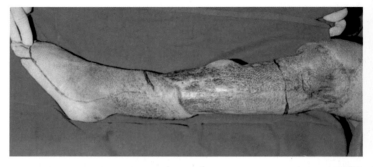

Fig. 6.84 Injury with pronounced skin abrasion and 3-cm tibial segment defect 1.5 years after autogenous bone grafting and a latissimus dorsi flap. There is now infected nonunion at the defect site with circular constriction caused by scar tissue.

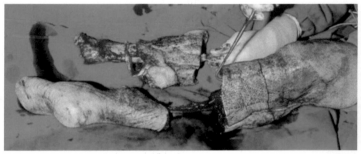

Fig. 6.85 Segment resection and dissection of the neurovascular pedicle.

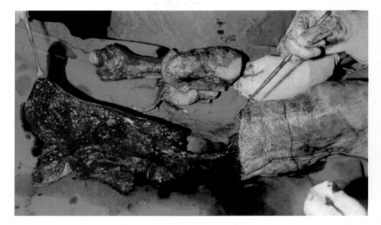

Fig. 6.86 Dissection of a pedicled neurovascular osteomyocutaneous calcaneus foot fillet.

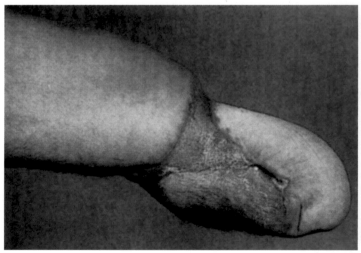

Fig. 6.87 The final result is a stump which can bear a prosthesis and has sensitive skin from the heel and sole of the foot.

Morbidity of the Donor Site

The indication for a muscle flap is only given after careful preoperative evaluation of possible complications at the donor site.

Survey articles cite the rate of severe complications (requiring revision) as 3%.

From the large number of available flaps, the following briefly discusses those most often used.

Latissimus Dorsi Flap

This flap is the most often used pedicle or microvascularly transplanted flap in reconstructive surgery. It is generally employed as a myocutaneous flap with a corresponding skin island. The skin island is primarily for monitoring flap perfusion during the acute phase and is often completely removed and replaced with a split-skin graft for matching purposes (thinning), although it plays an important role in lymph drainage.

Possible complications and morbidity at the donor site:

- Seroma
- Contour defect, problematic scar formation
- Lumbar hernia
- Nerve lesion
- Negligible functional change in shoulder mobility

Depending on the size of the harvested flap, seroma is the most frequent complication (approximately 80%). Numerous examinations have revealed no essential differences in seroma formation after using a scalpel or electrocautery.

To minimize shearing forces some authors recommend attaching the skin to the thoracic wall with resorbable sutures.

To achieve primary wound closure after harvesting a flap including a large island of skin, the wound edges must often be mobilized, resulting in a comparably large wound. For this reason, a Redon drain must be inserted in the anterior axillary and posterior sections of the donor site. Occasionally the wound must be aspirated several times after removing the drain. The seroma usually dries up gradually after a few weeks. In refractory cases 20% glucose solution has been instilled as an adhesive.

Contour defects and problematic scars often cannot be avoided. Follow-up examinations have shown that the scar is wider than 1.5 cm in 65% of cases despite intracutaneous suturing. Harvesting of a skin island should also be well planned in respect to scar-tissue formation. A transverse incision can be covered by a brassiere, while

NOTE

When choosing a suitable donor site, the surgeon must weigh the specific requirements of the tissue to be reconstructed against the defect at the donor site. Before every removal of a muscle or composite myocutaneous flap, a thorough anamnesis must be taken including handedness, profession, hobbies, etc.

NOTE

The complete muscle on one side of the body can be removed for transplantation.

incisions at the anterior edge of the muscle enable the patient to wear clothing with a deep décolleté at the back.

Neurotropic deficits are rare complications.

Paralysis of the brachial plexus can be due to incorrect positioning. This can be avoided if the arm remains abducted and not elevated.

Functional restrictions following loss of a muscle are principally negligible, as they can be compensated.

Rectus Abdominis Flap

In morbidity of the donor site it is necessary to differentiate between free and pedicle flaps and between those removed only at one end or at both ends. The muscle-saving technique in pedicled flaps offers no essential improvement in the function of the abdominal wall over harvesting the unilateral muscle. Age and adiposity have only a mild influence on donor-site morbidity on the abdomen. Severe concomitant diseases alone do not constitute a contraindication to harvesting a flap. There is, however, risk of ventilatory complications if the patient suffers from restricted respiratory function. Pregnancy and birth are possible after a flap has been harvested, but pregnancy is not recommended within 1 year after such an operation (**Table 6.2**).

There are no relevant data concerning problems with urination or defecation among older patients.

Disturbed sensibility at the donor site has been reported by two-thirds of the patients. Thirty percent of patients report such disturbances or even pain (which is only relevant on exertion) 1 year posoperatively.

Table 6.2 Possible complications and donor site morbidity

Complications	Incidence in %
Seroma	3
Umbilical necrosis	Often in smokers and adiposity
Contour irregularities	Up to 50
Abdominal wall hernia	Up to 18
Decreased muscle strength, relaxation of the abdominal wall	Up to 49
Impaired abdominal sensibility	Up to 65

Gastrocnemius Flap

After covering a defect with a medial or lateral gastrocnemius muscle head there is a deformity in the posterior thigh.

The deformity at the donor site of the lateral head is less severe. Some authors prefer the lateral head because it is easier to mobilize and to rotate due to its narrow anatomy. The deformity at the donor site is smaller.

Radial Flap

The cosmetic disadvantage at the donor site after harvesting this flap and covering the defect with a split-skin graft must be taken into consideration. Other disadvantages must also be taken into consideration. If the patient finds the grafted skin too hairy, this can be disturbing. Loss of the radial artery can cause intolerance of cold in the affected hand. There is often a slight loss of power in the muscles of the forearm.

NOTE

Closure of the abdominal wall with a synthetic net offers no advantage in avoiding hernias or relaxation of the abdominal wall.

It is recommended to perform a double-layer fascial closure with gathering of the opposing fascia.

NOTE

Functional deficits usually only remain for a few months. Training the soleus muscle and the remaining head of the gastrocnemius muscle quickly compensates the functional deficiency.

Bibliography

Anthony JP, Mathes J. Update on chronic osteomyelitis. In: Clinics in Plastic Surgery. Reconstruction of the Lower Extremity. London: Saunders; 1991

Arens P. Osteitis—immer noch ein Problem? Trauma Berufskrankh 2002;4:295–296

Biemer E. Free tissue transfer to the lower extremity—determination of its status. [Article in German] Chirurg 1986a;57(3):141–142

Biemer E. Dorsal foot flap (dorsalis pedis flap). Clinical use including management of the removal defect. [Article in German] Chirurg 1986b;57(3):137–139

Biemer E. Indications for free tissue transfer in comparison with alternative methods of coverage. [Article in German] Chirurg 1986c;57(3):113–114

Biemer E, Jaeger K. Drug treatment, after care and secondary interventions following lower leg reconstruction by free tissue transfer. [Article in German] Chirurg 1986;57(3):140

Böhm E. Chronische posttraumatische Osteomyelitis. Hefte zur Unfallheilkunde. Heidelberg: Springer; 1985

Brüser P. Die Osteomyelitis im Bereich der Finger. Oper Orthop Traumatol 1993;5:60–67

Burri C, Neugebauer R. Infektionen von Knochen und Gelenken. Aktuelle Probleme. In: Chirurgie und Orthopädie. Bern: Huber; 1990

Claudi BF, Oedekoven G. Biological osteosynthesis. [Article in German] Chirurg 1991;62(5):367–377

Diedrich O, Kraft CN, Sasse J, Zhou H, Lüring C. Primary subcutaneous hematogenous osteomyelitis in childhood. [Article in German] Unfallchirurg 2002;105(7):651–655

Esterhai JL Jr, Queenan J. Management of soft tissue wounds associated with type III open fractures. Orthop Clin North Am 1991;22(3):427–432

Friedrich PL. Die aseptische Versorgung frischer Wunden. Arch f. Klin Chir 1898;57:288–310

Godina M. Early microsurgical reconstruction of complex trauma of the extremities. Plast Reconstr Surg 1986;78(3):285–292

Grünert J, Brug E. Principles of secondary soft tissue reconstruction after open fractures of the tibia. [Article in German] Chirurg 1990;61(11):824–829

Habermeyer P, Schweiberer L. Soft tissue-plasty for the restoration of infected defects of the lower extremity. [Article in German] Orthopade 1983;12(4):205–217

Heppert V, Eckert P, Savic B. Septische Knochenchirurgie. Stuttgart: Schattauer; 1980

Heppert V, Wagner C, Glatzel U, Wentzensen A. Prinzipien der operativ-chirurgischen Therapie der Osteitis. Trauma Berufskrankh. 2002;4:321–328

Hesse UJ, Huber R, Rehm KE. Local muscle flap in soft tissue reconstruction following fracture and osteitis of the lower limb. [Article in German] Unfallchirurgie 1991;17(6):349–354

Jaeger K. Preoperative preparation and preliminary studies of free tissue transfer in lower leg reconstruction. [Article in German] Chirurg 1986;57(3):115–117

Kaiser E. Anatomic principles of free tissue transfer to the lower extremity. Latissimus flap—radialis flap—dorsalis pedis flap. [Article in German] Chirurg 1986;57(3):118–120

Ketterl R, Ascherl R, Steinau HU, Claudi B. Muskellappen bei infizierten Knochen. In: Rahmanzadeh R, Meißner A, eds. Störungen der Frakturheilung. 9. Steglitzer Unfalltagung. Heidelberg: Springer; 1991

Kinzl L, Suger G. Segmentresektion und Kallusdistraktion als unverzichtbare Elemente moderner Osteitistherapie. In: Hefte zu Der Unfallchirurg, Heft 255. Heidelberg: Springer; 1995

Knopp W, Steinau HU. Primary soft tissue treatment and soft tissue reconstruction. [Article in German] Chirurg 1991;62(5):378–387

Krettek C. Fracture and soft tissue damage. [Article in German] Chirurg 1998;69(6):684–700

Krupp S. Plastische Chirurgie. Klinik und Praxis. Landsberg: Ecomed-Verlag; 2002

Kutscha-Lissberg F, Hebler U, Kälicke T, Wingenfeld C, Arens S. Inzidenz, Diagnose, Manifestations- und Verlaufsformen der Osteitis. Trauma Berufskrankh. 2002;4:297–305

Lehnhardt M, Homann HH, Druecke D, Maslowski K, Muehlberger T, Steinau HU. Carl von Reyher's studies of wound therapy. [Article in German] Chirurg 2002;73(7):721–724

Masquelet AC, Gilbert A. Atlas der Lappenplastiken in der Chirurgie der Extremitäten. Stuttgart: Enke; 1998

Mathes SJ, Nahai F. Classification of the vascular anatomy of muscles: experimental and clinical correlation. Plast Reconstr Surg 1981;67(2):177–187

Mathes SJ, Alpert BS, Chang N. Use of the muscle flap in chronic osteomyelitis: experimental and clinical correlation. Plast Reconstr Surg 1982;69(5):815–829

Möllenhoff G, Buchholz J. Muscle power and shoulder joint function after removal of the latissimus dorsi muscle. Handchir Mikrochir Plast Chir 1994;26(2):75–79

Muhr G. Therapeutic strategies in fractures with soft tissue damage. [Article in German] Chirurg 1991;62(5):361–366

Oestern HJ, Tscherne H. Pathophysiology and classification of soft tissue damage in fractures. [Article in German] Orthopade 1983;12(1):2–8

Sauer H, Ritter G. Osteomyelitis und Osteitis im Kindesalter. Stuttgart: Gustav Fischer; 1986

Schmidt HGK, Wittek F, Fink B, Buck-Gramcko U. Treatment of chronic osteitis of the tibia. [Article in German] Unfallchirurg 1992;95(11):566–573

Schneider U, Böhm HJ, Hierholzer G. Aktuelle Anmerkungen zur posttraumatischen Osteomyelitis. Akt Chir 1997;32:154–159

Schnettler R, Lieser H, Klemm K. Chirurgische Behandlung der posttraumatischen chronischen Osteomyelitis. Akt Chir 1997;32:18–22

Spilker G. Removal technics for free tissue transfer to the lower extremity. Latissimus flap—radialis flap—dorsalis pedis flap. [Article in German] Chirurg 1986;57(3):121–125

Steinau HU. Microvascular latissimus dorsi transfer. Clinical use including management of the site of tissue removal. [Article in German] Chirurg 1986;57(3):126–133

Steinau HU, Biemer E, Feller AM, Hörl HW. Primary management and secondary reconstructive surgery of severe combined hand injuries. [Article in German] Chirurg 1988;59(11):740–748

Steinau HU, Feller AM, Hörl HW, Kunisch M, Klein B, Biemer E. Post-traumatic soft tissue defects of the heel. [Article in German] Chirurg 1989;60(4):287–294

Steinau HU, Biemer E. Stand der Replantations-Indikation und Grenzen in der Handchirurgie. Langenbeck Arch Chir. Suppl. II (Kongressbericht); 1990

Steinau HU, Germann G. Plastic reconstructive microsurgery in post-traumatic infection control and therapy. [Article in German] Chirurg 1991;62(12):852–860

Steinau HU, Askenazy L, Biemer E, Gradinger J. Bilateral arm amputation caused by high voltage burns in childhood: stump reconstruction by tissue expansion and fibula transfer. [Article in German] Chirurg 1991;62(5):426–429

Steinau HU, Germann G, Büttemeyer R, Hussmann J, Hebebrand D. Reconstructive surgery of knee para-articular amputation stumps. [Article in German] Unfallchirurgie 1993;19(5):272–277

Steinau HU, Hebebrand D, Vogt P, Peter FW, Tosson R. Reconstructive plastic surgery of thoracic wall defects. [Article in German] Chirurg 1997;68(5):461–468

Stock W, Wolf K. Radial artery grafts. Clinical use including management of the site of tissue removal. [Article in German] Chirurg 1986;57(3):134–136

Tiemann A, Bosse A, Muhr G. Das Fistelkarzinom als Komplikation der chronischen Osteomyelitis. Chir Praxis 1997/98;53:129–136

Vogt PM, Busch K, Peter FW, Möcklinghoff Ch, Torres A, Steinau HU. Plastische Rekonstruktion der bestrahlten Thoraxwand. Langenbecks Arch Chir Suppl. II (Kongressbericht); 1998

Vogt PM, Peter FW, Topsakal E, Torres A, Steinau HU. Use of growth factors in therapy of chronic wounds. Experimental, clinical and financial aspects. [Article in German] Chirurg 1998b;69(11):1197–1206

Weber A, Gisevius A. Bildgebende Verfahren in der Diagnostik der Osteitis. Was gibt es Neues? Trauma Berufskrankh 2002;4:306–313

Wick M, Kutscha-Lissberg F. Débridierungstechniken bei der operativen Sanierung der Osteitis. Trauma Berufskrankh 2002;4:358–362

7

Treatment of Infected Prostheses

Total Replacements of the Knee and Hip

T. Gehrke

Introduction

In its pathogenesis and specific disease progression, a periprosthetic infection is a peculiarity among inflammations in the human body. In contrast to many other infections of the soft tissues and the bones, a foreign body colonized by bacteria is the starting point of this disease (**Fig. 7.1**).

Therapy begins with the obligatory removal of all colonized foreign bodies in a consistent surgical and microbiologic procedure. It is of no importance whether the implant is changed in one-stage, two-stage, or even multiple-stage interventions. The decisive factor is that all infected foreign bodies are removed and surgical debridement of the soft tissues and bones is painstakingly and thoroughly performed. Necrotic portions of bone (sequestra) are radically removed because they must also be considered as foreign bodies liable to bacterial colonization (**Fig. 7.2**).

There is principally no difference in the diagnostic and therapeutic concept among the different joints. An infected hip prosthesis is subject to the exact same pathologic process as an infected total replacements of the knee or shoulder.

Classification

An infection occurring within the first 3 postoperative weeks is referred to as an **acute infection**.

An infection occurring after the third postoperative week is referred to as a **late infection**.

> **NOTE**
>
> Decisive factors for successful therapy of periprosthetic infections, regardless of their localization, are:
> - Removal of **all** foreign material
> - Complete surgical debridement of all infected tissues
> - Radical removal of **all** necrotic bone

Fig. 7.1 Periprosthetic infection caused by streptococci.

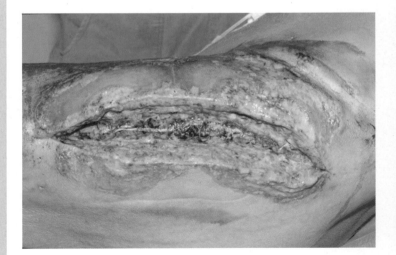

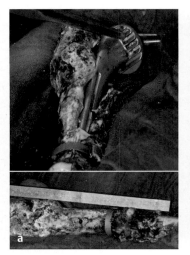
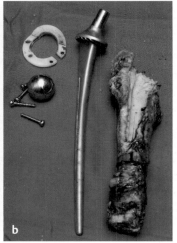

Fig. 7.2a, b Radical removal of foreign material, including the necrotic bone.

Diagnosis

Clinical Symptoms

- Pain (main symptom, often appearing after a painless interval)
- Redness
- Swelling
- Local warmth
- Wound dehiscence
- Fistulas
- Fever (rare, but an alarming sign): risk of sepsis!

Laboratory:
- C-reactive protein (CRP)
- Erythrocyte sedimentation rate (ESR)
- (Leukocyte count)

NOTE

The main clinical symptom of a periprosthetic infection is pain, which either persists after the operation or, in late infections, appears in the operated joint after a painless interval (see **Fig. 7.3**).

Any joint that is painful after implantation of a prosthesis is considered to have a periprosthetic infection until this has been definitely excluded.

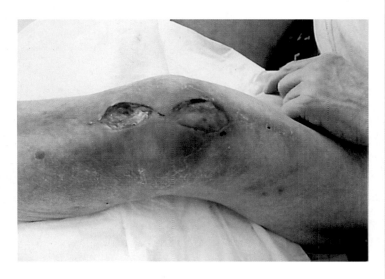

Fig. 7.3 Clinical picture of a periprosthetic infection of the knee joint.

NOTE

Both CRP and ESR always rise after an operation. The CRP level should have normalized after 2 to 3 weeks, while the ESR can remain elevated for up to a year. Therefore, controlling CRP values is of decisive importance. The leukocyte count has no or only very limited clinical relevance because it is generally within the normal range.

Radiologic Diagnosis

Plain films in standard planes should be taken and, if necessary, distance radiographs with a radiopaque scale.

Radiologic changes in periprosthetic infections:
- There are no pathognomic changes in the plain films.
- The bones show both areas of sclerosis and lysis (**Fig. 7.4**).

Scintigraphy: A bone scan is not recommended because it is very expensive, but has little clinical relevance.

Computed tomography (CT): Prosthetic materials create artifacts. This is only appropriate for individual implants with large bone defects.

Magnetic resonance imaging (MRI): Prosthetic materials create artifacts. The investigation is very expensive, but has little clinical relevance. It is appropriate to evaluate the condition of soft tissues (**Fig. 7.5**).

Distance radiographs with a radiopaque scale of the affected extremity with a precisely defined film-focus distance are often useful for planning an operation, especially if special implants or so-called megaprostheses (e.g., total femoral replacement) are required (**Fig. 7.6**).

NOTE

Radiologic Diagnosis is of secondary importance. Generally speaking, none of the techniques provide useful information. Late infections have typical signs in plain films, like periosteal reactions, ossifications, resorption margins, or osteolyses. Scintigraphy, CT, and MRI cannot differentiate septic loosening of a prosthesis from aseptic loosening. Artifacts in CT and MRI make it difficult to evaluate the condition of the bones.

Combined ^{111}In (indium) and ^{99m}Tc (technetium) leukocyte scintigraphy is superior to conventional scintigraphic procedures in making this differentiation, but is very expensive and can only be recommended in selected cases.

Fig. 7.4a, b Plain radiograph of a periprosthetic infection of the knee joint.

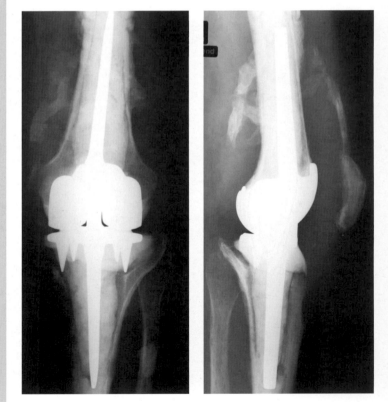

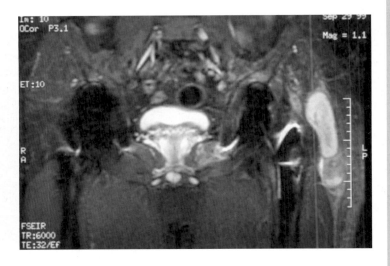

Fig. 7.5 MRI of the patient in **Fig. 7.6** showing a large soft-tissue abscess on the left greater trochanter.

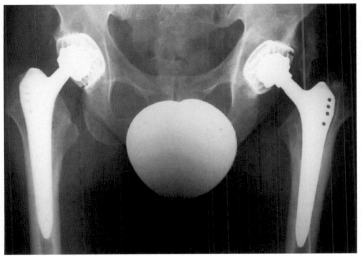

Fig. 7.6 Unremarkable radiograph of a periprosthetic infection of the left hip.

Joint Aspiration

Joint aspiration is the method of choice to obtain a representative sample to **determine the pathogen** (**Fig. 7.7**).

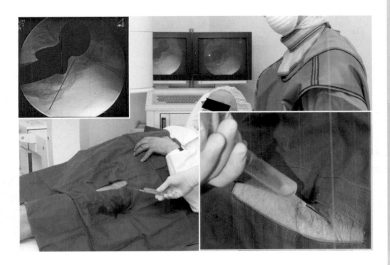

Fig. 7.7 Aspiration of a hip joint from anterior under fluoroscopic control.

NOTE

Discontinue systemic antibiotics 10–14 days before the aspiration.

Do not administer a local anesthetic during the aspiration (antimicrobial effect).

Do not irrigate or apply a contrast medium (dilution).

The obtained material must be incubated in the laboratory for at least 14 days.

Fig. 7.8 Sterile injection of aspirated fluid into a plain test tube.

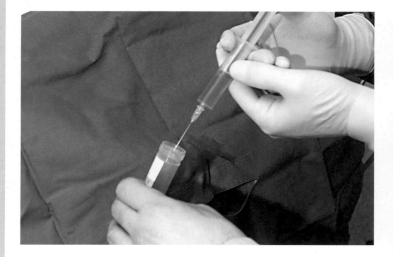

TIPS AND TRICKS

1. **Surrounding conditions:**
   - Conditions should be similar to those in the surgical theater.
   - Aspirations should only be performed under image intensifier or ultrasonic control.
   - Casting rooms and surgical anterooms are not suitable for aspirations.
   - Sterile gloves, masks, and caps are obligatory.
   - Skin must be disinfected according to general surgical disinfection standards.

2. **Aspiration site:**
   - A direct anterior approach from the groin is preferred for the hip joint. Be careful not to injure the femoral neurovascular bundle.
   - If there are periarticular calcifications, the lateral approach is more suitable.
   - If there is a total knee replacement (TKR), we prefer the so-called anterolateral arthroscopic approach.
   - If there is no TKR, the lateral approach below the proximal pole of the patella in the upper recess is suitable.
   - The aspiration needle is advanced until it touches the metal prosthesis. This indicates that the tip of the needle is definitely in the joint, and aspiration can be performed.
   - If no joint fluid can be aspirated, the surgical assistant bends and straightens the knee, which pumps fluid from the dorsal portions of the joint. A so-called dry aspiration can generally be avoided in this way and should only occur in very exceptional cases. It is not recommended to inject anything into the joint, as this can strongly dilute the intra-articular fluid aspirated and reduce the relative number of pathogens, making it difficult to identify them.

3. **Amount of fluid to aspirate:**
   - "The more the better," but at least 1 mL.
   - Larger amounts of aspirated fluid can be used as a "natural transport medium."
   - In addition to the amount of fluid aspirated, the composition of the fluid, like bloody, serous, or putrid, must be documented and reported on the form sent to the microbiologists.

4. **Material abraded from the fistula:**
   - After disinfecting the area surrounding the fistulous sinus, material is obtained by sharp curettage from deep within the fistulous tract and placed in a culture tube, for example, a bottle for anaerobic blood culture (**Fig. 7.8**).

5. **Transporting the sample:**
   - Samples must reach the laboratory within the shortest possible time to prevent sensitive pathogens (e.g., anaerobic bacteria) from dying.
   - If it is necessary to send the sample by courier or post, the sample must be protected for the duration of the transport. Special containers for anaerobic organisms (**Fig. 7.9**) or industrial transport mediums are suitable for this purpose.
   - If immediate transport is not possible, the medium should be conserved in a refrigerator at approximately 4 °C until it can be transported.

6. **Cultivation of samples:**
   - The cultivation and processing of the samples should fundamentally be performed by microbiologists who are experienced in diagnosing periprosthetic infections.

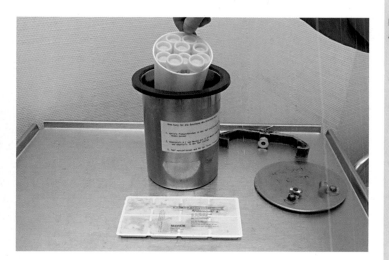

Fig. 7.9 Special container for transportation of an anaerobic sample.

Planning the Operation

Anesthesia

- Internists and anesthesiologists must evaluate the operative risk.
- There should be no preoperative autohemotransfusion or perioperative mechanical autotransfusion due to the risk of reinfection.
- At least eight units of banked blood should be available.

Radiographic Preparations

- In general, conventional radiographs of the affected joint in two to three planes in the standard position and exposure technique are sufficient (O'Neill and Harris 1984) (see above).
- Distance radiographs with a radiopaque scale of the affected extremity with a precisely defined film-focus distance may be required, particularly for special implants or so-called megaprostheses (e. g., total femoral replacement).

Informed Consent

- The success rate for operative replacement of an infected prosthesis is between 80% and 90%.
- This means there is a 10%–20% possibility of continuing or recurring infection.
- Disturbances in wound healing may require operative revision.
- The sciatic or femoral nerves could be damaged.
- There could be considerable blood loss, especially if the socket protrudes into the lesser (true) pelvis.
- There may be a loss of function and stability of the muscles surrounding the hip.
- The legs may differ in length.
- There is risk of an intraoperative and/or postoperative fracture
- The risk of aseptic loosening of the prosthesis or even early loosening is increased
- Large bone defects, especially of the acetabulum, will require another operation later to reconstruct the bone.
- There may be restriction of movement.
- The operated leg often cannot fully bear weight for up to 12 weeks postoperatively.
- If treatment of the infection is unsuccessful (persisting infection), amputation or exarticulation may be necessary.

Therapeutic Concept

Therapeutic Goals

- Eradication of the infection
- Maintenance of joint function

Therapeutic Options

- Conservative therapy (antibiotic suppression of pathogens)
- Surgical debridement without removing the prosthesis
- One-stage prosthesis exchange
- Two-stage prosthesis exchange
- Multiple-stage prosthesis exchange
- Arthrodesis
- Resection arthroplasty
- Amputation or exarticulation

Conservative Therapy
(Antibiotic Suppression of Pathogens)

Indication: inoperability due to high operative risk.

Disadvantages:
- Noneradication of the infection
- Danger of pathogen selection
- Development of resistant species
- Nonhealing fistulas as a permanent source of additional pathogen colonization

Exchange of Septic Hip Prosthesis

Surgical Preparations

- Identification of pathogens and availability of an antibiogram are prerequisites.
- Systematic and local antibiotics must be available.
- If there are large soft-tissue defects, a plastic surgeon must be called in.

Choice of Implants

- Implants of different lengths and shaft diameters must be available.
- If there is a loss of bone substance, intraoperative complications, like shaft fractures, perforations of the cortical layer and/or fenestration, and pelvic destruction are more likely. These must be taken into consideration when choosing an implant.
- In our hospital population we have been able to use a standard implant in approximately 60% of cases. In all other cases, we had to choose a longer stem to ensure sufficient anchorage in the bone.
- Large areas of pelvic destruction can cause difficulties because here the implantation of supportive cages or rings for the acetabular cup or in some cases even partial replacement of the pelvis is necessary.
- Allogenic shaft and socket reconstruction must not be performed if there is an infection because this means implanting another foreign body that is not protected from bacterial colonization by antibiotic bone cement.

- We only use megaprotheses, which generally replace two neighboring joints, when exchanging a prosthesis similar to the infected one (e.g., a periprosthetic infection of a total femoral replacement) because under certain circumstances the infection can spread to a healthy joint.
- If the pelvis is involved to the extent that the urinary bladder or iliac vessels could be injured, a vascular surgeon, abdominal surgeon, and an urologist should be called in.

Approach

The following approaches are recommended for surgical revisions or exchanging prostheses.

Suitable approaches to the hip joint for exchanging a prosthesis:
- Posterior
- Transtrochanteric
- Transgluteal
- Transfemoral

Less suitable approaches to the hip joint for exchanging a prosthesis:
- Anterolateral
- Anterior

We consider the main advantages of a posterior approach, also for operative revisions, to be the far-reaching protection of the abductor muscles, which are the most important pelvic stabilizers in the coronal plane. Nerves and vessels lying anterior are generally not traumatized, and even the relatively close sciatic nerve can be easily palpated and protected.

The increased danger of dislocation is considered a disadvantage, which, however, can be compensated by taking great care in the proper placement of the acetabular cup and reconstruction of the posterior soft tissues when closing the wound.

Incisions of the Skin and Fascia

Old scars which lie in the path of the skin incision are excised. If they are not directly in the planned incision, the surgeon must assure that there is sufficient distance between the new and the previous incision (**Fig. 7.10**).

Avoid crossing old scars at a sharp angle or changing directions.

NOTE

The dorsal approach provides better exposure of the cranial and cranioposterior portions of the acetabulum, which are most often affected by bone loss, and is also suitable for extensive reconstructive surgery. Lengthening the incision toward proximal exposes almost the complete pelvic wing.

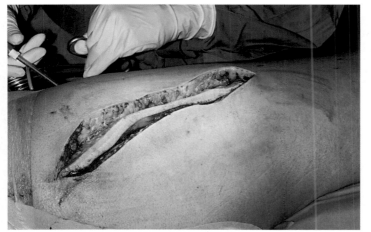

Fig. 7.10   Former incision scars are excised.

Fistulas should, whenever possible, lie in the line of incision and be radically excised by dissecting them down to the joint. If they are located too far anterior or posterior, they should be resected from a separate incision (**Fig. 7.11**).

After cleaving the fascia, all infected tissues, including muscle fasciae and infected portions of the muscle, are debrided (**Fig. 7.12**).

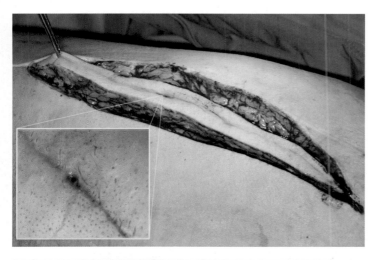

Fig. 7.11   Fistulas are included in the incision if possible.

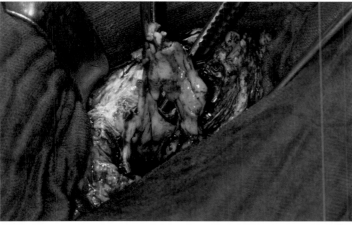

Fig. 7.12   Radical debridement of soft tissues.

This may require an L-shaped detachment of the vastus lateralis muscle to be able to dissect right down to the femoral shaft in a distal direction and remove infected tissue adjacent the bone. This also exposes perforations, fenestrations, and other infected defects in the cortical layer of the femoral shaft so that they can be removed and cleansed with sharp curettes, chisels, drills, Luer bone rongeurs, raspatories, burrs, etc. Especially defects in cortical bone or the small cortical openings for the perforating blood vessels can provide the starting point for extensive abscesses in the surrounding muscles.

Biopsies

Sample biopsies from all relevant areas must routinely be taken, labeled, and sent for microbiologic diagnosis.

Biopsies (routine):
- Joint capsule
- Shaft entrance
- Shaft interior
- Floor of the acetabulum

Biopsies (when necessary):
- Fistulous tracts
- Abscess contents

Technique for Explantation of Prostheses (Cemented Shafts)

Removing a cemented shaft is generally far easier and less complicated than removing cementless shafts.

The required instruments for removing cemented shafts are shown in **Fig. 7.13**.

Instruments for removal of the prosthesis (Fig. 7.14, 7.15, 7.16, 7.17, 7.18):
- System-specific extraction instruments
- Self-cutting cement extractors
- Taper extraction instrument
- Box-type stem extractor for firmly fixed or nonmodular heads

Chisels of different lengths and widths (Fig. 7.14):
- Sraight chisel
- Hollow chisel (sharpened on the inside and outside)
- Lambotte chisel
- Angled chisel

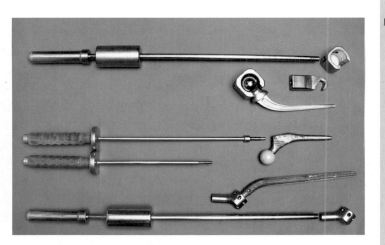

Fig. 7.13 Extraction instruments

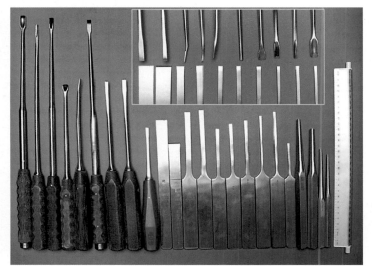

Fig. 7.14 Chisels of different lengths, forms, and widths.

Curettes (Figs. 7.15):
- Ball-headed reamers (diameter: 8–16 mm)
- Sharp curettes of different lengths and sizes
- Jet lavage

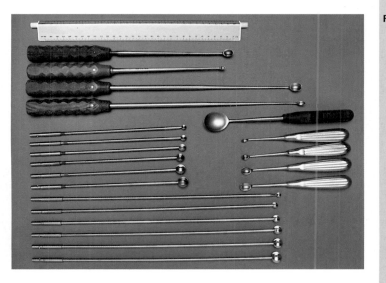

Fig. 7.15 Curetting instruments

Fig. 7.16 Clamps and forceps for removing bone cement.

Fig. 7.17 Thread cutters of different diameters for removing bone cement.

Fig. 7.18 Long drill bits (4.5 mm in diameter) for boring into the distal bone-cement plug.

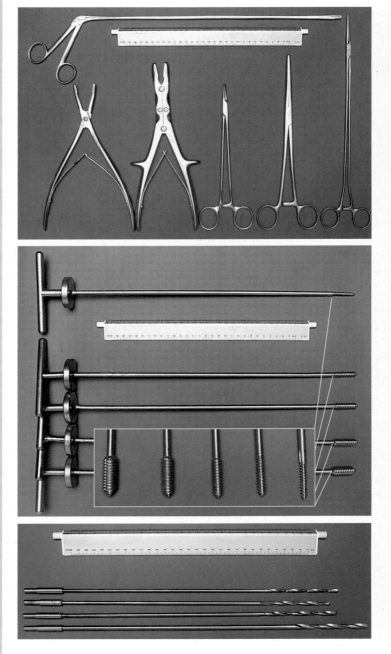

Removing a Prosthesis

1. Remove the bone cement between greater trochanter and the shoulder of the prosthesis.
2. Remove the cement between the prosthetic collar and the cortical bone of the femur.
3. Drive out the prosthetic shaft with a special taper extraction instrument. The punch is placed under the prosthetic collar. Use a box-type stem extractor for fixed, nonmodular heads.
4. Place the punch under the prosthetic collar.
5. Use a box-type stem extractor for rigid, nonmodular heads.

Removing the Cement

1. Remove the proximal portions of cement with narrow, straight chisels with symmetrical sharp blades.
2. Use a thread cutter in distal portions with a closed cement column.
3. Cement plugs remaining distal to the prosthetic shaft are drilled in the center and then removed with an appropriate tap (**Fig. 7.19**).

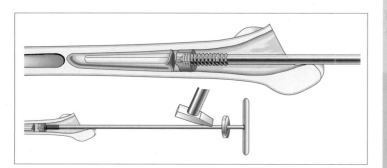

Removing Cementless Shafts

Cementless implants are often extremely difficult to remove. This is especially true because a large number of periprosthetic infections are so-called early infections, that is, they appear within the first year after the prosthesis was implanted. The following situation is often the cause: The infection started somewhere on the interface between the bone and the prosthetic shaft; the rest of the prosthesis is still well integrated in the bone.

Instruments for removing prosthetic cementless shafts:
1. **Extraction instruments:**
   - Systemic specific extraction instruments
   - Self-cutting cement extractors
   - Taper extraction instruments
   - Box-type stem extractor for firmly fixed or non-modular heads
2. **Chisels:**
   - Fine flexible osteotomes
   - Lambotte chisel
3. **Punch:**
   Drills and thin saw blades (for fenestration of bones).
   The prosthetic shaft is loosened with fine flexible or Lambotte chisels, which are driven between the bone and the prosthesis (**Fig. 7.20**).
   Place a self-cutting cement extractor device and drive out the prosthesis (**Fig. 7.21**).
   If necessary, fenestrate the bone or use a transfemoral approach.
   The prosthetic shaft can be circularly chiseled with a curved Lambotte chisel or sawn out with a curved

NOTE

The thickest possible thread cutter is twisted into the lumen with several turns until the resistance increases and there is a creaking noise.

The thread-cutting technique is only feasible and useful if the cement column is solid throughout. If one side is open, the thread cutter pierces the cancellous or cortical bone and may tear it open.

Fig. 7.19 Removal of bone cement with thread cutters.

NOTE

If the risk of drilling through the cortical bone is too great due to a cement plug which has broken off at an oblique angle or the femur has a strong anterior curvature, drilling must be performed under visual control through a window in the bone.

NOTE

When removing a cementless prosthetic shaft, the surgeon should decide to fenestrate the bone at a very early stage. In many cases fenestration is by far the more time-saving and gentle procedure. Windows should be cut in the anterior femur.

Fig. 7.20 Placing the fine flexible osteotomes at the prosthesis–bone interface.

saw blade from the bone window. Afterwards, it is usually possible to drive out the shaft with a punch after drilling into the shaft with a hard-metal drill bit (**Fig. 7.22**).

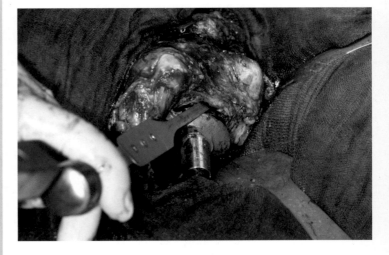

Fig. 7.21 Screwing in the taper extractor and driving out the prosthesis.

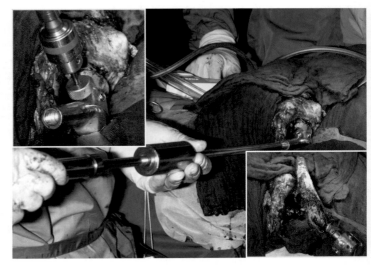

Fig. 7.22 Fenestration of the bone and sawing around the fixed prosthetic shaft.

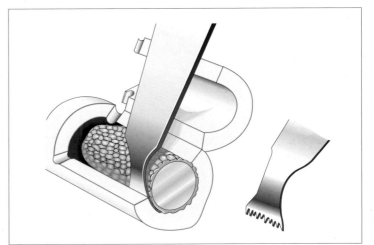

Curettage

Instruments for curetting the medullary cavity:
- Jet lavage, possible with Lavasept (Fresenius Kabi, Bad Homburg, Germany) (2%; **Fig. 7.23**)
- Ball-headed reamers
- Long sharp curettes

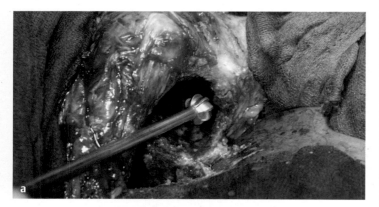

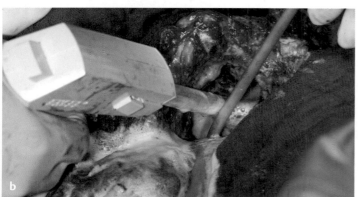

Fig. 7.23a, b Curetting the medullary cavity of the femur with a ball-headed burr and performing jet lavage.

Removal of the Acetabular Cup

Instruments for removing the acetabular cup:
- Special socket chisel
- Lambotte chisel
- Retrograde chisel
- Punch
- Bone-holding forceps
- 4.5-mm drill bit
- Thread cutter
- Sharp curette
- Ball-headed reamer

Removing Cemented Acetabular Cups

It is generally not very difficult to remove cemented acetabular cups. Cups which have been loosened are drilled in the middle with a 4.5-mm drill bit and then driven out in a retrograde direction with a thread cutter (**Fig. 7.24**).

Fig. 7.24a, b Removing a cemented acetabular cup.

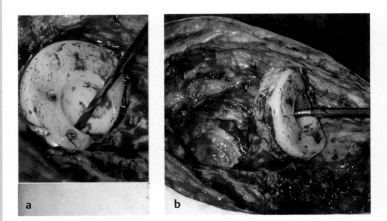

a   b

ERRORS AND RISKS

When loosening the acetabular cup with the chisel, take care not to destroy the bone, especially on the roof of the acetabulum.

TIPS AND TRICKS

If the acetabular cup cannot be removed whole with chisels, it must be divided like a pie with a flat, sharp chisel (e.g., Lambotte chisel).

TIPS AND TRICKS

A procedure which is very protective of the bone is to hook a retrograde chisel into the central hole in the floor of the acetabular cup and then drive it out (retrograde) (**Fig. 7.25**).

Fig. 7.25 Removing a cementless acetabular cup with a retrograde chisel.

If the cup is still well anchored, it can be loosened with a distally angulated and spherically curved chisel at the polyethylene (PE)–cement interface.

Remaining cement on the floor of the acetabular cup can be divided radially with the Lambotte chisel or scraped out with a sharp curette.

Removing Cementless Acetabular Cups

After exposing the edge of the cup and cutting it free, pry out the PE inlay with a straight chisel. Then loosen the screwed-in or press-fit cup circularly with a socket chisel whilst being extremely careful to protect the bone. The cup can then be removed with a bone-holding forceps or be driven out with a punch.

After removing all cement, carefully remove the floor of the acetabulum, which is usually covered with a loosening/infectious membrane (**Fig. 7.26**), with a sharp curette and scrape the bone clean with a ball-headed or crenated burr (**Fig. 7.27**).

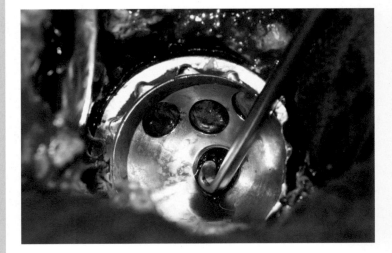

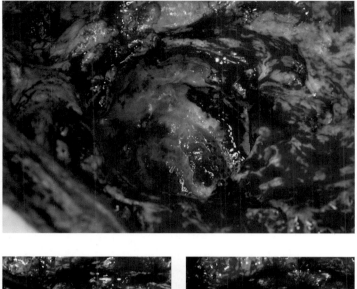

Fig. 7.26   Floor of the acetabulum lined with an infectious membrane.

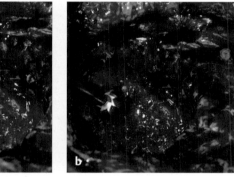

Fig. 7.27a, b   Curetting the acetabulum with a sharp curette and ball-headed burr.

One-Stage Prosthesis Exchange

After thorough debridement and removal of the implant, surgical gloves, abdominal pads, and contaminated instruments are exchanged. The acetabular and the shaft components are then implanted and fixed with antibiotic bone cement.

Fundamentals in the use of antibiotics in bone cement:

- Local and systemic antibiotics are chosen by an experienced microbiologist.
- Only antibiotics in powder form may be mixed with the bone cement (**Fig. 7.28**).
- Do not use watery solutions.
- The antibiotics must have sufficiently validated good elution characteristics from the bone cement.
- The total amount of antibiotic should not exceed 10% of the entire amount of bone cement. Otherwise the mechanical characteristics of the polymethylmethacrylate (PMMA) cement will be unacceptably weakened.
- The antibiotics should have a temporary bactericide effect on the cement surface.

NOTE

Reconstruction of the socket with allogenic or autogenic bone is contraindicated in one-stage exchange of an infected prosthesis because these bone grafts can be considered as foreign bodies and are not protected from renewed bacterial colonization by the surrounding antibiotic bone cement.

If there is no essential loss of bone substance in the acetabulum:

- Burr the acetabular cup with high-speed or ball-headed burrs.
- Drill anchoring holes with a 4.5-mm drill bit or calibrated drill (**Fig. 7.29**).
- Irrigate generously with jet lavage and perhaps even hydrogen peroxide.
- Affix the socket to the bone with antibiotic bone cement (see **Fig. 7.29**).

TIPS AND TRICKS

Under sterile conditions the circulating nurse hands the antibiotics in portions to the theater nurse, who then mixes them into the PMMA cement powder (Refobacin, Bone Cement R, Biomet, Berlin, Germany). The mixture should be as homogeneous as possible (see **Fig. 7.28**).

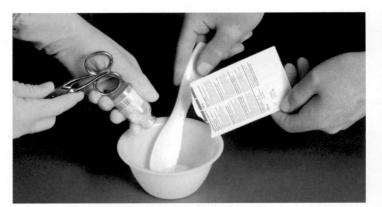

Fig. 7.28 Mixing an antibiotic into the bone-cement powder by hand for reimplantation of the acetabular cup.

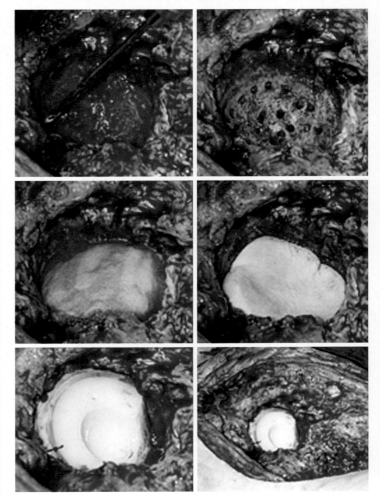

Fig. 7.29 Reimplantation of an acetabular cup with antibiotic bone cement after drilling anchoring holes and irrigation.

Cavernous defects with a closed protrusion:
- Revivify the bony floor of the socket.
- Drill anchoring holes with a 4.5-mm drill bit or calibrated drill.
- Irrigate generously with jet lavage and perhaps even hydrogen peroxide.
- Fill in the defects and affix the socket with antibiotic bone cement.

Craniolateral defect with a closed acetabular floor:
- Revivify the bony base of the socket.
- Drill anchoring holes with a 4.5-mm drill or calibrated drill.
- Irrigate generously with jet lavage and perhaps even hydrogen peroxide.
- Cancellous screws as support.
- Reimplant a collar socket whose collar is supported by cancellous screws with antibiotic bone cement.

Small perforations in the floor of the acetabulum:
This requires a two-stage cementing procedure in which the defects in the acetabular floor are first closed with cement disks and then the acetabular cup is cemented into place.

Craniomedial defects in the acetabulum with a large open protrusion:
- Depending on the size of the defect, fixate a protective cage or a protective socket ring with cancellous screws.
- Affix the acetabular cup with antibiotic bone cement.

Complete loss of the acetabulum with a large open protrusion:
Use a saddle prosthesis which is supported by the ilium. This, however, often leads to unsatisfactory results due to migration of the saddle prosthesis or recurrent infections because the cranial part of the saddle is insufficiently protected by the local antibiotics.

Reimplantation of the Shaft

The choice of shaft for reimplantation depends on the preoperative planning and bone defects discovered intraoperatively or the extent of required bone resections. Since this cannot always be planned in advance, a sufficient assortment of implants should be available.

The goal is a sufficient fixation of the prosthetic shaft in largely healthy and solid bone. The shaft should extend approximately 10 cm beyond the existing femoral defect or be at least as long as the resected femur (if it has been resected).

Principles of shaft reimplantation:
- The prosthetic shaft must be cemented.
- The prosthetic shaft must be anchored in at least 10 cm of healthy, solid bone.

- The length of the solid bone in which the prosthesis is to be anchored must be at least as long as the resected femur.
- If it is not possible to anchor the prosthesis in solid bone, a temporary, long-stem prosthesis must be implanted as a spacer. This will be exchanged for a total femoral replacement when the infection has definitely been eradicated (**Figs. 7.30a–c**).
- Intramedullary shaft reconstruction with allogenic bone grafts is not possible.

Fig. 7.30a–c
a Periprosthetic *Candida albicans* infection of a long-stem prosthesis with extensive bone involvement. One-stage prosthesis exchange was performed with considerable bone loss and insufficient anchoring of the prosthesis in the remaining bone. The new prosthesis is a total femoral replacement with reconstruction of the acetabulum after definite eradication of the infection.
b Temporary long-stem spacer prosthesis.
c Final result after eradication of the infection, total femoral replacement, and homologous reconstruction of the acetabulum.

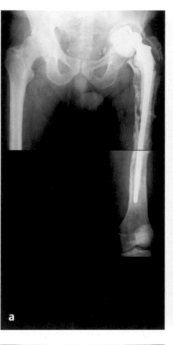
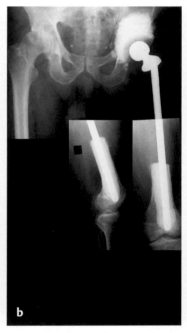
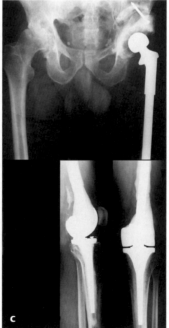

- The use of a PE sleeve to replace resected bone and prevent the shaft from sintering into the surroundings is contraindicated, as this would be a preferred site for pathogen colonization and is not protected by antibiotic bone cement.
- Resorbable cellulose gauze is recommended as a restrictor for the medullary cavity (**Fig. 7.31**).
- The distal end of the bone cement plug should end directly below the tip of the prosthesis to avoid complicating later reconstructive procedures.

NOTE

In a one-stage exchange of a septic prosthesis, the new prosthesis must be **cemented in**, since sufficient protection against renewed colonization of the implant by pathogens remaining in the site can only be ensured by antibiotic bone cement (**Fig. 7.32**).

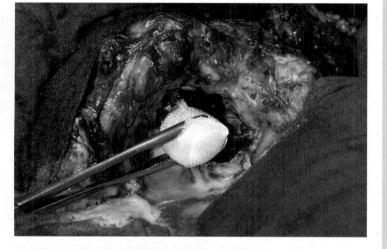

Fig. 7.31 Medullary cavity restrictor made of resorbable gauze.

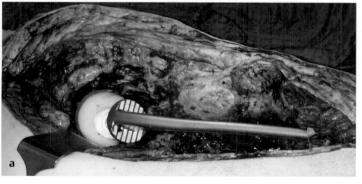

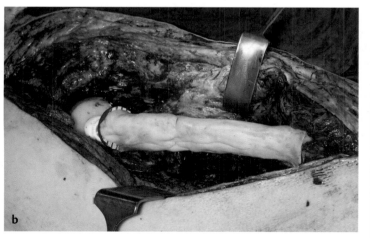

Fig. 7.32a, b Reimplantation of a shaft prosthesis with a sleeve of antibiotic bone cement to bridge the boneless space. The exposed parts of the prosthesis are encased in antibiotic bone cement to protect them from renewed bacterial colonization.

Wound Closure

Wound closure is generally primary and, as in the exchange of nonseptic prostheses, performed in layers.

Exchange of Septic Knee Prostheses

The diagnostic and therapeutic principles for septic knee prostheses are the same as for hip prostheses.

The problem in the surgical treatment of periprosthetic knee infections (**Fig. 7.33**) is the relative narrowness of the anatomical structures, including the posterior vascular and nervous pathways, as well as the considerably thinner soft-tissue coverage in comparison to the hip joint.

Despite these difficult circumstances, the knee joint must be debrided with the same radical thoroughness as in exchange of septic hip prostheses.

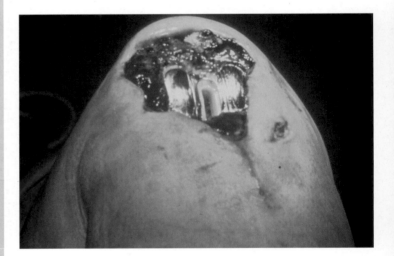

Fig. 7.33   Periprosthetic *Staphylococcus* infection of the knee joint.

NOTE

Debridement must be just as radical as in the exchange of a septic hip prosthesis.

Informed Consent

- The success rate of exchange of septic knee prostheses is 70%–80%.
- The possibility of persisting infection or recurrence is approximately 20%–30%.
- Disturbances in wound healing require surgical revision.
- The peroneal, tibial, and saphenus nerves could be damaged.
- There is a possibility of severe hemorrhaging, especially if arteries in the popliteal fossa are injured.
- If the extensor muscles are damaged, it may be necessary to stiffen the joint.

- There may be loss of function and stability of the muscles which stabilize the knee.
- The mobility of the knee may be restricted.
- There may be a limb-length discrepancy.
- There is danger of intraoperative and postoperative fractures.
- There is danger of aseptic loosening of the prosthesis, and the rate of early prosthetic loosening is increased.
- Full weight bearing is often not possible until the 12th postoperative week.
- If treatment is not successful and the infection persists, it may be necessary to perform an arthrodesis of the joint or amputate the limb.

Surgical Preparations

- Identify the pathogen(s).
- Prepare an antibiogram.
- Consult with microbiologists concerning the choice of local and systemic antibiotics.
- The operative risk should be clarified by an internist and an anesthesiologist.
- If there are large soft-tissue defects, call in a plastic surgeon.

Choice of Implant

The choice of a suitable implant depends on the extent of structural defects caused by the infection and necessary debridement.

Operative Technique

Figures 7.34, **7.35**, and **7.36** show gonarthrosis of the left knee with a fistulous periprosthetic infection with *Yersinia enterocolica* 1 year after implantation of a rotating hinge knee endoprosthesis due to rheumatoid arthritis.

Suitable approaches:
- Medial approach (parapatellar approach, subvastus approach) (**Fig. 7.37**)
- Lateral approach (usually combined with osteotomy of the tibial tuberosity)
- Anterior approach (slightly U-shaped, transverse Textor incision with osteotomy of the tibial tuberosity)

NOTE

Old scars within the incision should be excised.

Keep enough distance between the skin incision and old scars.

Do not incise across old scars or change directions.

Fistulous sinuses should be within the incision if possible.

Fig. 7.34a, b Postoperative radiograph after implantation of a rotating hinge knee-joint endoprosthesis.

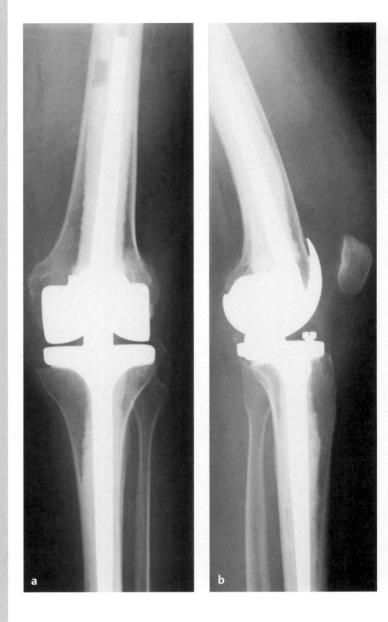

Fig. 7.35 Clinical picture 1 year after prosthesis implantation showing a fistula above the tibial tuberosity.

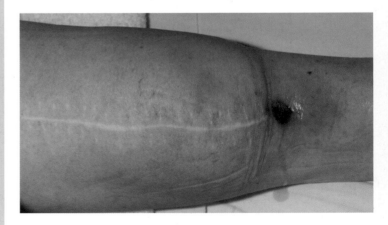

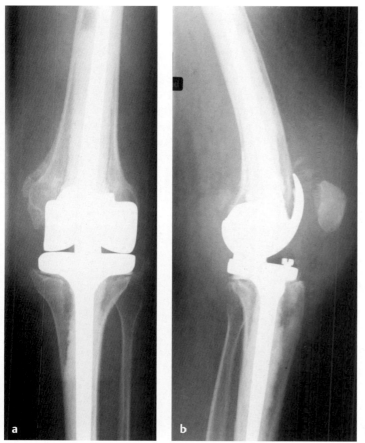

Fig. 7.36a, b Radiograph of a periprosthetic infection with periarticular calcifications.

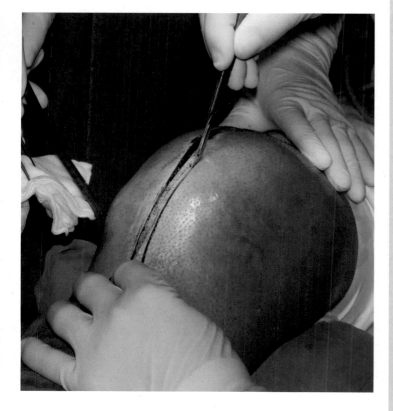

Fig. 7.37 Excision of the old surgical scar and the fistula.

Fig. 7.38 Debridement of the posterior portions of the joint.

Debridement

The infected tissues must be debrided thoroughly and radically, even in anatomically difficult regions like the popliteal fossa, with **complete** synovectomy. Debridement should be performed systematically.

In extensive periprosthetic infection the distal femur and the proximal tibia must be exposed so that any periosteal involvement or bone perforations can be cleaned out and curetted.

The medullary cavities are carefully curetted with a sharp curette and ball-headed burrs and then generously irrigated with jet lavage.

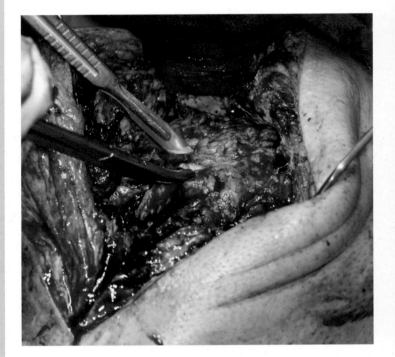

Removing the Implant

Cemented Prostheses

Removing cemented condylar prostheses:
1. Pry out the PE tibial inlay with a wide, flat chisel (**Fig. 7.39**).
2. Expose femoral components of the TKR as shown. First the cement fixation should be loosened with a flat Lambotte chisel or an oscillating saw wedged between the prosthesis and the cement (**Fig. 7.40**).

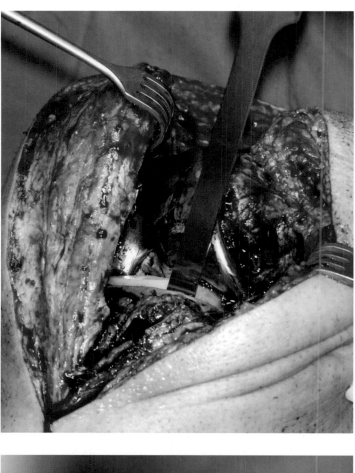

Fig. 7.39 Refer to text

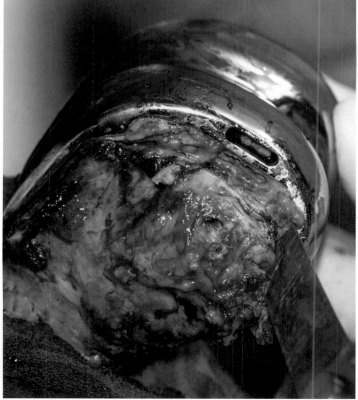

Fig. 7.40 Refer to text

3. Drive out the prosthesis with a punch or special extraction instruments (**Fig. 7.41**).
4. Curette the septic membrane covering the condyles with a Luer forceps, sharp curette, and ball-headed burrs (**Fig. 7.42**).
5. Bone cement can be removed with Lambotte chisels.
6. The anchoring holes are reamed out with a ball-headed burr.
7. Removal of cement used to anchor a prosthetic stem from the intramedullary cavity is the same as in a hip prosthesis.
8. The tibial prosthetic components are loosened with an oscillating saw or flat Lambotte chisel wedged between the prosthesis and the cement and then driven out with a punch, which is placed under the anterior edge of the prosthesis (**Fig. 7.43**).
9. Cement on the tibial plateau or in the proximal tibial medullary cavity is removed as described above (**Figs. 7.44 and 7.45**).

TIPS AND TRICKS

A narrow, hollow chisel is used to remove the cement from the anchoring holes. The cement is then extracted with clamps or forceps.

Fig. 7.41   Refer to text

Fig. 7.42   Refer to text

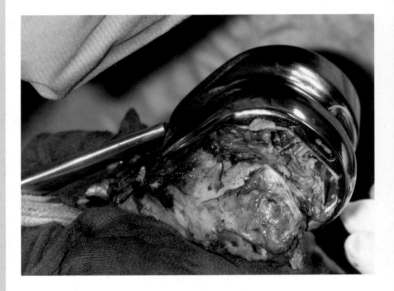

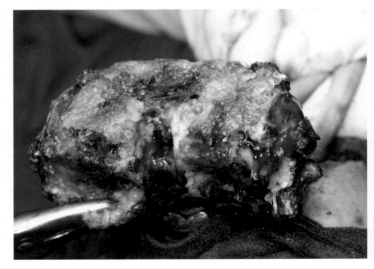

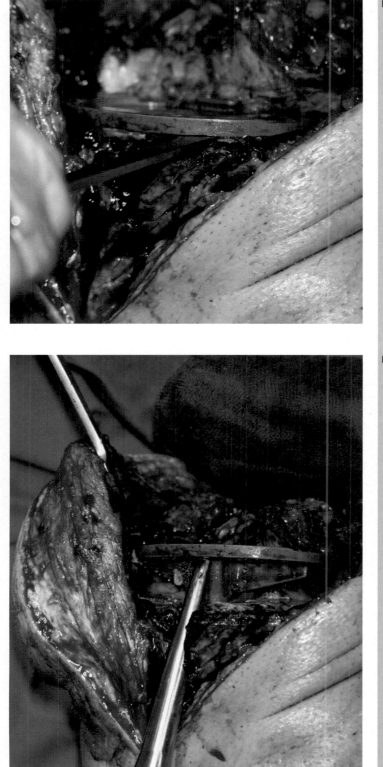

Fig. 7.43 Refer to text

Fig. 7.44 Refer to text

Fig. 7.45 Exposure of the distal femur and tibia and curettage of the perforations.

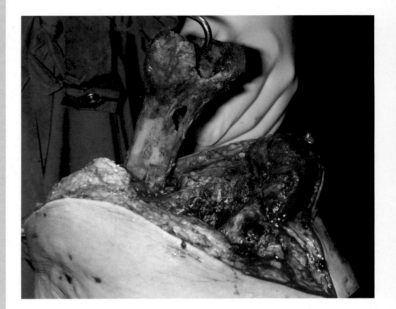

Cementless Condylar Prostheses

Removal of cementless TKR can be difficult because the firm attachment between the prosthesis and the bones can cause considerable bone defects or even fractures when the prosthesis is removed.

The least traumatic form of removal of firmly attached cementless condylar femoral components is with the Gigli saw. The prosthesis is sawed out of the bone. Afterwards the loosened prosthesis can be driven out with a punch or a special extraction instrument.

The tibial plateau can also be loosened either with a Gigli saw or a flat chisel and then be driven out with a punch.

Removing coarsely structured, cementless implants with stems is often hardly possible without causing considerable bone defects. In such cases, it is recommended to decide very early to fenestrate the bone. The femoral or tibial windows should be large enough to saw the prosthesis out with a curved oscillating saw or to chisel it out with Lambotte chisels.

The fundamental **choice of implant** for exchange of a septic prosthesis is generally simple, regardless of which procedure is used and whether replacement is done in one, two, or several stages. The required debridement, which almost always includes the stabilizing structures of the knee joint, like the ligaments, parts of the joint capsule, or muscles, demands reimplantation of a maximally stabilizing, hinged joint endoprosthesis affixed with bone cement. This model varies only in the length of the prosthetic stems, which must compensate bone defects and be adequately long if there is a great loss of bone (**Fig. 7.46**).

This can be achieved either with a prosthesis specially constructed according to preoperative distance radiographs with a radiopaque scale or by modular systems.

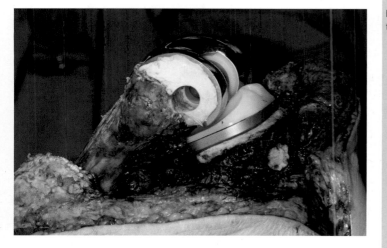

Fig. 7.46 Reimplantation of a hinged endoprosthesis with antibiotic bone cement.

Wound Closure

Primary wound closure is always preferable, even when exchanging a septic prosthesis of the knee joint. If this is not possible due to existing fistulas or abscesses, the skin coverage should adhere to procedures applied in plastic surgery (e.g., mesh graft, gastrocnemius flap).

Postoperative Care

There can be no uniform postoperative physiotherapeutic plan after exchanging a septic prosthesis because of the highly varied extent of the infections and the resulting different degrees of bone and soft-tissue damage.

The postoperative treatment plan must be individually tailored. This involves a compromise between any necessary immobilization of the patient due to structural damage and treatment of the infection, on the one hand, and the necessity of mobilization, especially among older, multimorbid patients on the other. Patients can generally begin mobilization within the first 8 postoperative days; weight bearing on the operated extremity should be adapted to intraoperative findings and substance defects (**Figs. 7.47 and 7.48**).

Systemic administration of antibiotics for 10–14 postoperative days (exception: streptococci—10 days penicillin G and oral administration of a basic cephalosporin for a further 14 days followed by depot penicillin for 6 months).

NOTE

The implant of choice for exchanging a septic prosthesis of the knee joint is the cemented rotating hinge or pure hinged endoprosthesis.
If the extensors are insufficient, perform arthrodesis with cemented arthrodesis nails.

Fig. 7.47a, b Postoperative radiograph

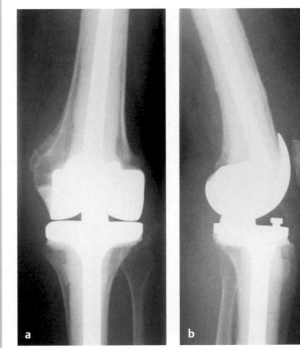

NOTE

The tips of the Redon drains must be sent in for microbiologic examination.

CRP values must be controlled regularly (every 3 days).

The CRP value should have regained its preoperative value by the 14th postoperative day.

If the CRP value rises or there is clinical suspicion of persisting infection, the joint should be aspirated immediately.

If there is wound dehiscence, hematoma, or a seroma leaking from the sutures, surgical revision must be performed immediately with suction/irrigation drainage.

Fig. 7.48a–d Functional result 1 year after surgery.

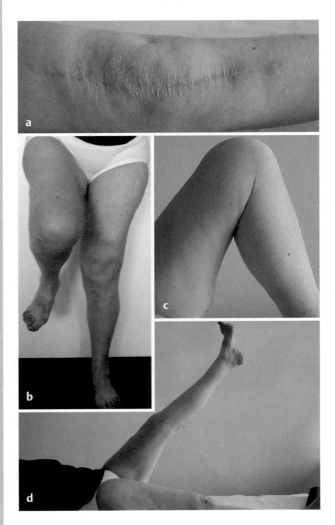

Case Study of Arthrodesis

An insufficient extensor system of the knee joint is an exceptional situation. If essential portions of the patellar ligament and/or the quadriceps muscle must be sacrificed during debridement, arthrodesis is indicated. Our preferred implant for a one-stage prosthesis exchange is the so-called arthrodesis nail. This involves a femoral and a tibial stem, which are interconnected by screws. The shafts are cemented, which offers the advantage of topical antibiotic administration. Risks, like infection of the pin or additional skin lesions, are avoided.

The patient was a 75-year-old female with a fistulous periprosthetic infection after a prosthesis of the knee joint had been exchanged and multiple soft-tissue revisions had been performed, including repeated plastic surgery to cover the wound and total insufficiency of the extensor system (**Figs. 7.49, 7.50, 7.51, 7.52**).

Pathogen: *Enterococcus faecalis*.

The infected prosthesis was removed, and an arthrodesis nail was implanted in a single operation. The antibiotic mixture per 40 g Refobacin Bone Cement R (Biomet, Berlin, Germany) consisted of 1 g ampicillin, 0.5 g gentamicin, and 2.0 g vancomycin. The systemic postoperative antibiotic therapy consisted of sultamicillin and gentamicin for 10 days.

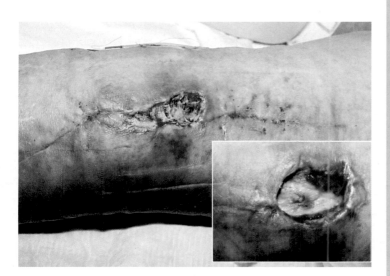

Fig. 7.49   Refer to text

Fig. 7.50a, b Preoperative radiographs

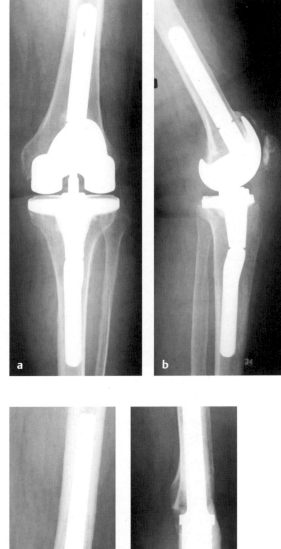

Fig. 7.51a, b Postoperative radiographs after arthrodesis with an arthrodesis nail.

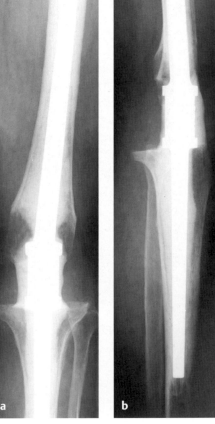

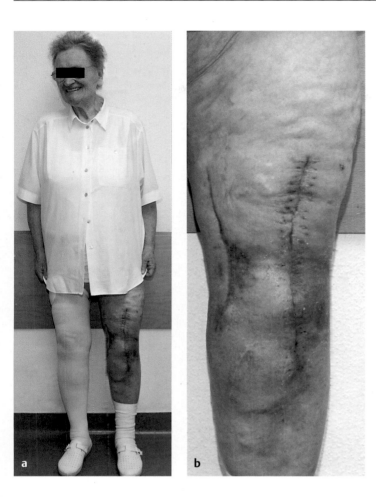

Fig. 7.52a, b Patient at discharge on the 18th postoperative day. The laboratory results on the day of discharge: CRP negative. Control aspiration: no pathogens detected.

Bibliography

Buchholz HW, Engelbrecht H. Depot effects of various antibiotics mixed with Palacos resins. [Article in German] Chirurg 1970;41(11):511–515

Buchholz HW, Engelbrecht E, Röttger J, Siegel A. Erkenntnisse nach Wechsel von über 400 infizierten Hüftendoprothesen. Orthop Praxis 1977;12:1117

Buchholz HW, Elson RA, Engelbrecht E, Lodenkämper H, Röttger J, Siegel A. Management of deep infection of total hip replacement. J Bone Joint Surg Br 1981;63-B(3):342–353

Charnley J. Postoperative infection after total hip replacement with special reference to air contamination in the operating room. Clin Orthop Relat Res 1972;87:167–187

Fitzgerald RH Jr, Nolan DR, Ilstrup DM, Van Scoy RE, Washington JA II, Coventry MB. Deep wound sepsis following total hip arthroplasty. J Bone Joint Surg Am 1977;59(7):847–855

Foerster VG, Buchholz HW, Lodenkämper H, Lodenkämper U. Antibiotika und Knochenzement—die lokaltherapeutische Bedeutung. In: Willert HG, Buchhorn G, eds. Knochenzement. Akt Probl Chir Orthop. Vol 31. Bern: Hans Huber Verlag; 1987:227–233

Frommelt L, Heinert K, Lodenkämper H, Buchholz HW. Lincomycin/Gentamicin-loaded PMMA bone-cement in the management of deep infection of total hip replacement by one stage exchange arthroplasty: a follow up study from 11 to minimum 3 years. Proceedings of the 4th International Congress on Clinical Microbiology; 1989; Nice, France. Abstract 767:40

Frommelt L, Gehrke T. Das infizierte Kunstgelenk: Mikrobiologische Aspekte. In: Hassenpflug J, Eulert G, eds. Praxis der Knieendoprothetik. Heidelberg: Springer; 2000

Gehrke T, Frommelt LV, Foerster G, Marx A. Pharmacokinetic study of a Gentamycin/Clindamycin bone cement used in one stage revision arthroplasty. In: Walenkamp GHIM, Murray DWE, eds. Bone Cement and Cementing Technique. Heidelberg: Springer; 2001

Gristina A, Costerton JW. Bacterial adherence, the glycocalix and musculoskeletal sepsis. Orthop Clin North Am 1984;15:517–535

Gristina AG. Biomaterial-centered infection: microbial adhesion versus tissue integration. Science 1987; 237(4822):1588–1595

Josefsson G, Lindberg L, Wiklander B. Systemic antibiotics and gentamicin-containing bone cement in the prophylaxis of postoperative infections in total hip arthroplasty. Clin Orthop Relat Res 1981;159(159):194–200

Lynch M, Esser MP, Shelley P, Wroblewski BM. Deep infection in Charnley low-friction arthroplasty. Comparison of plain and gentamicin-loaded cement. J Bone Joint Surg Br 1987;69(3):355–360

Nagai H, Wroblewski B, Gambhir A, et al. One stage revision total hip replacement for deep infection: 5- to 27-year follow-up study. AAOS, 70th Annual Meeting; February 5–9, 2003, New Orleans

Nieder E. Revisionsalloarthroplastik des Hüftgelenkes. In: Bauer R, Kerschbaumer F, Poisel S, eds. Orthopädische Operationslehre, Teil 1. Stuttgart: Thieme; 1994:255–370

Nieder E. Revisionsalloarthroplastik des Kniegelenkes. In: Bauer R, Kerschbaumer F, Poisel S, eds. Orthopädische Operationslehre, Teil 1. Stuttgart: Thieme; 1994:255–370, 619–673

Pietsch M, Wenisch C, Traussnig S, Trnoska R, Hofmann S. Temporary articulating spacer with antibiotic-impregnated cement for an infected knee endoprosthesis. [Article in German] Orthopäde 2003;32(6):490–497

Simmons TD, Stern SH. Diagnosis and management of the infected total knee arthroplasty. Am J Knee Surg 1996;9(2):99–106

Spangehl MJ, Masri BA, O'Connell JX, Duncan CP. Prospective analysis of preoperative and intraoperative investigations for the diagnosis of infection at the sites of two hundred and two revision total hip arthroplasties. J Bone Joint Surg Am 1999;81(5):672–683

Steinbrink K, Frommelt L. Treatment of periprosthetic infection of the hip using one-stage exchange surgery. [Article in German] Orthopäde 1995;24(4):335–343

Two-Stage Exchange of a Total Knee Replacement Using a Temporary Antibiotic Spacer Prosthesis

S. Hofmann, M. Piesch, Ch. Wenisch

Treatment Concept

Infection of an implanted total knee replacement (TKR) is a serious complication. Rare infections, which appear within the first 4–6 weeks after the operation (early infections), must be differentiated from the more common late infections, which often only appear years after the operation. The probability of an infection can be estimated according to the kind of intervention performed and the patient's individual risk factors (**Table 7.1**).

If an infection is present, further measures must be well planned and prepared. Immediate intervention with administration of an unspecific antibiotic combined with suction/irrigation drainage is only indicated for highly acute cases with systemic septic conditions and pyarthrosis after material has been taken for bacteriologic examination.

A two-stage prosthesis exchange is the most promising procedure for late infections (**Table 7.2**). The **two-stage prosthesis exchange** is performed in **four phases**:

Table 7.1 Probability of infections for different interventions

Intervention	Probability of infection in %
Surface replacement prosthesis	0.5–2
Revision procedures	2–5
Hinged prosthesis	4–10
High-risk patients (chemotherapy, HIV, chronic polyarthritis, diabetes mellitus, adiposity, trophic disturbances, history of infection, several previous operations)	5–15

Table 7.2 Alternative treatment possibilities for late infections and their chances of success

Intervention	Success rate in %
Permanent antibiotic suppression	20
Debridement alone	30
Resection arthroplasty	60
One-stage prosthesis exchange	70
Arthrodesis	80
Two-stage prosthesis exchange	90

1. First the infected soft tissues are debrided, the infected prosthesis is removed, and a spacer is implanted.
2. Systemic and local antibiotics are administered.
3. The spacer is removed, the site is again debrided, and a new TKR is implanted.
4. Systematic and local antibiotics are administered.

Indications

- An early infection is an acute infection appearing within 4–6 weeks after the primary implantation of a prosthesis.
- Debridement and exchange of the PE prosthesis alone are only appropriate for early infections.
- A late infection occurs later than 4–6 weeks after the primary implantation of a prosthesis.
- An exception is an acute onset of a late infection after primary implantation which shows no signs of infection for the first 2 postoperative years. An attempt can be made within 14 days after diagnosis to treat this like an early infection.
- The method of choice for a late infection is a two-stage exchange of the infected prosthesis. Remove the infected prosthesis, implant an antibiotic spacer prosthesis, and implant the new prosthesis after removing the spacer in a second operation.

Surgical Contraindications

- Multimorbid patient
- Life-threatening primary disease
- Inoperability due to poor patient condition
- No informed consent

Therapeutic Goals

- Eradicate the infection.
- Maintain mobility and joint function while eradicating the infection.
- Achieve a good functional outcome after implantation of the new prosthesis.

Diagnosis of a Late Infection

Acute infections are rare; subclinical, insidious infections are more common. Diagnosing an insidious infection is often difficult. Criteria are:
- High-risk patient

NOTE

Administer permanent antibiotic suppressive therapy only if surgery is contraindicated.

- Local and systemic signs of inflammation
- Pain at rest (night pain)
- Elevated CRP, ESR, and leukocytes
- Aspiration of the knee joint (positive bacteriologic result in 80%–90% of the cases)
- Early or progressive prosthetic loosening in radiographs
- CT (bone defects) and bone scans (combined dynamic bone scintigraphy with ^{99m}Tc- and ^{111}In-labeled leukocytes) as complementary methods

Surgical Preparations

- Take a thorough medical history, including all previous operations, previous medical reports, positive bacterial probes, antibiotics administered, and risk factors.
- Provide comprehensive patient information (therapeutic options, explanation of the advantages and disadvantages of one-stage versus two-stage procedures precise therapeutic plan and necessity for surgical revision, risks, and prospects of success).
- Document the patient information.
- Clarify the general surgical risk, including the necessity for surgical revision.
- Determine the peri- and postoperative antibiotic regime, including antibiotic bone cement, according to the antibiogram after consulting with a specialist in infectious diseases.
- Assure the availability of special instruments and implants.

Advantages of articulated spacer prostheses in comparison to rigid spacers:
- Joint function is maintained.
- Ligamentous contractures, muscle atrophy, shortening of muscles, and arthrofibrosis are limited.
- There is no additional bone loss.
- Reimplantation is facilitated.
- The functional outcome is better.
- The eradication rate is as good as that of fixed spacers (>90%).

ERRORS AND RISKS

The classic signs of inflammation (redness, warmth, and swelling) are often missed in low-grade infections.

The leukocyte count is often normal.

ESR and CRP may be normal in approximately 5% of cases.

Fever occurs only if the patient is septic.

Joint aspiration should not be performed during antibiotic administration (discontinue antibiotics at least 10 days before aspiration).

Minimum 14 days incubation of tissue probes. Nevertheless the aspiration result may be false-negative.

A positive bone scan does not confirm an infection, but a negative bone scan does exclude an infection.

There might be several other causes of pain when there is a TKR.

NOTE

If pain occurs in the presence of a TKR, an infection must always be suspected until it has been definitely excluded.

Crisis management includes intensive care by a trusted and responsible person (surgeon).

Clarify the care conditions in the patient's home, including physical therapy.

Therapeutic Concept in Placement of a Temporary Antibiotic Spacer Prosthesis

Articulated antibiotic spacer prostheses can prevent the negative effects of immobilization with a rigid spacer. An articulated spacer can be produced from antibiotic cement only or in a hybrid technique (antibiotic bone cement in combination with PE and metal).

- **Group I:** A temporary antibiotic spacer prosthesis (TASP) consists purely of bone cement. The tibial and femoral components are made of antibiotic bone cement only (formed manually in a mold on the table).
- **Group II:** Manually produced hybrid TASP. Antibiotic bone cement in combination with PE tibial insert and femoral metal component.
- **Group III:** Industrially produced hybrid spacer prosthesis (e.g., PROSTALAC prosthesis in combination with antibiotic-loaded acrylic cement, Smith and Nephew, USA).

We use a manually produced hybrid spacer prosthesis in a modified technique of the "Salt Lake City Concept" according to the original description by Aaron Hofmann et al. (1995).

Phase 1: Implantation of the Spacer Prosthesis

Step 1: Removal of the Infected TKR

- Use the tourniquet and do not use cell saver.
- Choose the right approach under consideration of old scars (no parallel incisions).
- Radically debride soft-tissues.
- Remove the prosthesis, including any patella replacement.
- Sterilize the cleaned femoral components and the PE inlay for later use as a spacer during the operation.
- Remove all remaining bone cement.
- Take tissue probes for bacterial and histologic examinations according to a standardized procedure (subcutaneous, intra-articular, implants, femur, tibia, and posterior capsule).
- After taking the probes, deflate the tourniquet, coagulate bleeders, and begin the preoperatively determined systemic antibiotic regime (two antibiotics).
- Check radical debridement of all joint surfaces again.
- Do not perform bone cuts or soft-tissue releases.
- Perform extensive jet lavage.

Step 2: Implantation of the Spacer Prosthesis

- Form a hybrid TASP using the sterilized PE insert and antibiotic-loaded cement for the tibia component.
- The femoral component consists of the sterilized femoral prosthesis and antibiotic-loaded cement.
- Both components are "press-fit" cemented.
- Mix the bone cement with antibiotics in therapeutic doses (e.g., Refobacin Revision, 1 g gentamicin + 1 g clindamycin in 40-g bone-cement powder, Biomet, Berlin, Germany) which is effective against 90% of the pathogens.
- Antibiotic bone cement can be mixed in the surgical theater according to the results of the antibiogram (4–6 g antibiotic in 40-g bone-cement powder; **Table 7.3**).
- The posterior surface of the patella is not replaced.
- The skin is closed over two drains without suction.

Table 7.3 Antibiotic bone cement according to the antibiogram

Antibiotic	Dose per 40 g bone cement (g)	Bacteria
Clindamycin	1.0	Staphylococci
Gentamicin	1.0	Staphylococci
	1.0	Streptococci
	1.0	Enterococci
	1.5	Enterobacteriaceae
	1.0	Propionibacteria
Cefuroxim	3.0	Staphylococci
Vancomycin	2.0	Staphylococci
	2.0	Enterococci
Oflaxacin	1.0	Staphylococci
Ampicillin	1.0	Enterococci
Cefotaxim	2.0	Enterobacteriaceae
Cefoperazon	2.0	*Pseudomonas*
Amikacin	2.0	*Pseudomonas*
Streptomycin	2.0	Mycobacteria

TIPS AND TRICKS

Use the original PE insert only if there is no macroscopic damage visible.

If the pathogens have not been identified, additionally mix 2 g vancomycin into the Refobacin Revision cement.

If the pathogens are resistant to gentamicin or clindamycin, additionally mix 2 g of an antibiotic which will be effective according to the antibiogram into the Refobacin Revision cement (**Table 7.3**).

If the pathogens are resistant to gentamicin and clindamycin, mix a maximal dose of an antibiotic which will be effective according to the antibiogram into the Refobacin Bone Cement R (0.5 g Refobacin [gentamicin] in 40-g bone-cement powder, Biomet, Berlin, Germany; **Table 7.3**).

The systemic antibiotic chosen should also be available for oral administration.

The bone cement should have a large surface area because the antibiotic is released from the surface only.

Consult the person responsible for the sterilization process when planning to implant a spacer.

Functional treatment begins early with the spacer prosthesis in place if the skin condition permits it.

ERRORS AND RISKS

- Discontinuing antibiotics early
- Immobilizing the leg with the spacer
- Reimplanting the prosthesis too early (infection not completely eradicated)
- Reimplanting the prosthesis after 12 weeks (the spacer itself becomes a foreign body when it no longer releases antibiotics)

Phase 2: Postoperative Interval

- Antibiotics are administered systemically for 5–10 days (effective antibiotic + rifampicin 2 × 600 mg) and changed according to the results of the antibiogram from the intraoperative probes if necessary.
- Rifampicin is ideal in combination with an effective monotherapy because it also has a bactericidal effect.
- Change to an oral antibiotic according to the antibiogram and oral bioavailability when the patient is discharged (effective antibiotic + rifampicin 1 × 600 mg) until the follow-up examination.
- Begin physical therapy on the first postoperative day with exercises and continuous passive motion (CPM) to a maximum of 90 °.
- For the first 5–10 postoperative days, the patient should be mobilized with an orthesis fixed in extension. After uncomplicated wound healing and if the patient feels stable when walking, remove the orthesis before the patient is discharged.
- Mobilize the patient with two crutches and 50 % weight bearing.
- The patient should perform daily exercises and build up the muscles at home.
- Regular training with a physiotherapist is necessary.
- The patient ingests two oral antibiotics until the first postoperative control at 6 weeks.
- Discontinue the antibiotics for 10 days and control whether the infection has been completely eradicated.
- Make an appointment for reimplantation of a prosthesis.

Criteria for eradication of an infection:
- Unremarkable local finding
- No night pain
- Normal or threshold CRP
- Routine aspiration not necessary
- Reimplant a revision prosthesis 6–12 weeks after the spacer implantation.
- If the infection persists, aspirate the joint again and continue antibiotics up to a maximum of 12 postoperative weeks. If infection persists go for another two-stage procedure.

Phase 3: Reimplantation of the TKR

Step 1: Removal of the Spacer Prosthesis

- Do not use the tourniquet but use the cell saver.
- Perform radical debridement.
- Remove the spacer prosthesis.
- Apply the standard procedure for taking tissue probes before starting antibiotics, as in phase 1 during spacer implantation.
- Administer a combination of two antibiotics (effective antibiotic + rifampicin 2 × 600 mg) systemically according to the previous antibiotic regime.

Step 2: Implantation of the New Prosthesis

- Correct the mechanical axis of the leg with correction bone cuts.
- Perform soft-tissue releases to balance the knee.
- Perform extensive jet lavage.
- Implant a new revision prosthesis with stem extensions.
- Use antibiotic bone cement according to the results of the previous antibiogram.
- Close the skin over two drains without suction.

Phase 4: Postoperative Interval

- Administer systemic antibiotics according to the previous antibiotic regime for 5–10 days.
- If there is still evidence of pathogens when the new prosthesis is implanted, adjust the antibiotics to the results of the antibiogram if necessary.
- Mobilize the patient as after primary prosthesis implantation.
- Administer oral antibiotics for 3–6 weeks after discharging the patient (an effective antibiotic + rifampicin 1 × 600 mg)
- Perform clinical, radiographic, and laboratory controls after 1, 3, 6, 12, and 24 months.

Surgical Procedure

Surgical revision of a septic TKR requires an experienced surgeon and a smoothly functioning team. These complicated operations should only be performed in centers with sufficient case numbers. Close cooperation with an experienced specialist in infectious diseases is a further essential prerequisite for success.

Few special instruments are required to implant a spacer prosthesis (microsaw, special chisels, universal extractor).

Phase 1: Implantation of the Spacer Prosthesis

Step 1: Removal of the Infected TKR (Figs. 7.53, 7.54, 7.55, 7.56)

Fig. 7.53 Careful approach with radical debridement (proximal, medial, and lateral recess and posterior capsule). The tibial tuberosity should only be removed in cases with extraordinarily stiff knees.

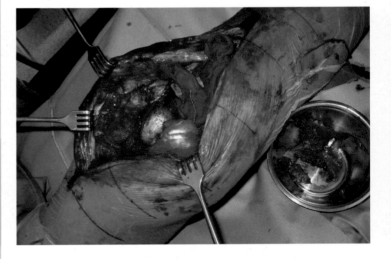

Fig. 7.54 Removal of the prosthetic components.

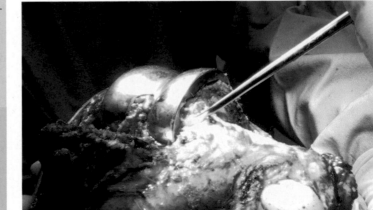

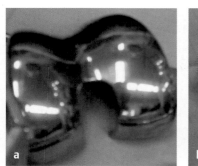

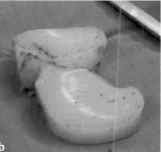

Fig. 7.55a, b Explanted components of the femoral prosthesis and PE inlay. After mechanical cleansing on the operating table, the prosthesis is sent for sterilization while the operation continues. If the PE has been mechanically damaged, a new PE joint surface must be used.

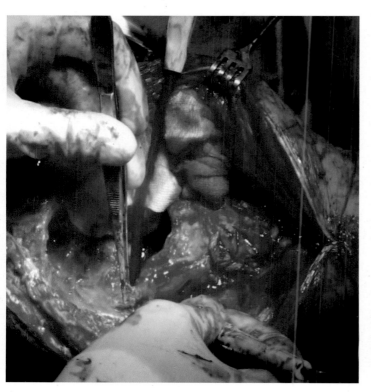

Fig. 7.56 Further radical debridement of the medial and lateral recess, the posterior joint capsule, and all insufficiently perfused tissues.

TIPS AND TRICKS

Perform generous jet lavage and hemostasis. Replace some of the surgical drapes and change the surgical gloves.

Step 2: Implantation of the Spacer Prosthesis (Figs. 7.57, 7.58, 7.59, 7.60, 7.61)

Produce a homogenous mixture of antibiotic and bone-cement powder using the "pharmaceutical mixture technique."

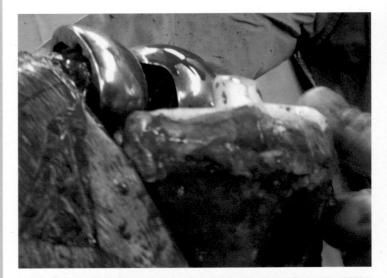

Fig. 7.57 Drill anchorage holes in the backside of the PE insert and mount the component with ample bone cement (cement consistency in a highly viscous stage). Bring in the femoral component without cement. Check the "flexion and extension gap." The cement hardens in extension with the leg under longitudinal traction. Ensure the straightest possible longitudinal axis. The cement is constantly reworked and finished.

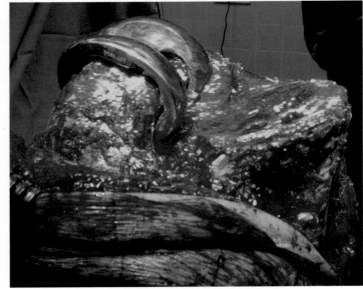

Fig. 7.58 Shortly before the cement hardens, the joint is moved once more and the tibial component removed. This represents the worst possible cementing technique (continuous reworking of the cement during the hardening process with blood and fluid on the interface) to prevent infiltration of the cement into the trabeculae.

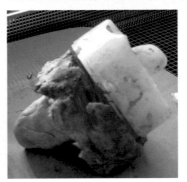

Fig. 7.59 The negative impression of the bone defects in the cement sufficiently anchors the tibial components without actually requiring cement fixation = "press-fit cementing."

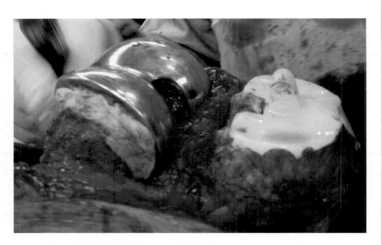

Fig. 7.60 Implantation of the femoral components with ample antibiotic bone cement and tibial components mounted with the same technique as described for the tibia.

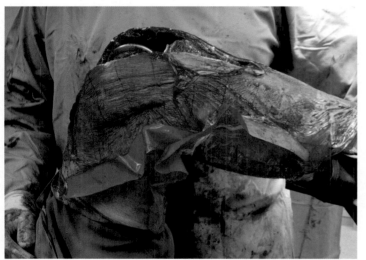

Fig. 7.61 Trial of function. No soft-tissue balancing. There should be relative stability in extension and sufficient stability in flexion to prevent dislocation of the components.

Phase 2: Postoperative Interval (Fig. 7.62)

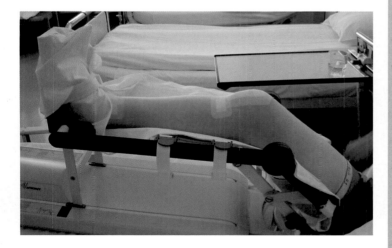

Fig. 7.62 Passive motion in the CPM machine. A maximum of 90° flexion is allowed, depending on the condition of the skin closure. An orthesis fixed in extension should be worn when walking until the wound has healed and afterwards only if the patient feels unstable.

Phase 3: Reimplantation of the TKR in the Absence of Clinical or Laboratory Signs of Infection

Step 1: Removal of the Spacer Prosthesis (Figs. 7.63, 7.64, 7.65)

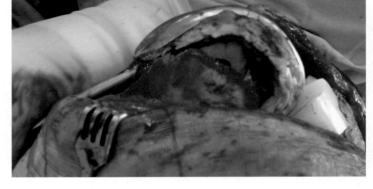

Fig. 7.63 Unproblematic extraction of the press-fit cemented femoral component with a universal extractor device without creating additional bone defects.

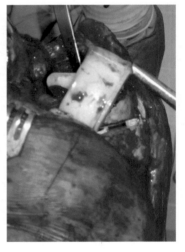

Fig. 7.64 Unproblematic extraction of the press-fit cemented PE tibial component with a universal extraction device without creating additional bone defects.

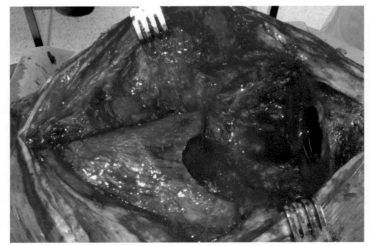

Fig. 7.65 Radical debridement of the medial and lateral recess and the posterior joint capsule.

Step 2: Implantation of the New Prosthesis (Figs. 7.66, 7.67, 7.68, 7.69, 7.70, 7.71, 7.72, 7.73, 7.74, 7.75)

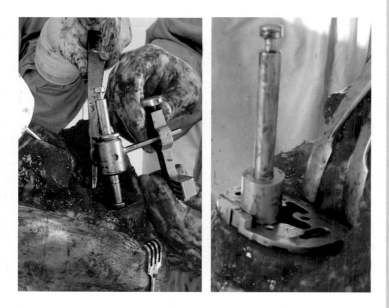

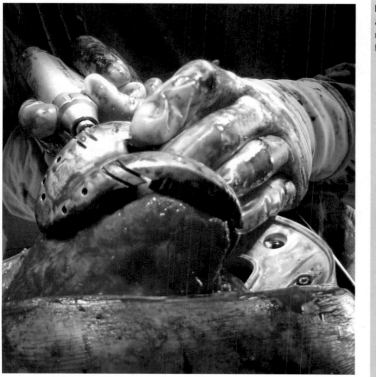

Fig. 7.66 Correction of the tibia alignment by a minimum correction cut in 90° to the neutral mechanical axis (caution: ensure the correct posterior slope and tibia rotation).

Fig. 7.67 Creating a stable tibia platform with stem extension (caution: in 90% of cases an offset stem is required).

Fig. 7.68 Correction of the femur alignment by a minimum correction cut in 90° to the neutral mechanical axis (caution: check and correct the femoral rotation parallel to the epicondylar line).

Fig. 7.69 Mount the femoral and tibial prostheses and attach the trial PE inlay. Check the alignment again and test the flexion and extension gaps. Perform soft-tissue releases when necessary.

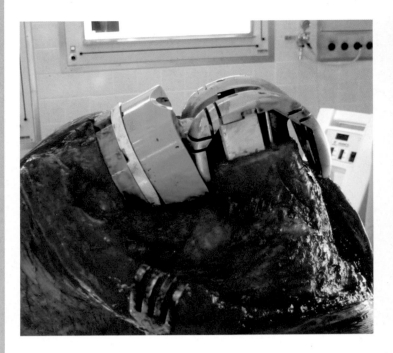

Fig. 7.70 Fill closed bone defects with bone grafts loaded with vancomycin (incubated in 2 g vancomycin to 500 ml NaCl) with the impaction technique.

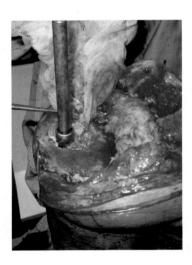

Fig. 7.71 Fill structural bone defects by using metal blocks or wedges.

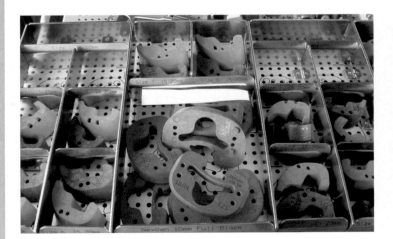

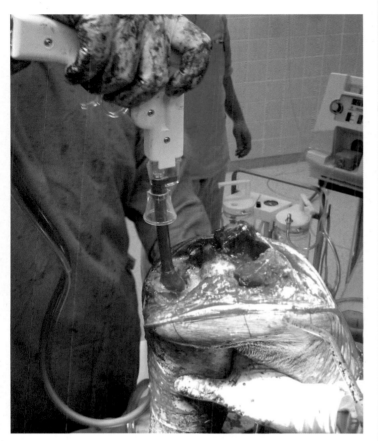

Fig. 7.72 After performing jet lavage and hemostasis, change the drapes and surgical gloves.

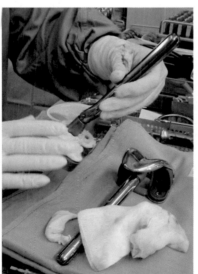

Fig. 7.73 Hybrid cementing technique for fixating the prosthesis with antibiotic bone cement (cement the components, but not the stem extensions).

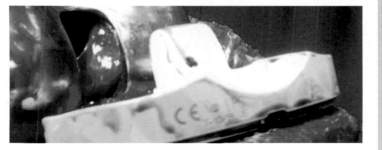

Fig. 7.74 If the medial and lateral ligaments are sufficient, use a semiconstrained articulating surface (posterior stabilized or rotating platform).

Fig. 7.75 If the medial or lateral ligament structures are insufficient or the flexion and extension gaps are not matched, use a constrained articulating surface (condylar constrained or rotating hinge).

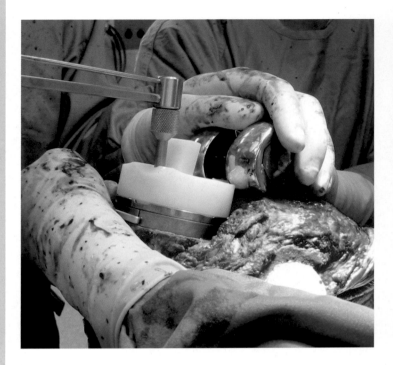

Case Study

See **Figs. 7.76, 7.77, 7.78, 7.79**.

Fig. 7.76 The radiograph shows signs of septic loosening of the revision prosthesis after a two-stage exchange procedure with a fixed antibiotic spacer as the last attempted revision.

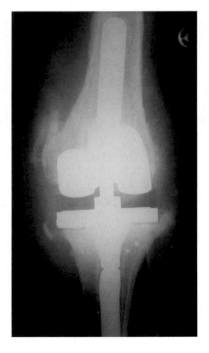

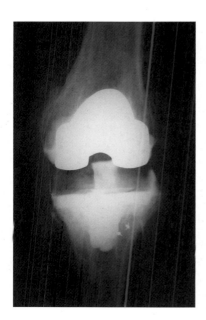

Fig. 7.77 Implantation of a TASP (2 g vancomycin to 40 g Refobacin Revision cement) with the standard technique.

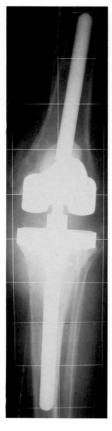

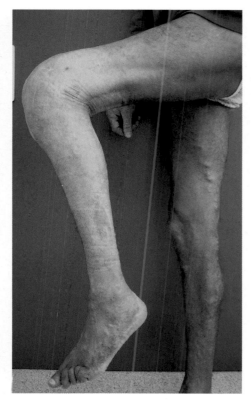

Fig. 7.78 Radiograph 6 weeks postoperative after reimplantation of a revision prosthesis. The implant is in place; femoral and tibial reconstruction has been performed. The prosthesis was fixed with a hybrid technique (components cemented, stems cementless). Laboratory tests (CRP, ESR, leukocyte count) and local findings were unremarkable.

Fig. 7.79 Clinical control 3 months postoperative. The patient has no pain and good function with active flexion 0-0-100°. There is no sign of a renewed infection.

Bibliography

Borden LS, Gearen PF. Infected total knee arthroplasty. A protocol for management. J Arthroplasty 1987;2(1):27–36

Cadambi A, Jones RE, Maale GE. A protocol for staged revision of infected total hip and knee arthroplasties: the use of antibiotic-cement-implant composites. Int Orthop 1995;3:133–145

Fehring TK, Odum S, Calton TF, Mason JB. Articulating versus static spacers in revision total knee arthroplasty for sepsis. The Ranawat Award. Clin Orthop Relat Res 2000;380(380):9–16

Frommelt L, Gehrke T. Das infizierte Kunstgelenk—mikrobiologische Konzepte. In: Eulert J, Hassenpflug J, eds. Praxis der Knieendoprothetik. Berlin: Springer; 2000:273–284

Goldstein WM, Kopplin M, Wall R, Berland K. Temporary articulating methylmethacrylate antibiotic spacer (TAM-MAS). A new method of intraoperative manufacturing of a custom articulating spacer. J Bone Joint Surg Am 2001;83-A(Suppl 2 Pt 2):92–97

Hofmann AA, Kane KR, Tkach TK, Plaster RL, Camargo MP. Treatment of infected total knee arthroplasty using an articulating spacer. Clin Orthop Relat Res 1995;321(321):45–54

Insall JN, Thompson FM, Brause BD. Two-stage reimplantation for the salvage of infected total knee arthroplasty. J Bone Joint Surg Am 1983;65(8):1087–1098

Masri BA, Kendall RW, Duncan CP, Beauchamp CP, McGraw RW, Bora B. Two-stage exchange arthroplasty using a functional antibiotic-loaded spacer in the treatment of the infected knee replacement: the Vancouver experience. Semin Arthroplasty 1994;5(3):122–136

McPherson EJ, Lewonowski K, Dorr LD. Techniques in arthroplasty. Use of an articulated PMMA spacer in the infected total knee arthroplasty. J Arthroplasty 1995;10(1):87–89

Pietsch M, Wenisch C, Traussnig S, Trnoska R, Hofmann S. Temporary articulating spacer with antibiotic-impregnated cement for an infected knee endoprosthesis. [Article in German] Orthopade 2003;32(6):490–497

Pietsch M, Hofmann S, Wenisch C. Treatment of deep infection of total knee arthroplasty using a two-stage procedure. Oper Orthop Traumatol 2006;18(1):66–87

Pietsch M, Wenisch C, Hofmann S. Treatment of infected total knee arthroplasty. 2-5-year results following two-stage reimplantation. [Article in German] Orthopäde 2009;38(4):348–354

Scott IR, Stockley I, Getty CJM. Exchange arthroplasty for infected knee replacements. A new two-stage method. J Bone Joint Surg Br 1993;75(1):28–31

Whiteside LA. Treatment of infected total knee arthroplasty. Clin Orthop Relat Res 1994;299(299):169–172

Thank You

The authors wish to thank Dr. Lars Frommelt, Hamburg for his help in creating the local antibiotic therapy concept with cement, as well as Prof. Reinhard Graf for his active support as Medical Director of the Stolzalpe Clinic in Austria.

8

Special Arthrodeses
for Infected Joints

V. Heppert

These increasingly hectic times are characterized by demands for limitless mobility. To keep pace, technical progress has also been made in the surgical theater in clinics. Continually improved implants and constant changes in artificial joints make it difficult for doctors to obtain long-term experience with one certain procedure. One must not, however, forget that a surgeon's or orthopedic surgeon's individual **learning curve** means the patient's **suffering curve**. Changing the implant used too often is counterproductive and increases the complication rate considerably.

Nonetheless, we surgeons nourish the patient's belief that just about everything can be corrected. Every trauma and every degenerating process in the joints which has been going on for decades is expected to be rectified by the physician's skill together with an optimal implant. Interestingly enough, both doctors and patients have contributed to the gradual development of this process in the clinical routine. For example, it is expected that a lower extremity which has suffered the severest traumatic injury can be salvaged and will even function after all reconstructive procedures have been applied. The surgeon is, of course, pleased and the patient happy when the leg need not be amputated. But, after getting used to the situation, instead of being satisfied both parties astoundingly became dissatisfied. Residual complaints are overrated, and new surgical procedures are considered. No one wants to remember the initial situation. This step, albeit well meant, often leads to complications. In individual cases the physician is well advised to say "no." But this must be learned.

In this difficult situation, arthrodesis—stiffening of the joint—is considered a relic of the distant past. It is expected to destroy the patient's mobility and create a permanent problem. If this procedure is recommended to a patient, the initial reaction is sudden doubt concerning the physician's professional competence. "You can just as well amputate my leg right now," is often the spontaneous reply. The patient has already suffered considerably. It is not taken into consideration that arthrodesis is often not the initial intervention, but is at the end of a long chain of operations and presents the possibility of painless or at least less painful use of the limb. If the individual case is critically analyzed from the physician's point of view, this step should actually have been taken earlier in the chain of interventions. A correctly performed arthrodesis offers undeniable advantages for the patient:

- Full weight bearing on the extremity
- Little or no pain
- No further operations planned in the future
- In the long run, no need for ortheses or orthopedic shoes

This can, however, only be achieved if sufficient bone substance remains in the knee or ankle when the arthrodesis is performed.

It makes little functional sense for the patient if one extremity is much shorter due to bone defects because then he or she will permanently have to rely on walking aids. A difference in length of up to 3 cm can easily be compensated in or on a shoe. The patient can even walk short distances barefoot without uncertainty. Greater limb-length discrepancies limit mobility and quality of life and can even be dangerous, especially among the elderly.

Depending on the localization of the arthrodesis and the patient's age and compliance, bone construction should be undertaken to equalize the difference in length. Whether bone grafting will be sufficient, callus distraction will be necessary, or an arthrodesis rod must be implanted (especially if there is a bone defect in the knee after numerous total knee replacements) to solve the problem, must be decided together with the patient and depends largely on the condition of the extremity. The goal must be to compensate the handicap of a stiff joint with optimal surrounding conditions.

An increasing number of total knee and ankle replacements are now being implanted worldwide. As the number of implants increases, so does the absolute number of complications. Under these circumstances, arthrodesis will revive. It offers patients the possibility to walk without pain in the majority of cases. If arthrodesis had been considered in the individual's chain of treatment at a time when there was still enough bone substance, far better functional outcomes would be possible.

Under these considerations, arthrodesis could even be a primary option for young patients with completely destroyed knee or angle joints as a result of extreme traumas. Implanting an artificial joint, which is a justified therapeutic option for older individuals in such situations, should not be considered for young patients. They experience the severe resulting problems while they are still relatively young. Remember the inventor of the total hip replacement, Sir John Charnley (1911–1982), who wisely said, "The surgeon implants a disease with every total joint replacement." This disadvantage does not exist with arthrodesis.

Knee Joint

Indications

- Septic joint destruction (bone, ligament) (**Fig. 8.1**)
- Widespread osteomyelitis of the distal femur
- Widespread osteomyelitis of the proximal tibia
- Infected prosthesis

Fig. 8.1 Stage 4 infection of the knee joint with extensive destruction of the bone and complete loss of cartilage.

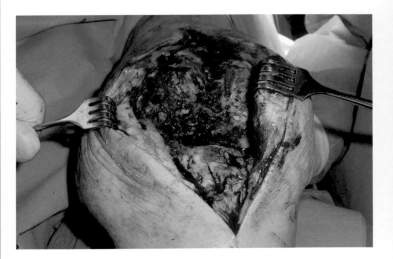

NOTE

A contraindication places the surgeon in a dilemma. One should always critically question the indication to amputate in such cases.

Older patients fare worse after an amputation than younger patients from a purely functional point of view. If the patient wishes to keep his/her leg in spite of considerable risk factors, there is no choice but to send the patient away or to comply with his/her (understandable) wish. In individual cases an arthrodesis rod which can bear weight early is a possible solution.

Providing information which cannot be misunderstood—for your own security—including all possible complications is an absolute necessity.

NOTE

A false assessment of the patient's compliance and especially of his/her subjective satisfaction after arthrodesis can cause the surgeon considerable problems afterwards. The patient often cannot imagine—despite sufficient verbal information—how life functions with a stiff knee. Medical guidance of the patient during the entire duration of treatment and thereafter is decisive. One possibility is to fit a brace for a few days preoperatively to give the patient an impression of what arthrodesis of the knee is like.

ERRORS AND RISKS

Axial malalignment: It is difficult to judge the axial alignment intraoperatively with an image intensifier. Varus deformities often result.

Persisting infections: It can make sense to perform a two-stage arthrodesis, especially in osteomyelitis of the adjacent areas (femoral condyle/tibial head).

Insufficient resection—to avoid extreme shortening of the leg—increases the danger of reinfection. If the infection is confined to the joint, this danger does not exist.

Nonconsolidation of the bone.

Functionally unsatisfactory shortening of the leg: especially after repeated infections of total knee replacements and final removal of the prosthesis, a shortening of the leg by > 4 cm is usually the result. Depending on the age of the patient and his/her risk factors, lengthening the shortened leg in the arthrodesis cleft can avoid this functionally unsatisfactory situation. For injury to nerves and vessels, see below.

Contraindications

- Multimorbid patient
- Lack of compliance
- Life-threatening disease
- Severe arterial occlusive disease

General Comments

The complex problems in destructive infectious joint disease of the knee are so multifaceted that different therapeutic options—arthrodesis versus total joint replacement—must always be discussed. The patient's wishes have priority. Even if these wishes in some cases make no sense medically, the physician is bound to respect them.

The surgeon's primary function is to offer advice; making demands or even applying pressure is simply not an option, regardless of contrary specialist opinion. The physician must never forget that any stiffening of the knee joint places considerable limitations on every patient. You can only try to convince the patient that a stiff knee joint is a safe option offering full weight bearing in the future, despite all functional restrictions.

If a patient is unsatisfied after successful arthrodesis, one should always consider whether the primary information and advice given to the patient was not sufficiently detailed.

Surgical Concepts

Eradication of the focus of infection and reconstruction by means of arthrodesis can be performed in either one- or two-stage procedures (**Table 8.1**). The decision is determined by the following situations:

- Extent of the infection
- Intensity of the infection
- Patient's condition
- Soft-tissue defects
- Bone grafting
- Stabilizing procedures

"Infection and metal are poor partners." This guiding principle, which is supported by every clinical routine when sepsis is involved, recommends a two-stage intervention for planned joint stabilization with an implant. After debridement (**Fig. 8.2**), a local antibiotic is inserted (spacer or polymethylmethacrylate [PMMA] chain). Immobilization is achieved with a cast or anterior clamps (fixator).

Table 8.1 Criteria for deciding whether to perform a one- or two-stage procedure

	One-stage procedure	Two-stage procedure
Extent of infection	Knee joint	Osteomyelitis
Intensity of infection	Chronic	Acute, purulent
Patient's condition	Healthy	Sick
Bone grafting	Not necessary	Necessary
Stabilization	Fixator	Plate/nail

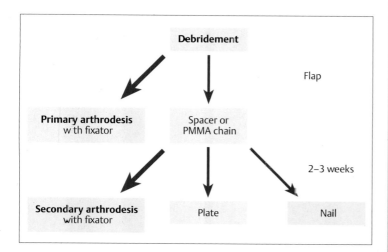

Fig. 8.2 Therapeutic concept for destructive infection of the knee joint.

Principal Signs and Symptoms

- Classical parameters of inflammation
- Fever
- Erythrocyte sedimentation rate (ESR) (leukocyte count is unspecific)
- C-reactive protein (CRP) is almost always elevated
- Pain on movement
- Fistulas may be present

Surgical Preparations

- Radiograph: Further imaging diagnostics are only required in exceptional situations.
- Smear: It is good policy to aspirate the joint before the operation so that adjuvant antibiotic therapy can be performed according to the most recent bacteriologic test results (e. g., methicillin-resistant *Staphylococcus aureus*, MRSA). In an acute emergency this may not be possible if it causes delay.
- Perform routine laboratory tests.
- Have four units of banked blood ready and available.
- Obtain informed consent from the patient, including:
  - General risks
  - The entire spectrum of problems, like "stiff knee"
  - Possible necessity of a blood transfusion
  - Axial malalignment
  - Rotational error
  - Shortened leg
  - Nerve damage, for example, peroneus, sciatic nerves
  - Vascular damage, for example, popliteal vessels
  - Failure of bone consolidation
  - Recurring infection

Special Instruments and Materials

- Oscillating saw
- Water-cooled round burr
- Broad chisel
- Jet lavage
- PMMA chains, Refobacin Bone Cement R, gentamicin sponge

NOTE

Possible complications must be written down. General comments like "damage to nerves or vessels" are not sufficient. It is important to be precise, for example "damage to the peroneal nerve."

Therapeutic Concept: Eradication of the Infection by Means of Primary Arthrodesis with an External Fixator

Soft Tissues

- Begin intravenous antibiotic administration approximately 30 minutes before the operation. Interrupt the blood supply. Inflate the tourniquet.
- Perform a central vertical incision to open the knee joint on the medial parapatellar side (**Fig. 8.1**).
- Take biopsies for bacteriologic and pathologic examination. Smears should no longer be taken without biopsies because the two together considerably increase identification of pathogens.
- Radically debride all infected soft tissues.
- Perform initial jet lavage (to reduce the number of pathogens).
- Eliminate existing or beginning soft-tissue defects with flaps (gastrocnemius or free flap).

Bones

- Consider the definitive leg axis when resecting the tibial and femoral joint surfaces (**Figs. 8.3 and 8.4**).
- Burr out any osteolytic foci in the tibial plateau or the femoral condyles.
- Resect all remaining cartilage.
- Resect the posterior surface of the patella and cut the remaining patella to size (**Fig. 8.5**).
- Mobilize the lateral and posterior aspects of the joint capsule with a curved raspatory on the tibial plateau or the femoral condyle to prevent later interposition by soft tissues during compression. Then debride the posterior portions of the capsule. (Be careful not to damage neighboring vessels!)
- Perform a second jet lavage (final cleansing).
- Insert one Steinmann pin approximately 10 cm proximal and one distal of the arthrodesis cleft (**Fig. 8.5**).
- Mount one AO fixator tube (Synthes, Inc., West Chester, PA, USA) equipped with six pin clamps medial and lateral. Steinmann pins are affixed to pin clamps 1 and 6, and the arthrodesis is performed after the leg has been repositioned. (Caution: avoid any rotational error!) (**Figs. 8.5 and 8.6**).
- Perform clinical and radiographic control of the axis of the leg and the arthrodesis (**Fig. 8.7**).

TIPS AND TRICKS

- Interrupting the blood supply facilitates the debridement of soft tissues.
- The leg is positioned on the operating table with the axis in the correct position and the knee in 10° flexion. Then two parallel incisions are cut with a saw in the femur and the tibia to one-third of the depth (**Fig. 8.3**). After repositioning the leg into 90° flexion, the bones are completely severed while protecting the soft tissues with Hohmann retractors (**Fig. 8.4**). When compression is later performed, the axis of the leg is automatically correct.
- If the infection has spread to differing degrees in the bone, this could cause nonlevel resection planes. In such cases it is better to perform two-stage spongiosaplasty than to perform a second resection, which would shorten the leg.
- After debriding the bone, the posterior soft tissues are again debrided because they are now easier to reach.
- Jet lavage afterwards is optional.
- The wound cavity is filled with Lavasept (caution: only apply the concentrate intended for internal use!). Allow it to take effect for several minutes, and then rinse it out with the remaining jet lavage irrigation fluid.
- The soft tissues may have suffered considerable trophic damage due to previous operations.
- Partial resection of the femoral condyles, which often protrude laterally over the remaining tibia, provides sufficient space to close the wound without tension.

- Implant two further Steinmann pins in the tibia and the femur approximately 2.5 cm from the arthrodesis cleft. Use a spot-film device and attach the Steinmann pins to pin clamps 3 and 4 on each side.
- Attach a clamp to each tube and apply compression to the arthrodesis.
- After radiographic control, the patella is fixed with a 4.5 AO traction screw (long threads) so that it bridges the arthrodesis cleft equally on both sides (**Fig. 8.7**).
- Mount one Schanz screw (two if there is severe dystrophy or extensive spongiosaplasty) from anterior in the femur and tibia and connect them with an AO tube with six pin clamps (**Fig. 8.6**).
- Now the remaining empty pin clamps are attached to the Steinmann pins (two medial and two lateral), producing a tentlike construction (**Fig. 8.6**).
- Remove the tourniquet, perform careful hemostasis, insert a local antibiotic, and close the wound in layers (**Fig. 8.8a, b**).

Fig. 8.3 The leg is in the correct position. Two parallel incisions are made with the saw in the femur and tibia to about one-third of the depth. To ensure the cuts are parallel, a saw blade is inserted in the first incision in the femur to demonstrate the correct direction for the incision in the tibia.

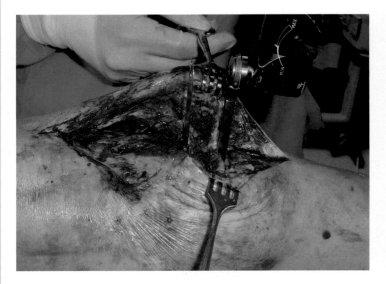

Fig. 8.4 The position of the leg is changed, and the femur and tibia are completely severed while protecting the soft tissues with Hohmann retractors.

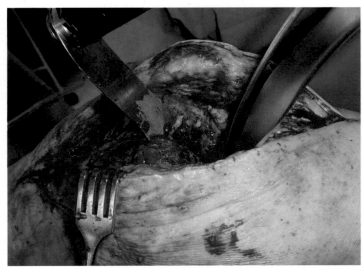

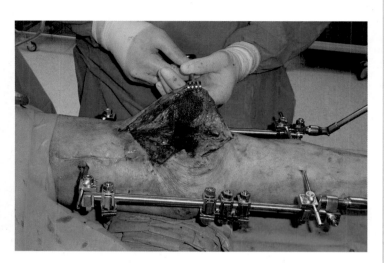

Fig. 8.5 The femur, tibia, and patella are dissected. Jet lavage has been performed. Two Steinmann pins are placed at a distance from the arthrodesis. Compression is applied to the arthrodesis with an AO fixator. Before closing the wound, check that no soft tissues are interposed in the cleft.

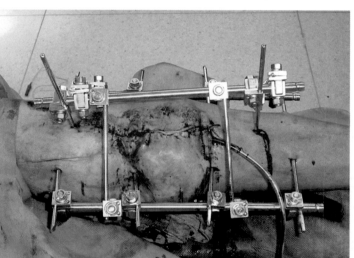

Fig. 8.6 The tent-shaped montage is finished. Protruding pins are shortened.

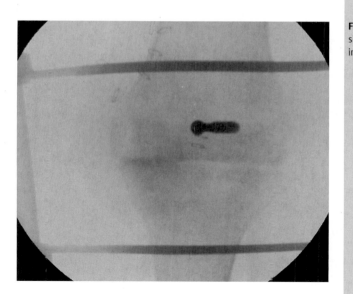

Fig. 8.7 The position of the arthrodesis compression screw is checked intraoperatively with an image intensifier.

Fig. 8.8a, b Radiograph of a healing arthrodesis of the knee after sepsis. An external fixator was applied.

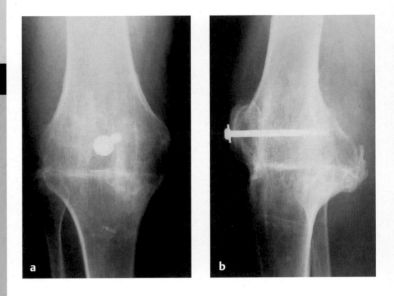

ERRORS AND RISKS

- Too much tension on the Steinmann pins causes early osteolysis. Too large a resection causes an unphysiologic shortening of the leg. Depending on the age of the patient, Ilizarov compression and distraction procedures can be discussed as alternatives.
- Soft tissues can become interposed in the arthrodesis cleft when compression is applied.
- If the traction screw protrudes too far behind the patella, nerves and blood vessels can be irritated. Careful adjustment under image-intensifier control is essential.
- Circulatory disturbances can arise if the leg is shortened too much. In such cases, the length must immediately be restored and the defect filled in with cancellous bone grafts (very rare occurrence).

Alternative Techniques of Bone Stabilization

All invasive procedures performed after an infection have an increased risk of persisting infection. For this reason, they should be performed in two stages after temporary placement of PMMA chains.

The nail system usually prevents shortening of the leg.

- Internal plate fixation
  Debridement is performed as described above. After removing the PMMA chains or spacer, jet lavage is reapplied to the operation site. The muscles are pushed aside just enough to allow a broad plate to be attached. After fixing the plane on one side, compression is applied to the arthrodesis, and the other side is fixed.
- The arthrodesis nail is shown in **Fig. 8.9**.

After removing the PMMA chains or spacer, the medullary cavity is opened with an awl. When viewed from antero-posterior (AP), the approach is in the middle. If viewed from the side, it is on the boundary between the first and second third of the tibial resection plane. The femur is opened in the middle. Both bones are drilled open to enable inner debridement to be performed. Then the site is cleansed with jet lavage. The medullary cavities of the femur and tibia are then prepared with an appropriate rasp (use a template). It is essential to perform a trial placement of the implant to check the axis, length, and rotation of the leg. Depending on the type of implant selected,

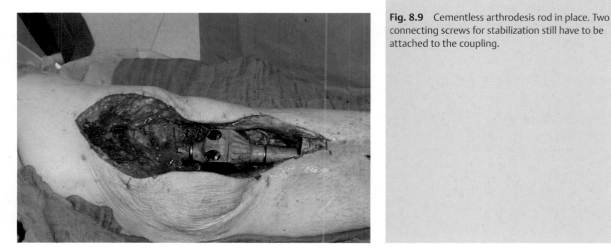

Fig. 8.9 Cementless arthrodesis rod in place. Two connecting screws for stabilization still have to be attached to the coupling.

both components are definitively implanted and fixed by special screws at the level of the former knee joint.

Follow-up

- The patient can apply partial weight bearing (20 kg) for 6 weeks, then increase weight bearing by 10 kg weekly. Full weight bearing should be achieved in the 12th week.
- The anterior clamps are removed 8–10 weeks after the operation to promote the joint dynamics (depending on the contact in the arthrodesis cleft).
- Remove the fixator 12–16 weeks after the operation. If spongiosaplasty was performed, leave the fixator for 16 weeks.
- If necessary apply a removable Neofract tutor for a further 4 weeks.
- Dress the pins daily.

Complications

- Pin-track infections, especially in the thigh, require careful clinical control and nursing care. Osteolyses are a late symptom! Exchange the pin early if there is persisting infection.
- If the bones fail to consolidate, perform spongiosaplasty and implant a new arthrodesis.

Further Reading

Garberina MJ, Fitch RD, Hoffmann ED, Hardaker WT, Vail TP, Scully SP. Knee arthrodesis with circular external fixation. Clin Orthop Relat Res 2001;382:168–178

Gossé F, Lazovic D, Peters G. Primary arthrodesis of the knee joint [Article in German] Orthopäde 1996;25(2):146–152

Hessmann M, Gotzen L, Baumgaertel F. Knee arthrodesis with a unilateral external fixator. Acta Chir Belg 1996;96(3):123–127

Incavo SJ, Lilly JW, Bartlett CS, Churchill DL. Arthrodesis of the knee: experience with intramedullary nailing. J Arthroplasty 2000;15(7):871–876

Kremer K, Lierse W, Platzer W, Schreiber HW, eds. Chirurgische Operationslehre: Posttraumatische Defekt- und Infektsanierung. Vol 10. Stuttgart: Thieme; 1997

Manzotti A, Pullen C, Guerreschi F, Catagni MA. Knee arthrodesis and limb lengthening in the treatment of infected total knee arthroplasty: case report. J Trauma 2002;52(2):359–363

Mutschler W, Haas N, eds. Praxis der Unfallchirurgie. Stuttgart: Thieme; 1999

Rockwood CA, Green DP, Bucholz RW, Heckman JD, eds. Fractures in Adults. 4th ed. Philadelphia: Lippincott Raven; 1996

Rüter A, Trentz O, Wagner M, eds. Unfallchirurgie. Munich: Urban & Schwarzenbeck; 1995

Wirth CJ, ed. Praxis der Orthopädie. 3rd ed. Stuttgart: Thieme; 2001

Ankle (Talocrural) Joint

Indications

- Septic joint destruction
- Extensive osteomyelitis of the distal tibia
- Extensive osteomyelitis of the talus (extremely rare)
- Infected total joint replacements

Contraindication

Multimorbid patient.

General Comments

The success of arthrodesis of the ankle joint does not depend on bone consolidation alone. The patient must understand before the operation that only the ankle joint will be stiffened. The patient initially considers him/herself mutilated and must therefore understand that permanent weight bearing of the affected leg with hardly any functional limitation **can** result after a technically correct operation. Especially in the early phase after removal of the external fixator there will be some complaints resulting from the dystrophy and increasing mobilization. The patient must be prepared for this.

Eradication of the infectious focus and reconstruction of the joint by means of arthrodesis can be performed in one or two stages (**Table 8.2**). The decision depends on:
- The extent of the infection
- The intensity of the infection
- Infection of the soft tissues
- Bone grafting
- Stabilizing procedures

Table 8.2 Criteria for deciding on a one- or two-stage procedure

	One-stage procedure	Two-stage procedure
Extent of infection	Ankle joint	Osteitis
Intensity of infection	Chronic, low-grade infection	Acute, purulent
Bone grafting	Not necessary	Required
Free flaps	Not required	Required
Stabilization	Fixator	Screw/nail

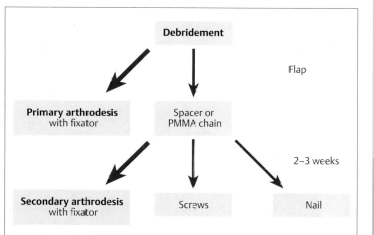

"Infection and metal are poor partners." This guiding principle, which is supported by every clinical routine when sepsis is involved, recommends a two-stage procedure for a planned joint stabilization. After debridement (**Fig. 8.10**), a local antibiotic is inserted (spacer or PMMA chain). Temporary immobilization is generally achieved with a cast.

Principal Signs and Symptoms

- Classical parameters of inflammation
- Fever
- ESR (leukocyte count is unspecific)
- CRP is almost always elevated
- Pain on movement
- Fistulas may be present

Surgical Preparations

- Radiograph in two planes (**Fig. 8.11**): Further imaging diagnostics are only required in exceptional situations.
- Smear: It is wise to aspirate the joint before the operation so that adjuvant antibiotic therapy can be performed according to the most recent bacteriologic test results (e. g., MRSA). In an acute emergency this may not be possible if it causes delay.
- Perform routine laboratory tests.
- Banked blood is generally not required.
- Informed consent of the patient includes:
  - General risks
  - The entire spectrum of problems, like a stiff ankle joint
  - Axial malalignment

NOTE

Arthrodesis is indicated if there is manifest joint destruction. Antibiotics alone or even injections are not appropriate therapy in such cases.

Adjuvant antibiotic administration according to the results of bacteriologic testing is correct therapy.

Soft-tissue defects are closed with a suralis-muscle flap, toe-extensor flap, or free flap immediately after debridement. The most common soft-tissue defects are treated by shortening the leg alone. If a free flap is transplanted, it should be temporarily secured with a fixator which **bridges the joint**.

ERRORS AND RISKS

Mistaken assessment of the patient's compliance and especially subjective satisfaction following arthrodesis; modern society demands movable joints.

- **Axial malalignment:** It is difficult to judge the axial alignment intraoperatively with an image intensifier. Varus deformities, like pes equines and pes calcaneus often result. If such deformities appear after removal of the fixator, everything should be disassembled and the joint resected.
- **Persisting infections:** Especially in osteomyelitis of adjacent bones (tibial pilon/talus), it is good policy to perform a two-stage arthrodesis. The bone may fail to consolidate.
- **Functionally unsatisfactory shortening of the leg:** A pronounced shortening of the leg results especially after osteomyelitis of the tibia or after infection of the total ankle replacement. Depending on the age of the patient and his or her risk factors, segment transfer can provide a solution.
- **Injury to blood vessels and nerves:** All three neurovascular bundles could be damaged because they lie near the bones in the ankle joint.

Fig. 8.11a, b Stage 4 infection of the talocrural joint after fracture.

- – Rotational error
- – Shortened leg
- – Failure of bone consolidation
- – Recurring infection

Special Instruments and Materials

- Oscillating saw
- Water-cooled round burr
- Broad chisel
- Jet lavage
- PMMA chains, Refobacin Bone Cement R, gentamicin sponge

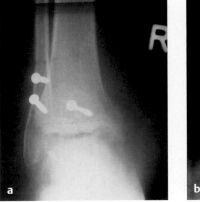
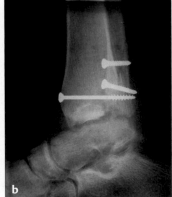

Eradication of Infection by Means of Primary Arthrodesis with an External Fixator and Charnley Clamp

Surgical Procedure

- Administer intravenous antibiotics 30 minutes before the operation begins.
- Interrupt the blood supply.
- Make a lateral longitudinal skin incision.
- Take biopsies for bacteriologic and pathologic examination. Smears should no longer be taken without biopsies because the two together considerably increase identification of pathogens.
- Perform an osteotomy of the fibula slanted toward the ankle joint using retractors (to protect the fibular artery) and resect the distal fibula.
- Radically debride all infected tissues from a lateral approach (**Fig. 8.12**).
- Perform a medial longitudinal incision and osteotomy of the medial ankle with a chisel while using Hohmann retractors (to protect the posterior tibial artery).
- Release the soft tissues anterior and posterior to the tibia near the arthrodesis using a curved raspatory.
- The foot is held by the surgical assistant in a correct 0° position (**Fig. 8.13**). Rotation in this phase is still unimportant.
- Place the Hohmann retractors from anterior and posterior around the tibia (to protect the anterior and posterior tibial arteries).
- Perform a vertical osteotomy of the tibia under image-intensifier control.
- Insert a saw blade in this cleft for orientation and perform parallel osteotomy of the talar joint plane (procedure analogous to that in **Fig. 8.3** for arthrodesis of the knee joint). The correct 0° position of the foot is essential in this phase (**Fig. 8.13**).
- Remove the saw blades and distract the foot.
- Complete the osteotomy using Hohmann retractors on the tibia and talus (**Fig. 8.13**).
- Edges may need to be corrected with a chisel.
- Perform jet lavage (to reduce pathogens) with the first half of the irrigation fluid.
- Burr out any possible foci of osteomyelitis in the talus and tibia.
- Mobilize the posterior part of the capsule with a curved raspatory on the talus and tibia to prevent later soft-tissue interposition when compression is applied.
- Perform a second jet lavage (final cleansing) with the remaining half of the irrigation fluid.
- Implant one Steinmann pin (3.2-mm drill bit) from medial in the anterior and one in the posterior talus under image-intensifier control (**Fig. 8.14**).

Fig. 8.12 Surgical site after resection of the lateral malleolus.

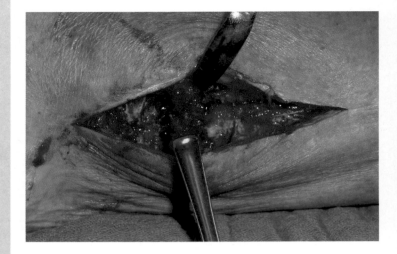

Fig. 8.13 Correct position of the foot. The tibial and talus joint surfaces have been resected in parallel and the wound has been cleansed with jet lavage.
The arrow pointing downward shows the arthrodesis cleft.
1 = distal tibia
2 = talus in the retro position

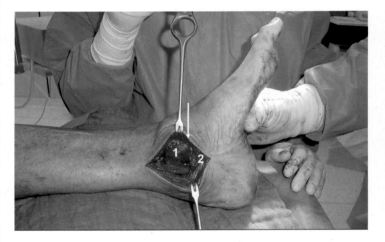

Fig. 8.14 Confirming the correct placement of the Steinmann pin in the talus with an image intensifier.

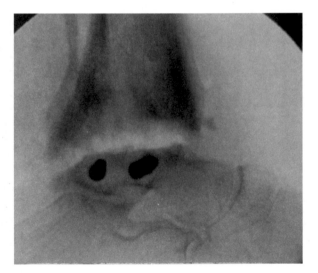

- Mount the assembly on the medial and lateral sides; a surgical assistant manually repositions the arthrodesis (slight retroversion, 10° lateral torsion).
- Implant one Steinmann pin from medial approximately 4 cm above the arthrodesis cleft (3.2-mm drill bit).
- After image-intensifier control to ensure that the arthrodesis is correct, apply compression by turning the threaded rods (Charnley) or using the clamps medial and lateral.
- Implant a second Steinmann pin from medial using a spot-film device approximately 8–10 cm above the arthrodesis cleft (4.5-mm drill bit). Apply compression as described above.
- Perform final image-intensifier control (**Fig. 8.15a, b**).
- Remove the tourniquet and wrap the leg in elastic bandages for 5 minutes.
- Then perform careful hemostasis, insert a gentamicin sponge (half medial and half lateral), place Redon drains, and close the wound (**Fig. 8.16**).
- Shorten the protruding Steinmann pins.

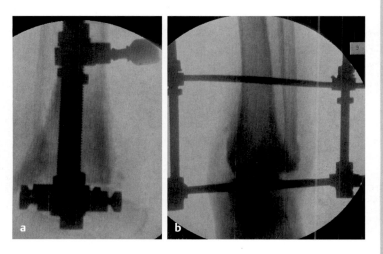

Fig. 8.15a, b
a Lateral view with image intensifier to confirm the placement before applying the proximal Steinmann pin. Correction can still be performed at any time without a problem.
b The same situation, AP control.

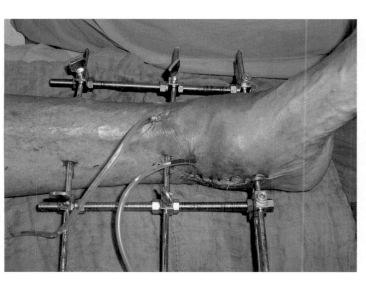

Fig. 8.16 The assembly is shown at the end of the operation. Steinmann pins must still be shortened.

Alternative Bone Stabilizing Procedures

All invasive procedures performed after an infection run an increased risk of persisting infection. For this reason they should be performed in two stages after temporary insertion of PMMA chains.

Debridement is performed as described above. After removing the PMMA chains/spacer, jet lavage is repeated at the operation site.

Screw Osteosynthesis

- Temporarily stabilize the arthrodesis in the correct position with Kirschner wires.
- Stabilization is achieved with Kirschner wires with three lag screws (short threads). Two are applied from proximal–medial and one from proximal–lateral.

Arthrodesis Nail

- Make a transpatellar incision and enter the tibial shaft with an awl.
- Stabilize the arthrodesis temporarily with Kirschner wires.
- Insert a guide wire through the arthrodesis cleft into the talus.
- Gently ream.
- Implant the nail with interlocking by means of transverse bolts in the talus.
- Attach a proximal interlocking bolt and apply compression to the arthrodesis (according to the system used).
- Then attach the second proximal interlocking bolt.

Follow-up

- The patient can apply partial weight bearing (20 kg) for 6 weeks and then increase weight bearing by 10 kg weekly. Full weight bearing should be achieved in the 12th week.
- Remove the fixator 12 weeks after the operation.
- Fit an orthopedic shoe to be worn for 4–6 months (**Fig. 8.17**).

TIPS AND TRICKS

- Interrupting the blood supply during the operation facilitates debridement of the soft tissues.
- Place the patient's foot on the operating table in the correct 0° position, then resect the tibia and talus in two parallel lines perpendicular to the bone to half the depth in each bone. Perform distraction and saw completely through the bones while protecting the soft tissues with Hohmann retractors. When compression is later applied, the axis is automatically correct.
- If the infection has spread to differing degrees in the bone, this could cause nonlevel resection planes. In such cases it is better to perform two-stage spongiosaplasty than to perform a second resection.
- There can be considerable trophic disturbance of the soft tissues as a result of earlier operations. Resection of the medial malleolus and the fibula provides enough space to close the wound without tension. This form of resection (in infected cases) also facilitates debridement because all regions in the ankle joint are optimally accessible and visible.
- The Charnley clamp is an ideal system for arthrodesis of the talocrural joint. The correct position of the pin in the talus is assured by the angular stability of the system. Primary placement of both pins in the talus can cause the threaded rods to no longer be parallel to the tibial axis later. In such cases it makes no sense to drill more holes in the talus. Instead, an AO fixator should be applied.
- If the level of resection makes correct placement of a second pin in the talus impossible (e. g., due to infection), it should be placed in the calcaneus and an AO fixator applied. The hybrid fixator cannot supply sufficient compression on the arthrodesis.

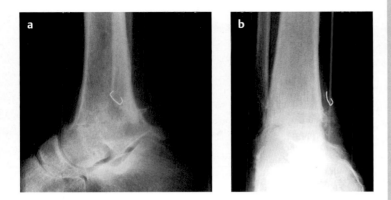

Fig. 8.17a, b Radiographic image of a healing arthrodesis of the ankle joint performed with a Charnley clamp 1 year postoperatively.

Complications

- Pin-track infections require careful clinical control and nursing care. Osteolyses are a late symptom (**Figs. 8.18 and 8.19**). Exchange the pin early if the infection persists. Pins may need to be placed in the calcaneus.
- If the bones fail to consolidate, perform spongiosa-plasty and renewed arthrodesis.

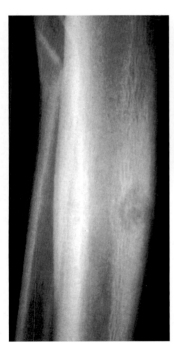

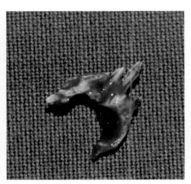

Fig. 8.18 Radiograph of the lower leg with a ring sequestrum after arthrodesis of the ankle joint with a fixator.

Fig. 8.19 Ring sequestrum after operative removal.

ERRORS AND RISKS

- Too much tension on the Steinmann pins causes early osteolysis on the side of the cortical bone subjected to pressure.
- Vascular damage: The three main blood vessels in the ankle joint all lie next to the bone. Perform careful dissection near the bone (curved raspatory) and use Hohmann retractors during the osteotomy to avoid direct injuries caused by the saw.
- Resecting too much bone causes an unphysiologic shortening of the leg. Compression-distraction procedures or Ilizarov segment transport are possible alternatives, depending on the age of the patient.
- Soft tissues could be interposed in the arthrodesis cleft when compression is applied.
- Circulatory disturbances can arise if the leg is shortened too much. In such cases, the length must immediately be restored and the defect filled in with cancellous bone chips (very rare occurrence).
- To avoid misalignment of the axis, the correct axis and rotation of the foot must be checked before mounting the fixator.

Further Reading

Berman AT, Bosacco SJ, Parks BG, et al. Compression arthrodesis of the ankle by triangular external fixation: biomechanical and clinical evaluation. Orthopedics 1999;22(12):1129–1134

Kitaoka HB. Arthrodesis of the ankle: technique, complications, and salvage treatment. Instr Course Lect 1999;48:255–261

Kremer K, Lierse W, Platzer W, Schreiber HW, eds. Chirurgische Operationslehre: Posttraumatische Defekt- und Infektsanierung, Vol 10. Stuttgart: Thieme; 1997

Mutschler W, Haas N, eds. Praxis der Unfallchirurgie. Stuttgart: Thieme; 1999

Pell RF IV, Myerson MS, Schon LC. Clinical outcome after primary triple arthrodesis. J Bone Joint Surg Am 2000;82(1):47–57

Richter D, Hahn MP, Laun RA, Ekkernkamp A, Muhr G, Ostermann PA. Arthrodesis of the infected ankle and subtalar joint: technique, indications, and results of 45 consecutive cases. J Trauma 1999;47(6):1072–1078

Rockwood CA, Green DP, Bucholz RW, Heckman JD, eds. Fractures in Adults. 4th ed. Philadelphia: Lippincott Raven; 1996

Rüter A, Trentz O, Wagner M, eds. Unfallchirurgie. Munich: Urban & Schwarzenbeck; 1995

Wirth CJ, ed. Praxis der Orthopädie. 3rd ed. Stuttgart: Thieme; 2001

Wu WL, Su FC, Cheng YM, Huang PJ, Chou YL, Chou CK. Gait analysis after ankle arthrodesis. Gait Posture 2000;11(1):54–61

Zwipp H, Grass R, Rammelt S, Dahlen C. Arthrodesis - nonunion of the ankle. Arthrodesis failed. [Article in German] Chirurg 1999;70(11):1216–1224

Index

Page numbers in *italics* refer to illustrations or tables